Clinics in Developmental Medicine
CHILDHOOD HEADACHE
2ND EDITION

Childhood Headache
2nd Edition

Edited by

ISHAQ ABU-ARAFEH
Fraser of Allander Neurosciences Unit, Royal Hospital for Sick
Children, Glasgow, UK

and

Consultant in Paediatrics and Paediatric Neurology, Forth Valley
Royal Hospital, Larbert, UK

2013
Mac Keith Press

© 2013 Mac Keith Press
6 Market Road, London, N7 9PW

Editor: Hilary M. Hart
Managing Director: Ann-Marie Halligan
Production Manager: Udoka Ohuonu
Project Management: Prepress Projects Ltd

First published in this edition in 2013

British Library Cataloguing-in-Publication data
A catalogue record for this book is available from the British Library

Cover image: Drawing by an 8-year-old girl depicting what her migraine feels like (see p. 312).

ISBN: 978-1-908316-75-2

Typeset by Prepress Projects Ltd, Perth, UK
Printed by Ashford Colour Press Ltd, Gosport, Hampshire, UK

Mac Keith Press is supported by Scope

CONTENTS

Contents

Contents

Contents

AUTHORS' APPOINTMENTS

Ishaq Abu-Arafeh   Consultant in Paediatrics and Paediatric Neurology, Forth Valley Royal Hospital, Larbert, UK; Fraser of Allander Neurosciences Unit, Royal Hospital for Sick Children, Glasgow, UK

Kamran A Ahmed   Department of Child and Adolescent Neurology, Mayo Clinic, Rochester, MN, USA

Mas Ahmed   Consultant in Paediatrics, Paediatric Department, Queen's University Hospital, Romford, UK

Frank Andrasik   Distinguished Professor and Chair of Psychology, Department of Psychology, University of Memphis, Memphis, TN, USA

Benedetta Bellini   Department of Pediatrics and Child and Adolescent Neuropsychiatry, Faculty of Medicine and Odontoiatrics, "La Sapienza" University, Rome, Italy

Alessandra Cescut   Department of Psychology, Faculty of Medicine and Psychology, "La Sapienza" University, Rome, Italy

Francesca Craba   Department of Psychology, Faculty of Medicine and Psychology, "La Sapienza" University, Rome, Italy

Jean-Christophe Cuvellier   Division of Paediatric Neurology, Department of Paediatrics, Lille Faculty of Medicine and Children's Hospital, Lille, France

Peter J Goadsby   Headache Group—Department of Neurology, University of California, San Francisco, San Francisco, CA, USA

Vincenzo Guidetti   Professor of Child and Adolescent Neuropsychiatry, Department of Pediatrics and Child and Adolescent Neuropsychiatry, Faculty of Medicine and Odontoiatrics, "La Sapienza" University, Rome, Italy

Mirja Hämäläinen   Department of Pediatric Neurology, Hospital for Children and Adolescents, Helsinki University Central Hospital, Helsinki, Finland

Andrew D Hershey   Professor of Paediatrics and Neurology, Headache Center, Division of Neurology, University of Cincinnati, College of Medicine, Cincinnati Children's Hospital Medical Center, Cincinnati, OH, USA

David P Kernick   General Practitioner, St. Thomas Health Centre, Exeter, UK

Giorgio Lambru   Clinical Research Associate, Institute of Neurology, The National Hospital for Neurology and Neurosurgery, London, UK

Donald Lewis[†]   Professor of Pediatrics, Department of Pediatrics, Children's Hospital of The King's Daughters, Norfolk, VA, USA

Franco Lucchese   Department of Psychology, Faculty of Medicine and Psychology, "La Sapienza" University, Rome, Italy

Kenneth J Mack   Professor of Child and Adolescent Neurology, Department of Neurology, Mayo Clinic, Rochester, MN, USA

Stewart Macleod   Consultant Paediatric Neurologist, Fraser of Allander Neurosciences Unit, Royal Hospital for Sick Children, Glasgow, UK

Manjit Matharu   Consultant Neurologist, Headache Group, Institute of Neurology, The National Hospital for Neurology and Neurosurgery, London, UK

Susanne Osterhaus   Clinical Child and Adolescent Psychologist, Practice for Psychotherapy, Diagnosis and Training in Cognitive Behavioural Therapy, Haarlem, the Netherlands

----

[†]Deceased.

Scott W Powers
Professor and Director of the Center for Child Behavior and Nutrition, Division of Behavioral Medicine and Clinical Psychology, Cincinnati Children's Hospital Medical Center, and Department of Pediatrics, University of Cincinnati, College of Medicine, Cincinnati, OH, USA

Vicky Quarshie
Headache Specialist Nurse, Headache Service, Hull and East Yorkshire Hospitals NHS Trust, Hull, UK

Amanda Rach
Department of Psychology, University of Memphis, Memphis, TN, USA

George Russell†
Emeritus Professor of Child Health, University of Aberdeen, Aberdeen, UK

Michael Bjørn Russell
Professor and Consultant Neurologist, Head and Neck Research Group, Research Centre, Akershus University Hospital, Oslo, Norway

Shashi S Seshia
Clinical Professor, Department of Pediatrics, Division of Pediatric Neurology, University of Saskatchewan, Saskatoon, SK, Canada

Sepideh Taheri
Consultant Paediatrician, Royal Hospital for Sick Children, Edinburgh, UK

William P Whitehouse
Clinical Associate Professor and Honorary Consultant Paediatric Neurologist, Academic Division of Child Health, University of Nottingham, Queen's Medical Centre, Nottingham, UK

Andrew N Williams
Consultant Community Paediatrician, Virtual Academic Unit, CDC, Northampton General Hospital, Northampton, UK

Paul Winner
Professor in Child Neurology, Palm Beach Headache Center, Premiere Research Institute, Palm Beach Neurology, Nova Southeastern University, West Palm Beach, FL, USA

Çiçek Wöber-Bingöl
Professor of Clinical Neurology, Head and Founder of the Headache Outpatient Clinic for Children and Adolescents, Department of Child and Adolescent Psychiatry, Medical University of Vienna, Vienna, Austria

---

†Deceased.

DEDICATION

This book is dedicated to Professor George Russell and Professor Donald Lewis, both of whom contributed immensely to our knowledge of childhood headache in general and to this book in particular. We are saddened by their unexpected deaths, shortly before this book was completed.

FOREWORD

Knowledge of childhood headache among general practitioners, paediatric specialists and child psychiatrists is not perfect. Unfortunately, this is sometimes also true of paediatric neurologists at specialist clinics. For this reason, this second edition of *Childhood Headache* will serve as a major resource not only for trained doctors but also for medical students and paramedical professionals, including nurses, psychologists, social workers and physiotherapists, who will all benefit from the complete and well-structured information it contains.

Headache is sometimes a symptom of an underlying brain dysfunction, but it can also be a result of extracerebral or extracranial causes. Discussions of headache in children (aged up to 18y) mainly involve migraine and tension-type headache. Included here are important syndromes related to migraine such as colic in infancy, benign paroxysmal torticollis, benign paroxysmal vertigo, cyclical vomiting syndrome and abdominal migraine.

It is important to recognise that the overall prevalence of headache in children is about 60%, with a preponderance in females. About 20% of schoolchildren complain of headache more than once a week and around 10% more than 2 days a week. About 5% of children with headache will suffer moderate or severe impairment.

This second edition of *Childhood Headache* provides a thorough account of the spectrum of symptoms that come under the collective term 'headache'. Its 31 chapters, written by well-known experts in the field, are comprehensive in illustrating all conceivable aspects of childhood headache.

The first seven chapters deal with the background to headache including the history, pathophysiology, genetics and epidemiology. In many chapters the importance of taking a careful history, including family history, is stressed, and this cannot be overemphasised. The basis of one chapter is classification using the current International Classification of Headache Disorders, 2nd edition (ICHD-II). As with all classifications, it has raised many questions, and this is why the forthcoming 3rd edition (ICHD-III) will be much appreciated.

Another chapter deals with the important topic of headache and quality of life. Two chapters describe the assessment and investigation of headache, highlighting the importance of 'red flags' in alerting physicians and guiding investigations. Childhood migraine is the topic of the following four chapters.

There are then four important chapters on headache comorbidity and migraine-related syndromes. Next are four chapters on tension-type headache and chronic headaches with key differential diagnoses. A description of symptomatic headache, especially that due to brain tumours, as well as idiopathic intracranial hypertension, follows, together with, in the next four chapters, a description of the craniofacial causes of headache and post-traumatic headache. The investigation of headache with suspicion of brain tumour is fundamental, and the 'red flags' must be borne in mind.

The psychological aspects and treatment of childhood headache are presented in two chapters and point to the need for a multidisciplinary approach to the topic.

One chapter deals with dietary management of migraine in particular, while two chapters are devoted to the management of childhood headache in general practice and at specialist clinics. The last chapter describes children's expression of migraine symptoms through drawing.

The content of this book is easy to read and understand. In most chapters interesting case reports are included, and the comprehensive reference lists also include web information, which is a real advantage. I have no doubt that this book will become an appreciable asset for all clinicians dealing with childhood headache.

Orvar Eeg-Olofsson
Professor of Child Neurology
Department of Women's and Children's Health
Uppsala University
Uppsala, Sweden

PREFACE

The second edition of *Childhood Headache* comes 11 years after the first was published in 2002 and follows a huge increase in interest in headache in children and adolescents and a monumental increase in the amount of research published on the subject.

Experts from around the world have contributed to this edition of *Childhood Headache* in order to provide a global view of the subject. It is hoped that the book will provide global agreement on how to approach, manage and treat children with headache, wherever they happen to live. The impact of headache on the child's life and education continues to be universal, but unfortunately it is poorly recognised or under-reported in many parts of the world. An emphasis on the impact of headache on children is therefore present across the chapters of the book.

The first edition received many positive and encouraging reviews. The inclusion of case studies and clinical examples was suggested as an area in which the first edition could improve, and therefore in this edition readers will notice that, wherever possible, authors have given clinical cases to illustrate an issue related to a difficult diagnosis, unusual or atypical presentation, management issues or treatment options. I hope this addition to the book will enhance the clinical nature of the discussion and will put the child with headache at the centre of the learning process.

Other reviewers described the first edition as 'too scientific', so a balance of science and clinical practice was sought in this edition. I hope that we have been able to provide enough material to satisfy the needs of both the busy clinician and the research-active reader.

Ishaq Abu-Arafeh
Glasgow, January 2013

ACKNOWLEDGEMENTS

As editor I am grateful for how much I have learnt over the past 10 years about 'headache' from both my patients and influential paediatric headache specialists (many of whom have contributed to this book). I am also grateful for the support of my wife (Ghada) and children (Ahmad and Hashem) in allowing me the time to spend on this book. I am also indebted to my colleagues, who made it possible for me to make changes to my working schedule and helped in seeing this book through. I am especially grateful to Lauryn, Robert and Stephanie for providing the drawings for Chapter 31 and the book cover.

The author of Chapter 2 (Andrew N Williams) would like to thank Professor Robert Arnott, Professor Timothy Chappell, Dr Dharval Dave, Mr Colm Harte, Professor Mark Geller, Dr Sue Hawkins, Dr Katherine Hunt, Professor Hansruedi Isler, Professor Steve King, Dr MA McShane, Professor Kenneth Mack, Dr Hannah Newton, Dr Richard Newton, Dr Jonathan Reinarz, Dr Robert Sunderland, Dr Andrea Tanner, Professor Giorgio Zachin, the Unit for the History of Medicine, the University of Birmingham, the archive at Northampton General Hospital and the Richmond postgraduate library, and Northampton General Hospital for their assistance and comments.

The author of Chapters 5, 8 and 20 (Shashi S Seshia) is grateful for continuing support from the Faculty of Medicine and Department of Pediatrics, University of Saskatchewan, Saskatoon, Canada. He thanks Dr Ishaq Abu-Arafeh for his insightful suggestions.

Much of the information in Chapter 20 is similar to that in two recent publications, Seshia et al (2010a) and Seshia (2012).

1
INTRODUCTION

Ishaq Abu-Arafeh

Headache as a symptom has been reported over the ages, but interest in headache as a health issue and as a set of specific clinical disorders has taken a huge leap over the past half-century, especially in children. Increased awareness of the misery that headache can cause to sufferers and the need for effective treatment have enhanced the drive to explore the science of headache over the past 30 years, with the volume of research output increasing exponentially. A MEDLINE search of headache in children will return thousands of results, mostly published over the past 20 years, but despite the huge amount of research and the volumes written on the subject, there is still a gap in our knowledge which needs to be filled in order to obtain reliable evidence for making recommendations in management of headache in general and in paediatrics in particular.

There is no doubt that man has suffered from headache throughout recorded history and all over the world, but it is only in modern times that headache has taken a prominent position in research circles, and also in service provision, because of the accumulating knowledge of its impact on the lives of sufferers. Ancient writings and folk literature have described different types of headache, different causes and also remedies that vary from the use of simple natural herbs to the most complex physical interventions. Early attempts on classification of headache disorders may be dated back some 5000 years to the ancient Egyptians (Isler 1987), which shows how people in the past were just as fascinated or distressed with headache as we are in contemporary times. In this book, a review of the history of headache with a focus on children does not only provoke curiosity and fascination but also shows how the science of headache has come through many stages, beginning as a mere puzzling story or anecdote.

The art and science of treating children with headache have evolved greatly over the past century, alongside the developments in medical specialisation of childhood medicine and the emergence of paediatrics as an independent medical speciality, making way for the ever-increasing space given to headache in paediatric literature and textbooks. The discussion of headache as a childhood disorder has increased from the mere mention of the condition in passing, to a short description in a paragraph or two, to a full chapter and finally to books dedicated to the condition such as this book and its first edition in 2002 (Chapter 2).

Paediatricians, paediatric neurologists, child psychiatrists, paediatric headache specialists and others all played their part in enriching the paediatric literature on the subject. Bo Bille, working in Sweden, is credited with pioneering work on headache in schoolchildren in the 1950s (Bille 1962), and all through the rest of the twentieth century (Bille 1981, 1997), which

1

made him the true father of modern childhood headache research. The advances in clinical research on childhood headache have helped in enabling an evidence-based approach to the understanding of its epidemiology, classification, diagnosis and management. However, much more research is still needed in order to support 'expert opinions' and avoid idiosyncratic recommendations. In this book, a comprehensive discussion of current practice and research provides an adequate basis to support clinicians in their day-to-day practice and also researchers in appraising the most current theories and areas of controversy.

The need for a scientific approach to headache in general, and migraine in particular, emerged in the middle of the last century with attempts on classification and defining criteria for the diagnosis of migraine in children, such as those suggested by Vahlquist (1955). This was followed by a more comprehensive attempt on the classification of headache disorder by an ad hoc committee established for that purpose (Friedman 1962). These two attempts were an important prelude to the first International Headache Society (IHS) classification of headache disorders in 1988 (Headache Classification Committee of the International Headache Society 1988). The success of the IHS classifications and their wide acceptance across the world provoked a stream of debate and discussions, which enriched the classification with important details and sophistication, as seen in the second edition of the International Classification of Headache Disorders (Headache Classification Subcommittee of the International Headache Society 2004). The standardisation of the classification and diagnosis of headache disorders, though not perfect, has helped researchers and clinicians to debate, assess and modify many aspects of the criteria for the diagnosis of headache disorders, enabling better understanding and management of headache. It has also helped in moving knowledge and expertise on the subject from the pure art of clinical acumen to a standardised scientific approach.

There is no doubt that the International Headache Society with its, so far, two editions of headache classification has positively promoted headache to the forefront of world medical, social and political interest. However, headache in children has, unfortunately, continued to lag behind and is often presented as a subtitle or a footnote in the classification of headache disorders, which is derived from experience in adult patients and aimed at the adult population (apart from a small section on migraine in children). Therefore, in Chapter 5, the classification of headache disorders has been given an extensive analysis from the paediatric perspective, aiming to show the differences in clinical presentations of headache disorders in children and adults and proposing an operational methodology to help practising clinicians in making diagnoses and clinical decisions.

The epidemiology of headache and migraine has been extensively researched in many parts of the world, and the introduction of the International Headache Society's classification and criteria for the diagnosis of headache disorders made it easier to compare populations and also to systematically review the evidence and provide a global view of the prevalence of headache in children, as shown in Chapter 6. Such analysis allowed better understanding of the sex and geographic differences in the prevalence of headache worldwide.

The assessment of the child with headache has always been a source of anxiety to paediatricians, with serious neurological disorders being at the back of their minds. In order to help with planning a methodical and reliable approach to assess the child with headache, several chapters of this book have looked at the roles of different healthcare professionals, including the general practitioner (Chapter 28), the paediatrician (Chapter 9), the paediatric neurologist (Chapter 8), the child psychologist (Chapters 26 and 27) and the headache specialist in the setting of a dedicated headache clinic (Chapter 29). A holistic approach to the child with headache is, therefore, encouraged and a full assessment should include an appraisal of the child's lifestyle. Also of importance is the assessment of the impact of headache on child and family life using recognised tools for assessment, monitoring of progress and response to management as described in Chapter 7.

As the majority of children who seek medical advice for their headaches suffer from migraine and tension-type headache, the emphasis in this book is on these two important aspects of headache, whilst also recognising the changing pattern of clinical presentations, with many children seen with chronic daily headache, mixed types of headache and some less common types of headache. Accurate diagnoses continue to be paramount and therefore an emphasis on recognition of 'red flags' and appropriate investigations for children with possible serious secondary headaches are highlighted in several chapters of this book, but without unnecessary alarm.

As the child with headache may present in many different settings and may be assessed by several specialists, it was important that in this book we addressed the management issues in primary care, hospital medical clinics, and child psychiatry and highlighted the important nursing roles in management. We have also addressed several aspects of management including lifestyle issues, medications, dietary intervention, and psychological and psychiatric assessment and treatment.

This book aims to provide clinicians with up-to-date evidence on childhood headache and its treatment, but unfortunately there will always be a lag period between writing and publishing in print, a problem that may become less important in the future as electronic publishing becomes the norm. This book also aims to provide researchers with up-to-date analysis of areas in childhood headache that are supported by research evidence, scientific explanations and hypothesis generation. It also provides discussions on areas of uncertainty in childhood headache, areas lacking in evidence and areas in which a test of hypothesis needs to be addressed in future research.

REFERENCES

Bille B (1962) Migraine in schoolchildren. *Acta Paediatr* 136(Suppl 51): 14–151.

Bille B (1981) Migraine in childhood and its prognosis. *Cephalalgia* 1: 71–5. http://dx.doi.org/10.1111/j.1468-2982.1981.tb00012.x

Bille B (1997) A 40-year follow-up of school children with migraine. *Cephalalgia* 17: 488–91. http://dx.doi.org/10.1046/j.1468-2982.1997.1704488.x

Friedman AP (Chairman), Ad Hoc Committee on Classification of Headache (1962) Classification of headache. *Arch Neurol* 6: 173–6. http://dx.doi.org/10.1001/archneur.1962.00450210001001

Headache Classification Committee of the International Headache Society (1988) Classification and diagnostic criteria for headache disorders, neuralgias and facial pain. *Cephalalgia* 8(Suppl 7): 1–96.

Headache Classification Subcommittee of the International Headache Society (2004) The international classification of headache disorders: 2nd edition. *Cephalalgia* 24(Suppl 1): 9–160.

Isler H (1987) Retrospect: the history of thought about migraine from Aretaeus to 1920. In: Blau JN, editor. *Migraine*. London: Chapman & Hall, pp. 659–74.

Vahlquist B (1955) Migraine in children. *Int Arch Allergy Appl Immunol* 7: 348–355. http://dx.doi.org/10.1159/000228238

2
HISTORY OF HEADACHE IN CHILDHOOD: FROM HEADACHE TABLETS TO HEADACHE TABLETS

Andrew N Williams

Childhood headache research has been called the 'Cinderella' of paediatric neurology and has previously been totally eclipsed by that of headache in adulthood (Howells 2010, Zanchin 2010). Any history of a paediatric condition must be viewed through the lens of historical context. From the medical perspective, this involves the changing understanding, development and subsequent evolution of specialist children's services and the significant change in the epidemiology of paediatric conditions, particularly within the Western world over the last half century. From the sociological perspective, the increasing recognition of children and childhood must also be considered.

> In considering the subject of headaches in children, I may reasonably be accused of selecting a symptom which in some cases is the leading feature of intracranial change, and at others merely an indication of passing functional disturbance.
>
> Day (1872)

> Migraine occurs in children – as only the inexperienced will deny – very nearly as often as on adults, and with pretty much the same symptoms.
>
> Henoch (1889)

The history of headache in childhood

Cases of headache in childhood are infrequently scattered throughout the historical medical literature, and many great works, such as those of Ambroise Paré (1510–90), have no record of childhood headache at all, although Paré is aware of migraines, which he calls 'Megrim' (Paré 1634, Larner 2010).

The earliest known description of headache in childhood dates from the Mesopotamian era and is an incantation called 'AmarSuen's Headache' (Fig. 2.1). Its exact age remains unknown, possibly as early as the third millennium BC (Zayas 2007).

Mesopotamian physicians considered headache as a disease rather than a symptom and believed spirits caused headaches (Nemet-Nejat 1998).

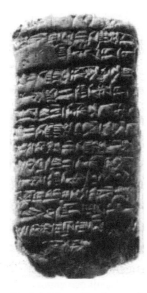

This text translates as follows:

The headache (-demon) is directed towards the man.

The headache-demon is set to distress the neck muscles.

There is no small opening which can ensnare the galla-demon.

No binding can be tied on the headache (-demon).

It is the young lad who is seized by the headache-demon.

It is the young maiden whose diseased neck twitches.

Fig. 2.1 The earliest known description of headache in childhood, which dates from the Mesopotamian era and is an incantation called 'AmarSuen's Headache'. The author would like to thank Professor Geller for providing the photograph of the tablet (van Dijk and Geller 2003).

Trephination was first performed around 5000 BC with the logic for this procedure, other than for head injuries, remaining a cause for ongoing debate (Verano and Finger 2010). There are very few trephined children's skulls, even if we take into account the fact that children's skulls are not as durable as those of adults, especially if mutilated. Thus we can no more than speculate for the reasons for this surgery. However, two cases of child trephination in Harappan civilisation, 2450 to 1900 BC, have been discovered; one child died shortly after surgery and the other child had hydrocephaly (Arnott 2011).

The *Second Book of Kings* relates how a child was resuscitated following collapse after headache. However, this is generally considered to be a case of sunstroke rather than another more serious intracranial pathology (Rosner 1976).

There are well-documented adult cases: one example from a stone tablet tells of Agestratos whose headache was relieved by sleeping overnight in the temple of Epidaurus (Guthrie 1945). Concerning the use of votives (a model or mask of the head that is left as an offering) for the treatment of headache, it is not possible to prove or refute their use for children (Celli 1933, Wells 1985, Morel 1989, Blomerus 1999).

Further complexities can arise through problems in mistranslation or looking too narrowly through a modern lens. Jowett's paraphrase translation from Plato's *Republic* 'when a student imagines that philosophy gives him a headache' (Plato 1888) against a more recent one of 'brain strain' (TDJ Chappell, personal communication 2011).

The *Midrash Rabbah,* the homiletical commentary on the Bible, describes a King addressing his convalescing son, 'here we slept, here we cooled ourselves, here you had a headache' (Genesis, Rabbah).

Within the Medieval period, Râazi (otherwise known as Rhazes, 860–940 CE) described a case suggestive of basilar migraine: 'I visited a young girl who suffered from aphasia following a severe headache attack, washing her head with warm water, she spoke again' (Gorji and Ghadiri 2002).

The birth of child neurology and neurodisability

An extremely important contribution was made by Felix Würtz (or Wuertz) of Basel (1518–74), who was a friend of Paracelsus (Morton 1970, Isler 2010a). Würtz wrote, in German, *Ein schönes und nutzliches Kinderbuechlin* (1616) and its English translation, *A Beautiful and Useful Children's Booklet* (1656) (Wuertz 1563, Würtz 1656, Morton 1970). Writing from his own experience of headaches, Würtz stated that children who complain of headache should be taken seriously and protected from exacerbating and provoking factors, such as light (Isler 2010a).

Charles Le Pois (1563–1633), a migraineur himself, in 1618 described *hemicraniae insultus*, attacks of migraine associated with stroke-like features from age 12 to 17:

> At 12 she experienced a severe left temporal headache followed by bilious vomiting. The headache was preceded by a sense of numbness, stiffness, and a sensation resembling the movement of ants crawling from her left little finger, across her other fingers and hand, and up the arm *aurae cujusdam instar ascendentism* like an ascending breeze.
>
> (Le Pois 1616)

Diagnosis and potential misdiagnosis remain perennial problems in headache management. One example of misdiagnosis is seen in the published record of the English physician John Hall (1575–1635), the son-in-law of William Shakespeare (1564–1616). He records how he treated a 13-year-old girl, Mary Comb, on 15 February 1631, who presented with a 'light convulsion'. As well as being treated for epilepsy, Mary was also treated with ointments for hysteria, the rationale being that some form of displacement of the womb had occurred. The treatment was successful: 'by this it returned to its place' (Fig. 2.2) (Hall 1679, Lane 2001a). A contemporary reading would suggest the case was of migraine rather than epilepsy (I Abu-Arafeh, personal communication 2011). However, the case does illustrate the ongoing debate, originating from the late nineteenth century, of the relationship between migraine and epilepsy (Jackson 1876, Gowers 1907, Brett 1991).

John Wepfer (1620–95) of Schaffhausen, Switzerland, provided the earliest known description of hemiplegic stroke (Fig. 2.3) following migraine as a 12-year-old child (Wepfer 1727).

Thomas Willis (1621–75) was the first to write about paediatric neurology and neurodisability, with specific chapters on childhood epilepsy and mental retardation[a], using case histories and post-mortem studies (Williams 2003a).

Willis made important inroads into our understanding of headache, relating his lack of faith in treatments such as mercury craniotomy (Rapoport 2000). Willis also introduced the

---

[a]UK usage: learning disability.

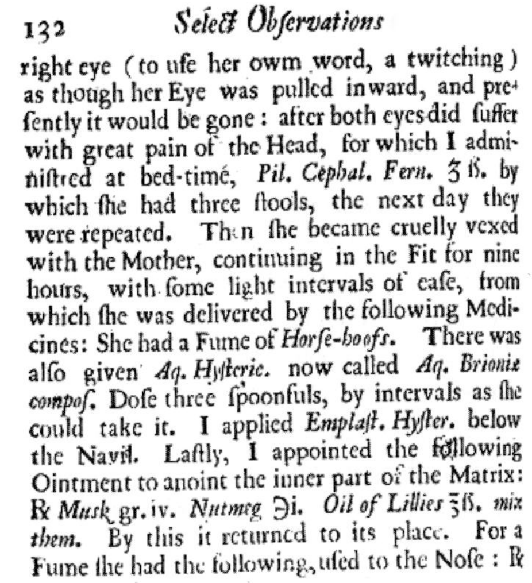

132   *Select Observations*

right eye (to ufe her owm word, a twitching)
as though her Eye was pulled inward, and pre-
fently it would be gone : after both eyes did fuffer
with great pain of the Head, for which I admi-
niftred at bed-time, *Pil. Cephal. Fern.* ʒ ß. by
which fhe had three ftools, the next day they
were repeated.   Then fhe became cruelly vexed
with the Mother, continuing in the Fit for nine
hours, with fome light intervals of eafe, from
which fhe was delivered by the following Medicines: She had a Fume of *Horfe-hoofs.*   There was
alfo given *Aq. Hyfteric.* now called *Aq. Brioniæ
compof.* Dofe three fpoonfuls, by intervals as fhe
could take it.   I applied *Emplaft. Hyfter.* below
the Navil.   Laftly, I appointed the following
Ointment to anoint the inner part of the Matrix:
Ṛ *Mufk* gr. iv. *Nutmeg* Ǝi.   *Oil of Lillies* ʒ ß. *mix
them.*   By this it returned to its place.   For a
Fume fhe had the following, ufed to the Nofe : Ṛ

Fig. 2.2 Mary Comb as related by Dr John Hall in 1631.

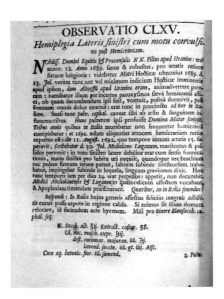

Wepfer (1727), with permission of the Archive
Northampton General Hospital.

The son of the most noble knight and proconsul N.N. among the people of Uri: he was 12 years anno 1689, healthy and hefty, and of longish stature for his age: he seemed to his mother to be subject to hectic disorder on 13th July 1689 but then I could not perceive even the least sign of imminent hectic on him when I was in Altdorf among the Uri people: it was told that he was affected by irregular paroxysms of fierce hemicrania, from which he had to lie down, he vomited, then slept, after sleep all the pain vanished: he was then preparing to travel to Italy. But in the summer of 1692 he again experienced several times terrible hemicrania: on 11th August 1692, when he came into his 15th year, it was written that he came from Milan to Lugano, meager and pallid, : in his whole left side he was weaker, with a feeling of formication,he could not use his left hand as he wanted, and sometimes he could not hold fast neither arm, nor foot, and his lip was retracted to the left, which distressed his speech, he said that his tongue was heavy...'
This condition remained until 1693.

(Translated by Professor H. Isler)

Fig. 2.3 Wepfer stroke following migraine.

first effective migraine drug, caffeine (Isler 2010b). However, Willis did not make a distinction between headaches at different ages, although he does mention headaches that first started in childhood.

Willis describes his post-mortem experience of headache (Willis 1672). In this context, Willis relates the case histories of two Oxford scholars who died of headache: one was found to have a thrombosis in the venous sinus on post-mortem; the other a ruptured intracranial abscess (Hughes 1989, Williams 2003b). The former had been treated under Galenic principles with 'Blooding, Clysters, Playsters, Revulsives, Vesicatories, also, inward Remedies for withdrawing the course of the Blood and Humours from the Head' (Willis 1685).

Commonplace books, medical correspondence and other literature

From the seventeenth century, commonplace books survive. They include recipes for headache, but the age of the sufferer is not mentioned.

Surviving medical correspondence allows a further perspective. One example is the correspondence addressed to Sir Hans Sloane (1660–1753), dated 14 September 1723, and written by Mr Isaiah Farrington about his unnamed 21-year-old daughter. He relates that she had, from about 10 years of age, suffered from violent headaches. She was seen by the local oculist and by local physicians for a long time: 'most of the remedies have not helped, but the steel ones have relieved her headaches' (Sloane 1723). Steel pills, *Chalybs Praeparata*, were rust. Iron or steel filings were moistened in vinegar and exposed to air until they turned to rust (Lane 2001b).

Eighteenth century onwards

In the mid-eighteenth century, Robert Whytt (1714–66) wrote about 'periodical headache' but omitted children's cases (Whytt 1751). More influential were Whytt's 1768 *Observations on the Dropsy in the Brain*, in which he related his experience of 20 cases of internal hydrocephalus in children, which we now know to be tuberculous meningitis (Whytt 1768). 'They complain of a pain in the crown of their head, or in the forehead above their eyes' (Ruhräh 1904).

The physician and poet Erasmus Darwin (1731–1802) is noted among adult headache historians for having suggested a centrifuge of headache (Silberstein et al 2005). The influence of Whytt is seen in late eighteenth-century medical correspondence (see letter below) between Erasmus Darwin and his son Robert (1766–1848), also a physician, concerning the case of Penelope Boothby, a 7-year-old girl (King-Hele 2007). Penelope was the much-loved only child of the linguist and minor poet Sir Brooke Boothby (1744–1824), who was the subject of a notable portrait by Sir Joshua Reynolds (1723–92). Her headache symptoms proved unremitting and she died on 13 March 1791, most likely of otitis media progressing to cerebral venous thrombosis via petrous osteitis.

To Robert Darwin, 9 March 1791

I am here attending Miss Pen. Boothby, who has I think the Hydrocephalus – or if not so, an abscess or other extraneous pressure on or within the brain.

About 3 weeks ago she began to scream out with pain on the left side of her head, or ear; or eye and temple, of that side <u>only</u>, which was succeeded by vomiting. And

---

both these (viz pain of head and vomiting) recur'd about thrice in 24 hours, sometimes in her sleep. And was apparently well at the intervals; pulse regular 104 or 6. She is 7 years old.

This continued a week, and seem'd to give way to one or two calomel purges;.... and zi of unguent caerul. Once a day for 3 days on her head amongst her hair, and lastly a blister on her back and bark in extract every six hours. About a week ago she appear'd quite well, pulse always 104 or 6. On the next day, she became so sleepy and torpid that for two days and half, nothing roused her.

During the first 10 days or fortnight she seem'd rather too sensible to light and complained of it. Now she seem'd to lose all sensibility. By having her head shaved, and a blister apply'd on the left bregma, this sleepyness ceased, but the pain and vomiting recur'd with great violence. A blister apply'd on her back next day did not relieve the pain and sickness. Last night the pain was relieved by filling her affected ear with laudanum- and again this morning by a mixture of laudanum and ether. The calomel has been twice repeated and the mercurial unction on her head.......

Now as the pain is so long confined on one side, can this be Hydrocephalus? Could the trephine be justify'd? As she is a much humour'd child the quantity of pain cannot be ascertain'd by her so frequently screaming out.

If it was an abscess in the brain, would there not be shivering fits? This return of violent pain and total cessation of stupor is not usual, as [you] will see in Whytt's treatise on Hydrocephalus.

I have read Quin's treatise on Hydrocephaulus, but see no observations but what are more clearly given in Whytt. Her pulse was as slow as 80 once this morning immediately after her sleep, but she was then crying out.....

Yours most affectionately,
E. Darwin.

P: I am going to put leeches on the left parietal bone and afterwards apply a blister on Miss P. Boothby

Another illustration of practice is seen in the early nineteenth-century case of Harry Tremayne (1814–1823). John Tremayne wrote about his son Harry's progressive illness and different, often extremely distressing, medical treatments. Harry had an increasing number of bilious attacks, headaches and a squint from the age of 6 years, and died despite the best medical advice available. Harry was seen by an oculist as well as by the notable surgeon Sir Astley Cooper (1768–1841), the latter having 'great fears for him' (James and Williams 2008).

The textbooks of the late eighteenth century up to the late nineteenth century generally have no record of 'headache', 'cephalalgia' or 'migraine' concerning children, even though Tissot made the distinction between migraine and common headache (Tissot 1783). It is either omitted completely (Underwood 1799, Darwall 1830, Dewees 1833, Hunter 1837, Smith

1879) or given as a general chapter making no distinction between adults and children (Buchan 1798). One notable exception is Henry Good Wright's obscure *Headaches Their Causes and Their Cure* in which there is a short section on childhood headache (Wright 1867). Wright sees the principal causes being 'disordered digestion', presaging a measles/scarlet fever infection, poor ventilation, poor dentition, head injury and excessive hours of study. The general view, though, where given, would be seeing childhood headache as part of a continuum into adult life, generally becoming milder in older age (Heberden 1816).

> The most violent headaches will frequently harass a person for the greatest part
> of his life, without shortening his days or impairing his faculties, or unfitting him,
> when his pains are over, for any of the employments of active or contemplative life.
>
> Heberden (1816)

This is reflected when we consider, as an illustrative case, one eminent nineteenth-century paediatrician, Charles West (1816–98). Charles West was instrumental in founding Great Ormond Street Hospital and was its chief physician when it opened in 1852 (Lomax 1996). West's *Lectures on the Diseases of Infancy and Childhood* (1854) does not include any mention of 'headache', 'cephalalgia' or 'migraine' (West 1854). Even in his later Lumelian lectures, *On Some Disorders of the Nervous System* (1871), there were only three mentions of 'headache' in the entire text (West 1871). Reviewing the Great Ormond Street Hospital archive for the period between 1852 and 1914, there were 79 admissions ascribed to 'cephalalgia' and 'headache'. There was but one death, the remainder being discharged, cured or relieved (HHARP 2011).

It must be recalled that the context of this record is of poor patients freely admitted on a background of high infant mortality, child malnutrition and cholera epidemics.

The 1870s were a very interesting period for the history of childhood headache. Edward Liveing's (1832–1919) *Observations on Megrim or Sick-Headache* was first published in the *British Medical Journal* (*BMJ*) and later as a book (Liveing 1872, 1873). Liveing did not see headache in childhood as distinct from headache in adulthood, other than 'a patient suffers from typical migraine, one of his children from the same malady' (Liveing 1872). He discussed cases of migraine with an onset during childhood. Nevertheless, by writing 'the malady is essentially one of the nervous system… the paroxysms may be described as nerve storms', Liveing started a debate which continues to the present day (Liveing 1873). Latham (1832–1923) writing on 'The Pathology of Sick-Headache' in the *BMJ* also makes no mention of children (Latham 1873). Later that year, William Henry Day (1830–1907) wrote the earliest known paper on headaches in children and gave the first child headache classification (Table 2.1), using a modification of an earlier 1835 adult classification of G. Hume Weatherhead (Day 1872, Harms 1967).

> In considering the subject of headaches in children, I may reasonably be accused
> of selecting a symptom which in some cases is the leading feature of intercranial
> change, and at others merely an indication of passing functional disturbance.
>
> Day (1872)

TABLE 2.1
Day's classification of headache in children (1872)

Cerebral headache, attributable to injury
Gastric or sick headache
Headache from anaemia and neuralgia
Headache depending on plethora or fullness of blood
Headache depending on some intricate change in the cerebral membranes or tissues of the brain – a condition amenable to treatment at an early stage
Epileptic headache
Headaches of fever, such as typhus, relapsing fever and typhoid

This and later works, *On Irritable Brain and Congestion of the Brain of Children*, were not cited by contemporary authors and passed into obscurity (Day 1873, 1886). Interestingly, Day does not mention childhood migraine, nor do later nineteenth-century authors (Holt 1899, Goodhart 1902). However, Henoch strongly disagreed, seeing migraine as a significant child health problem, and included a detailed description (Henoch 1889).

From this period childhood headache starts to be explicitly mentioned in literature. Henrik Ibsen's *Ghosts* is one example: 'I thought they were only the ordinary headaches that I used to get so badly when small' (Ibsen 1881); and Henoch's *Lectures on Children's Diseases* (1889) another: 'Migraine occurs in children – as only the inexperienced will deny – very nearly as often as on adults, and with pretty much the same symptoms' (Henoch 1889).

A fictional description of hallucinations in childhood migraine is said to be related in Lewis Carroll's *Alice's Adventures in Wonderland* (Todd 1955). By the early twentieth century childhood migraine was accepted, but, as Still related, it was 'not very common, but I have seen a good many instances' (Still 1924).

Later twentieth century

From the 1930s onwards, and especially after the Second World War, there was a growing interest in headache in childhood and childhood migraine (Riley 1937, Vahlquist and Hackzell 1949, Krupp and Friedman 1953, Vahlquist 1955, Burke and Peters 1956, Apley 1958). However, as late as 1949, some authors still did not consider it worthy of any comment (Ellis 1949). From this time, discussions of childhood migraine at paediatric meetings began to be recorded (Friedman 1953). This growing understanding led to the first symposium and specialist monograph on childhood headache in 1962 (Bille 1962). Friedman and Harms edited the first book on headaches in children (Friedman and Harms 1967). Over the coming decades, further books followed (Barlow 1984, Hockaday 1988, McGrath and Hillier 2001, Winner and Rothner 2001, Abu-Arafeh 2002, Guidetti et al 2002, Winner et al 2008). A similar trend is seen with paediatric neurology books now giving a separate chapter in later editions (Brett 1991, Wilson 1997). More widely, the 1980s omission from within paediatrics of the developing world was later reversed (Coovadia 1988, Coovada and Wittenberg 1998).

Recent developments in headache and migraine

There has been a vast increase in knowledge over the past 30 years on many aspects of headache and migraine in children and adolescents. Areas of new knowledge span over epidemiology, clinical classification of headache disorders, understanding of pathophysiology, use of modern imaging technology, pharmacology and therapeutics, as well as the prognosis of headache disorders and their impact on patients and society at large. Many of these aspects will be discussed in appropriate chapters in this book.

Dedication

The author would like to dedicate this chapter to Dr William Whitehouse and the late Dr Stuart H. Green, both exemplary as children's physicians, consultant paediatric neurologists, inspirational teachers and friends.

REFERENCES

Abu-Arafeh I (ed.) (2002) *Childhood Headache. Clinics in Developmental Medicine*. London: Mac Keith Press.
Apley J (1958) A common denominator in the recurrent pains of childhood. *Proc Roy Soc Med* 51: 1023–4.
Arnott R (forthcoming 2011) Health and the origins of urban society: the archaeology of disease, medicine and public health in the Harappan Civilisation, New Delhi, Chapter 7
Barlow CF (ed) (1984) *Headaches Migraine in Childhood. Clinics in Developmental Medicine No 91*. Oxford: Blackwell Scientific Publications.
Bille B (1962) Symposium on headache in childhood. *Acta Paediatr* 51(Suppl): 1–151.
Blomerus ALL (1999) *The Anatomical Votive Terracotta Phenomenon: Healing Sanctuaries in the Etrusco-Latial-Campanian Region during the Fourth through First Centuries B.C.* Master of Arts theses: University of Cincinnati.
Brett EM (1991) *Pediatric Neurology*, 2nd edn. Edinburgh: Churchill Livingstone, pp. 556–9.
Buchan W (1798) Chapter XXXIV of the head-ach. In: *Domestic Medicine Sixteenth Edition*. London: Balfour and Creech, 352–7.
Burke EC, Peters GA (1956) Migraine in childhood, a preliminary report. *Am J Dis Child* 92: 330–6.
Celli A (1933) *The History of Malaria in the Roman Campagna from Ancient Times*. London: J. Bale, Sons & Danielsson, Ltd. reprinted Scarborough 1969, p 16 and 82.
Coovadia HM (1988) *Paediatrics & Child Health – A Manual for Health Professionals in the Third World*. Cape Town: Oxford University Press.
Coovada HM, Wittenberg DF (eds) (1998) *Paediatrics & Child Health – A manual for Health Professionals in the Third World*. Cape Town: Oxford University Press.
Darwall J (1830) *Plain Instructions for the Management of Infants with Practical Observations on the Disorders Incident to Children*. London: Whittaker, Treacher, and Arnot.
Day WH (1872) Headaches in children – an abstract of a paper read before the Harveian Society of London. *BMJ* 2: 523. http://dx.doi.org/10.1136/bmj.2.619.523
Day WH (1873) *Essays on Diseases of Children*. London: J & A Churchill.
Day WH (1886) *On the Irritable Brain and Congestion of the Brain of Children*. London: Bailliere, Tindall, & Cox.
Dewees WP (1833) *A Treatise on the Physical and Medical Treatment of Children*, 5th edn. Philadelphia: Carey, Lea & Blanchard.
Ellis BRWB (ed.) (1949) *Child Health and Development*. London: Churchill.
Friedman AP (1953) Migraine in children. *Trans Am Neurol Assoc* 3 (78th Ann Meeting): 101.
Friedman AP, Harms E (eds) (1967) *Headaches in Children*. United States: Charles C Thomas.
Goodhart JF (1902) *The Diseases of Children*, 7th edn. London: WB Saunders, pp. 613–15.
Gorji A, Ghadiri MK (2002) History of headache in medieval Persian literature. *Lancet Neurol* 1: 510–15. http://dx.doi.org/10.1016/S1474-4422(02)00226-0
Gowers WR (1907) *The Borderland of Epilepsy*. London: Churchill.
Guidetti V, Russell G, Sillanpää M, Winner P (eds) (2002) *Headache and Migraine in Childhood and Adolescence*. London: Martin Dunitz.

Guthrie D (1945) *A History of Medicine.* London: Thomas Nelson and Sons, p. 44.

Hall J (1679) Observation XLIV *Select Observations on English Bodies of Eminent Persons in Desperate Diseases.* London: William Marshall at the Bible in Newgate-street, pp. 131–3.

Harms E (1967) Historical retrospect. In: Friedman AP, Harms E, editors. *Headaches in Children.* Springfield, IL: Charles C Thomas, pp. 5–9.

Heberden W (1816) Capitis dolor. In: *Commentaries on the History and Cure of Diseases,* 4th edn. London: Payne and Foss, pp. 77–83.

Henoch E (1889) *Lectures on Childrens' Diseases. A Handbook for Practitioners and Students, Volume 1* (translated from the 4th edition 1889*).* London: New Sydenham Society, pp. 349–52.

HHARP (Historic Hospital Admission Records Project) (2011) (http://www.hharp.org), Kingston University, London.

Hockaday J (1988) *Migraine in Childhood.* London: Butterworths.

Holt LE (1899) General and functional nervous disorders. In: *The Diseases of Infancy and Childhood.* London: Thomas Lewin, pp. 689–90.

Howells R (2010) Headaches in childhood and adolescence. *Adv Clin Neurosci Rehabil* 10: 27–9.

Hughes JT (1989) Thomas Willis: the first Oxford neuropathologist. In: Rose FC, editor. *Neuroscience Across the Centuries.* London: Smith-Gordon. pp. 93–4.

Hunter J (1837) *The Works of John Hunter.* London: Longman, Rees, Orme, Brooke, Green and Longman.

Ibsen H (1881) In: Baldick R and Radice B 1973 *Ghosts.* London: Penguin Classics, p. 73.

Isler H (2010a) Neurology and the neurological sciences in the German-speaking countries. *Handb Clin Neurol* 95: 668.

Isler H (2010b) The development of neurology and the neurological sciences in the 17th century. *Handb Clin Neurol* 95: 91–106. http://dx.doi.org/10.1016/S0072-9752(08)02108-8

Jackson JH (1876) In: Taylor J, editor. (1931) *Selected Writings of John Hughlings Jackson.* London: Hodder and Stoughton, p. 153.

James RM, Williams AN (2008) Two Georgian fathers: diverse in experience, united in grief. *J Med Humanit* 34: 70–9. http://dx.doi.org/10.1136/jmh.2008.000281

King-Hele D (2007) *The Collected letters of Erasmus Darwin.* Cambridge: Cambridge University Press, p. 378.

Krupp GR, Friedman AP (1953) Recurrent headache in children, a study of 100 clinic cases. *N Y State J Med* 53: 43–6.

Lane J (2001a) *John Hall His Patients. The Medical Practice of Shakespeare's son-in law.* Stratford upon Avon: The Shakespeare Birthplace Trust, pp. 262–8.

Lane J (2001b) *John Hall his Patients. The Medical Practice of Shakespeare's Son-in-law.* Stratford upon Avon: The Shakespeare Birthplace Trust, p. 81.

Larner AJ (2010) Neurological literature: headache (part 7): megrim. *Adv Clin Neurosci Rehabil* 10: 16.

Latham PW (1873) The pathology of sick-headache. *BMJ* 1: 113. http://dx.doi.org/10.1136/bmj.1.631.113

Le Pois C (Piso, Carolus) Selectorium observationum et consiliorum de praeteritis hactenus morbis effecti-busque praeter na'turam ab aqua, seu serosa colluvie et diluvie, orbis liber singularis. Lugduni Batavorum (Ponti ad Monticulum: 1618). Cited in: Isler H, Clifford Rose F (eds) (2000) Historical background. In: Olensen J, Tfelt-Hansen P and Welch KMA, editors. *The Headaches,* 2nd edn. Philadelphia: Lippincott Williams & Wilkins, p 3.

Liveing E (1872) Observations on megrim or sick-headache. *BMJ* 1: 364–6. http://dx.doi.org/10.1136/bmj.1.588.364-a

Liveing E (1873) *Observations on Megrim, Sick- headache, and Some Allied Disorder: A contribution to the Pathology of Nerve Storms.* London: J and A Churchill.

Lomax E M (1996) Small and special: the development of hospitals for children in Victorian Britain. *Med Hist Suppl* 16: Wellcome Trust.

McGrath PA, Hillier LM (eds) (2001) *The Child with Headache: Diagnosis and Treatment. Progress in Pain research and Management,* Vol. 19. Seattle: IASP Press.

Morel JP (1989). Aspects économiques d'un sanctuaire: Fondo Ruozzo à Teano, Campanie. *Sc Ant* 3–4. 509.

Morton LT (1970) *A Medical Bibliography,* 3rd edn. London: André Deutsch.

Nemet-Nejat KR (1998) *Daily Life in Ancient Mesopotamia.* Westport, Connecticut: Greenwood Publishing Group, pp. 80 and 130.

Paré A (1634) The works of Ambrose Paréy Translated out of Latine and compared with the French. By Th. Johnson. London: Th. Cotes and R. Young.

Plato (1888) Republic III 407b9-c2. In: Jowett B, editor. *The Republic of Plato.* Oxford: Clarenden.

Rapoport A (2000) Migraine, the evolution of our knowledge. *Arch Neurol* 57: 1221–3. http://dx.doi.org/10.1001/archneur.57.8.1221

Riley HA (1937) Migraine in children and the mechanism of the attack. *Bull Neurol Inst New York* 6: 387–402.

Rosner F (1976) A biblical headache. *JAMA* 235: 1327. http://dx.doi.org/10.1001/jama.1976.03260390013012

Ruhräh J (1904) The history of tuberculous meningitis. *Med Library Hist J* 2: 160–5.

Silberstein SD, Stiles MA, Young WB (eds) (2005) *Atlas of Migraine and Other Headaches*, 2nd edn. London: Taylor & Francis.

Sloane H (1723) *The Correspondence of Sir Hans Sloane*. London: British Library.

Smith JL (1879) *A Treatise on the Diseases of Infancy and Childhood*. Philadelphia: HC Lea.

Still GF (1924) *Common Disorders and Diseases of Childhood*, 4th edn. Oxford: Oxford Medical Publications, pp. 718–33.

Tissot SA (1783) Traité des nerfs et de leurs maladies. De la catalepsie, de l'exstase, de l'anesthésie de las migraine et des maladies du cerveau. In: *Oeuvres de Monsieur Tissot, Vol 13*. Paris: Lausaunne, pp. 133–173.

Todd J (1955) The syndrome of Alice in Wonderland. *Can Med Assoc J* 73: 701.

Underwood M (1799) *Treatise on the Disease of Children*. London: J. Matthews.

Vahlquist B, Hackzell G (1949) Migraine of early onset. A study of thirty one cases in which the disease first appeared between one and four years of age. *Acta Paediatr* 38: 622–36. http://dx.doi.org/10.1111/j.1651-2227.1949.tb17914.x

Vahlquist B (1955) Migraine in children. *Int Arch Allergy Immunol* 7: 348–55. http://dx.doi.org/10.1159/000228238

van Dijk, Geller JM (2003) Ur III incantations from the Frau Professor Hilprecht-Sammlung Collection, Jena. Wiesbaden: Harrasowitz Verlag, p. 12

Verano JW, Finger S (2010) Ancient trepanation. *Handb Clin Neurol* 95: 3–14. http://dx.doi.org/10.1016/S0072-9752(08)02101-5

Wells C (1985) A medical interpretation of the votive terracottas: an appendix to a sanctuary at ponte di nona. *J Br Archaeol Assoc* 138: 41–7.

West C (1854) *Lectures on the Diseases of Infancy and Childhood*. Philadelphia: Blanchard and Lea. http://dx.doi.org/10.1037/12108-000

West C (1871) *On Some Disorders of the Nervous System in Childhood*. London: Blanchard and Lea.

Wepfer J (1727) Observationes Medico-practicae de Affectibus capitis…. Scaphaeii. J A Ziegler Schaffenhausen. Obs CLXV pp. 798–802.

Whytt R (1751) *An Essay on the Vital and Involuntary Motions of Animals*. Edinburgh: Hamilton Balfour, pp. 620–622 and 709–12.

Whytt R (1768) *Obervations on the Dropsy in the Brain*. Edinburgh: J. Balfour.

Winner P, Rothner AD (eds) (2001) *Headache in Children and Adolescents*. Hamilton, Ontario: BC Decker.

Winner P, Lewis DW, Rothner AD (2008) *Headache in Children and Adolescents. Second edition*. Hamilton, Ontario: BC Decker.

Williams AN (2003a) Thomas Willis' practice of paediatric neurology and disability. *J Hist Neurosci* 12: 350–67. http://dx.doi.org/10.1076/jhin.12.4.350.27910

Williams AN (2003b) Thomas Willis' understanding of cerebrovascular disorders. *J Stroke Cerebrovasc Dis* 12: 280–4. http://dx.doi.org/10.1016/j.jstrokecerebrovasdis.2003.09.012

Willis T (1672) *De anima brutorum quae hominis vitalis ac sensitiva est*. Oxford: Richard Davis.

Willis T (1685) *The London Practice of Physick*. London: Basset and Crooke 1685.

Wilson J (1997) Headache in childhood. In: Brett EM, editor. *Paediatric Neurology Third Edition*. London: Churchill Livingstone, pp. 589–97.

Wright HG (1867) Headaches in childhood and youth. *Headaches Their Causes and their Cure*. Philadephia: Lindsay and Blakeston, pp. 14–20.

Wuertz (also Wirtz) F. (1563) Practica der Wund-Arzney. Basel, apud Petrum Pernam. Basel, Sebastian Henricpetri (1616): including the posthumous first edition of the tract on pediatric surgery by Wuertz "Ein schÖnes und nutzliches Kinderbuechlin."

Würtz F (1656) *An Experimental Treatise of Surgerie in 4 Parts*. London: Gartrude Dawson, pp. 352–3.

Zayas V (2007) On headache tablets: headache incantations from Ur III (2113- 2038 BC). *Med Health R I* 90: 46–7.

Zanchin G (2010) Headache a historical outline. *Handb Clin Neurol* 95: 375–86. http://dx.doi.org/10.1016/S0072-9752(08)02125-8

3
PATHOPHYSIOLOGY OF MIGRAINE AND OTHER HEADACHES

Peter J Goadsby

Headache is a ubiquitous problem and, as such, very commonly leads to referral to paediatricians or neurologists when it becomes intrusive. Migraine is very clearly the most common form of disabling headache to present to any level of medical care, be it primary or secondary care. Because paediatric and adolescent presentations of primary headache disorders are, as expected, somewhat less phenotypically rich, one needs to consider the entire biology and natural history to make the diagnosis and plan management. Books written by and aimed at the adult headache specialist or neurologist, albeit with paediatric coverage, provide a very substantial account of the disorders (Silberstein et al 2002, Lance and Goadsby 2005, Olesen et al 2005, Lipton and Bigal 2006), even to the detail of frequent headache (Goadsby et al 2005).

Adolescent and childhood coverage is limited by two very broad problems: first, there seems to be a disproportionate preoccupation with the differences between adult and childhood migraine and, second, there is an understandable limitation on research in childhood headache. It is the author's experience that, although the clinical manifestations are more subtle and recognition of the syndromes requires a more searching clinical approach, the similarities in the underpinning themes are stunning. Migraine is a disorder for life, from the more unsettled child (Guidetti et al 1984) with colic (Gelfand et al 2012b), to the late-life migrainous accompaniments. Its disability is no less devastating for the child, who cannot enjoy the most precious years, than for the adult, whose productive years are blighted. This chapter will cover the broad basis of the current understanding of the biology of primary headache disorders. The pain pathways are somewhat generic in that head pain is just that, head pain. The central modulatory systems and the inherited background of the problems are what almost certainly dissect out the particular problems and allow clinical differentiation of the syndromes.

The essential elements to be considered (Table 3.1) in understanding migraine are as follows:
- anatomy of head pain: the large intracranial vessels and dura mater, and their trigemino-vascular innervation;
- physiology and pharmacology of activation of the peripheral branches of the ophthalmic branch of the trigeminal nerve;
- physiology and pharmacology of the trigeminal nucleus, in particular its most caudal part, the trigeminocervical complex;

TABLE 3.1
Neuroanatomical processing of dural and vascular head pain

Target innervation	Structure	Comments
Cranial vessels, dura mater	Ophthalmic branch of trigeminal nerve	
First	Trigeminal ganglion	Middle cranial fossa
Second	Trigeminal nucleus (quintothalamic tract)	Trigeminal n. caudalis and C1/C2 dorsal horns
Third	Thalamus	Ventrobasal complex
		Medial nucleus of posterior group
		Intralaminar complex
Final	Cortex	Insulae
		Frontal cortex
		Anterior cingulate cortex
		Basal ganglia

- central nervous system activation in association with pain in thalamus and cortical areas; and
- brainstem and diencephalic modulatory systems that control trigeminal pain processing.

Trigeminovascular anatomy – structures that produce, or are perceived to produce, pain

Surrounding the large cerebral vessels, pial vessels, large venous sinuses and dura mater is a plexus of largely unmyelinated fibres that arise from the ophthalmic division of the trigeminal ganglion (McNaughton 1966) and in the posterior fossa from the upper cervical dorsal roots (Arbab et al 1986). Trigeminal nerve fibres innervating cerebral vessels arise from neurons in the trigeminal ganglion that contain substance P and calcitonin gene-related peptide (CGRP) (Uddman et al 1985), both of which can be released when the trigeminal ganglion is stimulated in either humans or cats (Goadsby et al 1988). Stimulation of the cranial vessels, such as the superior sagittal sinus, is certainly painful in humans (Feindel et al 1960, McNaughton and Feindel 1977). Human dural nerves that innervate the cranial vessels largely consist of small-diameter, myelinated and unmyelinated fibres that almost certainly subserve a nociceptive function (Cushing 1904).

What is the source of the pain in migraine? The pain process is likely to be a combination of direct factors, i.e. activation of the nociceptors of pain-producing intracranial structures, in concert with a reduction in the normal functioning of the endogenous pain control pathways that normally gate that pain (Goadsby et al 1991). If the carotid artery is occluded ipsilateral to the side of headache in migraineurs then two-thirds will experience relief; this does not account for the other one-third and is what one might expect if the problem is a dysmodulation of normality (Drummond and Lance 1983). Moreover, distension of major cerebral vessels by balloon dilatation leads to pain referred to the ophthalmic division of the trigeminal nerve, which makes it likely that intracranial structures are the primary targets of the dysmodulation (Martins et al 1993, Nichols et al 1990, 1993). There is little doubt that sufficient changes in vascular diameter produce pain. However, are the changes in migraine that are much less pronounced, inconsistent from patient to patient and indeed not always present (Friberg et al 1991) sufficient in themselves to produce pain? When considering the contribution of the periphery and the brain, one must keep an open mind; we accept photophobia and phonophobia without any hint that there is peripheral change, so why should a peripheral change be important for the pain? This remains a fundamental question without obvious resolution.

Trigeminovascular physiology – peripheral connections

A considerable amount of experimental work on animals and humans has been carried out to understand the physiology of the activation of trigeminal nociceptive afferents. These data allow us to build up a picture of what might happen during migraine and some plausible explanation of how the current acute antimigraine compounds might work (Goadsby 2000).

PLASMA PROTEIN EXTRAVASATION

Moskowitz (1990) has performed a series of experiments suggesting that some component of the pain of migraine may be a form of sterile neurogenic inflammation. Neurogenic plasma extravasation can be seen during electrical stimulation of the trigeminal ganglion in the rat (Markowitz et al 1987). Plasma extravasation can be blocked by ergot alkaloids (Buzzi and Moskowitz 1991), indometacin (Buzzi et al 1989), acetylsalicylic acid (Buzzi et al 1989) and the serotonin 5-HT$_{1B/1D/1F}$ agonist sumatriptan (Buzzi and Moskowitz 1990). The pharmacology of current abortive antimigraine drugs in the context of plasma protein extravasation has been reviewed in detail (Cutrer et al 1997). In addition, trigeminal ganglion stimulation results in structural changes in the dura mater, including mast cell degranulation (Dimitriadou et al 1991) and changes in postcapillary venules including platelet aggregation (Dimitriadou et al 1992). While it is generally accepted that such changes, and particularly the initiation of a sterile inflammatory response, would cause pain (Strassman et al 1996, Burstein et al 1998), it is not clear whether this is sufficient of itself or requires other stimulators or promoters. In the context of migraine it seems clear that the model has very distinct limitations. First, the idea that migraine involves repeated inflammatory insults yet brain function, even into late life, is normal seems incongruent (Kurth et al 2011). Second, there is a very significant body of literature on at least 10 candidate migraine treatments that work in the model and are ineffective in migraine (Peroutka 2005).

It has been shown that, although plasma extravasation in the retina, which is blockable by sumatriptan, could be seen after trigeminal ganglion stimulation in the rat, no changes are seen with retinal angiography during acute attacks of migraine or cluster headache (May et al 1998b). A limitation of this study was the probable sampling of both retina and choroid elements in rats, given that choroidal vessels have fenestrated capillaries (Steuer et al 2004). Clearly, the blockade of neurogenic plasma protein extravasation is not predictive of antimigraine efficacy in humans, as evidenced by the failure in clinical trials of substance P, neurokinin-1 antagonists (Goldstein et al 1997, Connor et al 1998, Norman et al 1998, Diener and The RPR100893 Study Group 2003), specific plasma protein extravasation (PPE) blockers, CP122,288 (Roon et al 2000) and 4991w93 (Earl et al 1999), an endothelin antagonist (May et al 1996) and a neurosteroid ganaxolone (Data et al 1998). Indeed, substance P (neurokinin-1) receptor blockers also have no role in the preventive management of migraine (Goldstein et al 2001). The role of dural neurogenic plasma extravasation has recently been reviewed (Peroutka 2005) and, as a basis for thinking about migraine in inflammatory terms, seems both outdated and irrational.

NEUROPEPTIDE STUDIES

Electrical stimulation of the trigeminal ganglion in both humans and cats leads to increases in extracerebral blood flow (Goadsby and Duckworth 1987, Tran-Dinh et al 1992) and local cranial release of both CGRP and substance P (Goadsby et al 1988). In the cat, stimulation of the more nociceptive specific structure, the superior sagittal sinus, increases cerebral blood flow to a greater extent than trigeminal ganglion stimulation (Goadsby et al 1997). A substantial component of the trigeminovascular activation is mediated by a pathway traversing the superior salivatory nucleus (Knight et al 2005) and projecting through the greater superficial petrosal branch of the facial nerve (Lambert et al 1984), again releasing a powerful vasodilator peptide – vasoactive intestinal polypeptide (VIP) (Goadsby and Macdonald 1985).

Glucagon–secretin family peptides

VIP, peptide histidine isoleucine (methionine), pituitary adenylate cyclase-activating polypeptide (PACAP), helodermin and helospectin I and II are all part of the glucagon–secretin superfamily of peptides (Harmar et al 2012). PACAP is known as PACAP38, as it has 38 residues (Arimura 1992). PACAP is found in the trigeminocervical complex (Christiansen et al 2004), and is a potent cerebral vasodilator (Uddman et al 1993). VIP and PACAP exert their effects through G-protein coupled receptors: PAC_1, $VPAC_1$ and $VPAC_2$. PAC1 receptors are selective for PACAP, whereas $VPAC_1$ and $VPAC_2$ bind VIP and PACAP. VIP-ergic innervation of the cerebral vessels is predominantly anterior rather than posterior (Matsuyama et al 1983). This may contribute to this region's vulnerability to spreading depression and in part explain why the aura is so very often seen to commence posteriorly. In humans, VIP invokes only minimal headache (Hansen et al 2006), while invoking marked vasodilation (Rahmann et al 2008), whereas PACAP, which is also elevated after superior sagittal sinus stimulation (Zagami et al 1995), triggers migraine and vasodilation (Schytz et al 2009). PACAP38 also triggers headache in healthy individuals (Amin et al 2012).

Calcitonin gene-related peptide

Stimulation of the more specifically vascular, pain-producing superior sagittal sinus increases cerebral blood flow and jugular vein CGRP levels (Zagami et al 1990). Evidence from humans suggests that CGRP is elevated in the headache phase of migraine (Goadsby et al 1990, Gallai et al 1995), cluster headache (Goadsby and Edvinsson 1994, Fanciullacci et al 1995), chronic paroxysmal hemicrania (Goadsby and Edvinsson 1996) and in throbbing exacerbations of 'chronic tension-type headache' (Ashina et al 2000), whose phenotype might more usefully be considered part of chronic migraine (Olesen et al 2006). An exception is what seems to be less well-developed migraine, in which CGRP is not elevated (Tvedskov et al 2005). In the round, these data support the view that the trigeminovascular system may be activated in a protective role in these conditions. It is of interest in this regard that compounds that have *not* shown activity in human migraine, notably the conformationally restricted analogue of sumatriptan, CP122,288 (Knight et al 1999), and the conformationally restricted analogue of zolmitriptan, 4991w93 (Knight et al 2001), were *ineffective* inhibitors of CGRP release after superior sagittal sinus stimulation in the cat. A clear answer for the importance of CGRP comes from clinical studies of potent, specific CGRP receptor antagonists, such as olcegepant (Doods et al 2000) or telcagepant (Miller et al 2010). These compounds have no vascular actions (Petersen et al 2004, 2005, Van der Schueren et al 2011). At least four compounds have been shown to be effective in the treatment of acute migraine: olcegepant (Olesen et al 2004), telcagepant (Ho et al 2008, Connor et al 2009), MK-3207 (Hewitt et al 2011) and BI44370TA (Diener et al 2011).

CGRP alone does not mediate plasma protein extravasation
There is no direct evidence that CGRP alone will produce increased vascular permeability in the dura mater (Brain and Grant 2004). In a study in mice, CGRP was not active in the plasma extravasation assay (Tam and Brain 2004) but was a potent vasodilator (Grant et al 2004). Consistent with this, and in contrast to the mice which have a neurokinin-1 receptor knockout (Kandere-Grzybowska et al 2003), animals in which the CGRP gene is disrupted still have a plasma extravasation response to the application of mustard oil to the ear, which in turn can be blocked by a neurokinin-1 receptor antagonist (Grant et al 2005). Maltos and colleagues (2004) dropped substance P or CGRP onto exposed dental pulp, after first drilling into the tooth and then 'sticking' a probe through the cavity onto the pulp. Given the prestimulus of the drilling, CGRP by virtue of vasodilation, but not acting alone, may have promoted Evans blue leakage. Taken together, it seems clear in the experimental setting that CGRP alone does not promote plasma extravasation, and that the efficacy of CGRP receptor antagonists in migraine does not provide any evidence for a role for plasma protein extravasation in the disorder.

Trigeminovascular physiology – central connections

THE TRIGEMINOCERVICAL COMPLEX
The sites within the brainstem that are responsible for craniovascular pain have been mapped in experimental animals including the monkey (Fig. 3.1). Using Fos immunohistochemistry, a method for looking at activated cells after meningeal irritation with blood, Fos expression is reported in the trigeminal nucleus caudalis (Nozaki et al 1992). After stimulation of the superior sagittal sinus, Fos-like immunoreactivity is seen in the trigeminal nucleus caudalis and in the dorsal horn at the C1 and C2 levels in the cat (Kaube et al 1993c) and monkey (Goadsby and Hoskin 1997). Fos-like immunoreactivity can be observed bilaterally after unilateral stimulation of the peridural tissue around the meningeal artery (Hoskin et al 1999). Activation in the high cervical cord is consistent with similar data using 2-deoxyglucose measurements with superior sagittal sinus stimulation (Goadsby and Zagami 1991) and consistent with the observations of Kerr (Kerr 1961, Kerr and Olafson 1961), and recent human studies (Piovesan et al 2001). Direct evidence for activation of neurons in the high cervical cord from

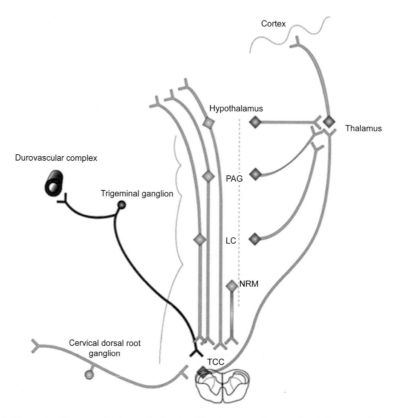

Fig. 3.1 Elements of the neurobiology of migraine. The durovascular complex is innervated dominantly by branches of the ophthalmic (first) division of the trigeminal nerve that pass to the trigeminal ganglion and project to a complex of second-order neurons in the trigeminal nucleus caudalis and dorsal horns of the C1 and C2 spinal cord, the trigeminocervical complex (TCC). There is a convergent input from the C2 upper spinal root afferents onto these TCC neurons (Bartsch and Goadsby 2005). TCC neurons project to the contralateral trigeminothalamic neurons via the quintothalamic tract that decussates in the brainstem. TCC neuronal activity can be modulated by projections from nucleus raphe magnus (NRM), locus coeruleus (LC), ventrolateral periaqueductal grey (PAG) and hypothalamus, each of which, save NRM, can also directly modulate thalamic activity. Migraine is likely to represent a dysfunction of these diencephalic and brainstem modulatory systems (Akerman et al 2011).

stimulation of both forebrain dura mater and regions innervated by the greater occipital nerve has been provided (Bartsch and Goadsby 2001, 2002). Taken together, these data suggest a view of the trigeminal nucleus extending beyond the traditional nucleus caudalis boundary to the dorsal horn of the high cervical region in a functional continuum that includes a cervical extension. The entire group of cells could be regarded functionally as the *trigeminocervical* complex and probably accounts for the largest part of the pain phenotype of primary headaches (Bartsch and Goadsby 2005).

These data demonstrate that a substantial portion of the trigeminovascular nociceptive information comes by way of the most caudal cells. This concept provides an anatomical explanation for the referral of pain to the back of the head in migraine. Moreover, experimental pharmacological evidence suggests that some abortive antimigraine drugs, such as dihydroergotamine (Hoskin et al 1996), acetylsalicylic acid (Kaube et al 1993b), sumatriptan after blood–brain barrier disruption (Kaube et al 1993a), eletriptan (Goadsby and Hoskin 1999), naratriptan (Goadsby and Knight 1997, Cumberbatch et al 1998), rizatriptan (Cumberbatch et al 1997), zolmitriptan (Goadsby and Hoskin 1996) and the CGRP receptor antagonists (Storer et al 2004), can have actions at these second-order neurons. Such an effect would reduce neuronal activity, providing a clear site for therapeutic intervention in migraine.

Higher-order processing

THALAMUS

Following transmission in the caudal brainstem and high cervical spinal cord, information is relayed in a group of fibres (the quintothalamic tract) to the thalamus (Fig. 3.1). Processing of vascular pain in the thalamus occurs in the ventral posteromedial thalamus, medial nucleus of the posterior complex and intralaminar thalamus (Zagami and Goadsby 1991). Zagami and Lambert (1991) have shown, by application of capsaicin to the superior sagittal sinus, that trigeminal projections with a high degree of nociceptive input are processed in neurons, particularly in the ventral posteromedial thalamus and in its ventral periphery. These neurons may be a target for preventive treatments; certainly they are inhibited by β-adrenoceptor blockers, such as propranolol (Shields and Goadsby 2005), valproate through a $GABA_A$ mechanism (Andreou et al 2010) and topiramate through a glutamate kainate-GluR5 mechanism (Andreou and Goadsby 2011). Remarkably, they may also be a target for acute treatments such as triptans – $5-HT_{1B/1D}$ receptor agonists – as microiontophoresis of naratriptan on venteroposteromedial thalamic neurons inhibits their activation by trigeminal nociceptive afferent stimulation (Shields and Goadsby 2006), and gepants – CGRP receptor antagonists (Summ et al 2010). Human imaging studies have confirmed activation of thalamus contralateral to pain in acute migraine (Bahra et al 2001, Afridi et al 2005a), cluster headache (May et al 1998a) and SUNCT (short-lasting unilateral neuralgiform headache with conjunctival injection and tearing) (May et al 1999).

CORTICAL PROCESSING

Pain in general is a complex phenomenon that is mediated by a network of neuronal structures, including cingulate cortex, insulae and thalamus (Melzack and Casey 1968, Jones et al 1991a, Derbyshire et al 1997). One framework proposes *medial* (thalamus, anterior cingulate cortex and prefrontal cortex) and *lateral* (primary and secondary somatosensory cortex) *pain systems*, and these have been investigated using functional imaging techniques (Jones et al 1991b). Most functional imaging studies demonstrate activation in these structures with clinical or experimental pain and recent reviews are available (Chen 1993, Derbyshire et al 1997). Recently, the amygdala (Bernard et al 1992, Hsieh et al 1996, Derbyshire et al 1997), basal ganglia (Chudler and Dong 1995, Derbyshire et al 1997) and posterior parietal cortex (Dong et al 1996) have also been implicated in central nervous system responses to pain.

It has been shown that, in migraine, anterior cingulate cortex, frontal cortex, and visual and auditory association cortex are activated during acute attacks (Weiller et al 1995, Bahra et al 2001, Sprenger et al 2012). Similarly, in cluster headache, cingulate cortex, insula, prefrontal cortex and basal ganglia are activated during pain (May et al 1998a). The activation of these non-specific areas during acute migraine and cluster headache is neither surprising nor unusual in pattern. How these areas relate to each other, as well as the processing, is unknown and will require challenging and technically difficult experiments to work out. A recent functional imaging study suggests that cortical regions, particularly the orbitofrontal cortex, may be important in medication overuse headache (Fumal et al 2006). This problem is both widespread and in need of study in some detail.

Central modulation of trigeminal pain

A key observation, perhaps the crucial observation of functional imaging in migraine, has been that brainstem areas are active during pain and that after successful treatment this activation persists (Weiller et al 1995, Bahra et al 2001, Denuelle et al 2004, Afridi et al 2005a,b). The areas active are in the dorsal midbrain and the dorsolateral pons. The dorsal midbrain activation corresponds with the brain region that Raskin et al (1987) initially reported, and Veloso et al (1998) confirmed, to cause migraine-like headache when stimulated in patients with electrodes implanted for pain control. Moreover, lesions, for example from multiple sclerosis (Haas et al 1993) or a developmental venous anomaly (Goadsby 2002), also produce migraine. A pressing question is: what are the roles for these areas in the disorder, initiation, maintenance or termination of the attack?

It has been shown in experiments on animals that stimulation of a discrete nucleus in the brainstem – nucleus locus coeruleus (the main central noradrenergic nucleus) – reduces cerebral blood flow in a frequency-dependent manner (Goadsby et al 1982) through an α_2-adrenoceptor-linked mechanism (Goadsby et al 1985). This reduction is maximal in the occipital cortex (Goadsby and Duckworth 1989). While a 25% overall reduction in cerebral blood flow is seen, extracerebral vasodilatation occurs in parallel (Goadsby et al 1982). In addition, the main serotonin-containing nucleus in the brainstem, the midbrain dorsal raphe nucleus, can increase cerebral blood flow when activated (Goadsby et al 1991). Following stimulation of the superior sagittal sinus, Fos expression is increased in the ventrolateral periaqueductal grey matter (PAG) in cats and monkeys (Hoskin et al 2001). Similarly, stimulation of this region will inhibit sagittal sinus-evoked trigeminal neuronal activity in cats (Knight and Goadsby 1999). The ventrolateral PAG would certainly have been included within the area of activation on the human neuroimaging studies outlined above, so its physiology and interactions with the trigeminovascular system are of particular interest. These aminergic brainstem neurons are an attractive site to host the basic defects in migraine and require detailed study and further human neuroimaging as we try to define the detail of the biology of migraine.

Pathophysiology of childhood periodic syndromes

A more particular issue in childhood headache is understanding the periodic syndromes that are accepted precursors of migraine in adulthood, such as cyclical vomiting, abdominal migraine and benign paroxysmal vertigo of childhood. The author would add benign paroxysmal torticollis of infancy (Giffin et al 2002) and perhaps infantile colic (Gelfand et al 2012a) to this list. The evidence for the association of these syndromes and childhood migraine is mainly based on the epidemiological and clinical studies with some medium- to long-term follow-up of patients (Chapters 15, 16 and 17). We have recently seen a 2.6-fold increase in colic in infants whose mothers have migraine compared with mothers who do not (Gelfand et al 2012a). Biochemical, physiological and genetic evidence of association is hard to obtain, but the description of a common genetic mechanism between familial hemiplegic migraine (FHM) and paroxysmal torticollis of infancy, viz. involvement of the *CACNA1A* gene (Giffin et al 2002) that is clearly involved in FHM (Ophoff et al 1996), implicates paroxysmal torticollis of infancy in the precursor spectrum. Vertigo in migraine is very common, and provides a link to the childhood vertigo syndrome (Dieterich and Brandt 1999). One sees cyclical vomiting in adults, although uncommonly, and the abdominal pain syndrome is much less obvious. One could speculate that, as brainstem modulatory systems mature, their targets alter and thus the syndromes change. Attacks associated with excitement, thus particular for ruining many an enjoyable childhood experience, may have their origin again in aminergic systems, such as locus coeruleus, implicated in migraine by functional imaging studies, and from the basic science literature (Foote et al 1991, Fureman and Hess 2005).

Summary

An understanding of the basic anatomy and physiology of the cranial circulation facilitates the assessment and management of patients with migraine. Physiological processes clearly mature and change in childhood and adolescence, so it should not be a surprise that migraine evolves and changes, maturing to its adult form during adolescence. It seems likely that it is the brain control mechanisms that alter and mature (Akerman et al 2011); perhaps this explains why the disease has the same flavour all through life but runs at different temperatures. Indeed, changes in the aminergic nuclei with age (Amaral and Sinnamon 1977) may explain much about why migraine tends to abate with age. It has become clear that migraine is *not* a *vascular* headache *but* that the trigeminovascular and parasympathetic innervation of the cranial circulation drives the vascular changes of migraine, which is in essence *neurovascular* in expression. Migraine involves a disease process of the central nervous system at its core (Sprenger and Goadsby 2010, Sprenger et al 2010). Migraine may be considered an episodic aminergic systems dysfunction with predominantly sensory consequences. The pain may well share more with photophobia and phonophobia, in being a perceived as opposed to a peripherally generated phenomenon, than has been appreciated. As therapy evolves towards the next century such a concept will drive new treatments and an understanding of the basic anatomy and physiology of headache will aid clinical management at every level, from explaining the problem to the patient, to initiating treatment.

REFERENCES

Afridi S, Giffin NJ, Kaube H et al (2005a) A PET study in spontaneous migraine. *Arch Neurol* 62: 1270–5. http://dx.doi.org/10.1001/archneur.62.8.1270
Afridi S, Matharu MS, Lee L et al (2005b) A PET study exploring the laterality of brainstem activation in migraine using glyceryl trinitrate. *Brain* 128: 932–9. http://dx.doi.org/10.1093/brain/awh416

Akerman S, Holland P, Goadsby PJ (2011) Diencephalic and brainstem mechanisms in migraine. *Nat Rev Neurosci* 12: 570–84. http://dx.doi.org/10.1038/nrn3057

Amaral DG, Sinnamon HM (1977) The locus coeruleus: neurobiology of a central noradrenergic nucleus. *Prog Neurobiol* 9: 147–96. http://dx.doi.org/10.1016/0301-0082(77)90016-8

Amin FM, Asghar MS, Guo S et al (2012) Headache and prolonged dilatation of the middle meningeal artery by PACAP38 in healthy volunteers. *Cephalalgia* 32: 140–9. http://dx.doi.org/10.1177/0333102411431333

Andreou AP, Goadsby PJ (2011) Topiramate in the treatment of migraine: a kainate (glutamate) receptor antagonist within the trigeminothalamic pathway. *Cephalalgia* 31: 1343–58. http://dx.doi.org/10.1177/0333102411418259

Andreou AP, Shields KG, Goadsby PJ (2010) GABA and valproate modulate trigeminovascular nociceptive transmission in the thalamus. *Neurobiol Disease* 37: 314–23. http://dx.doi.org/10.1016/j.nbd.2009.10.007

Arbab MA-R, Wiklund L, Svendgaard NA (1986) Origin and distribution of cerebral vascular innervation from superior cervical, trigeminal and spinal ganglia investigated with retrograde and anterograde WGA-HRP tracing in the rat. *Neuroscience* 19: 695–708. http://dx.doi.org/10.1016/0306-4522(86)90293-9

Arimura A (1992) Pituitary adenylate cyclase activating polypeptide (PACAP): discovery and current status of research. *Regul Pept* 37: 287–303. http://dx.doi.org/10.1016/0167-0115(92)90621-Z

Ashina M, Bendsten L, Jensen R, Schifter S, Jansen-Olesen I, Olesen J (2000) Plasma levels of calcitonin gene-related peptide in chronic tension-type headache. *Neurology* 55: 1335–40. http://dx.doi.org/10.1212/WNL.55.9.1335

Bahra A, Matharu MS, Buchel C, Frackowiak RSJ, Goadsby PJ (2001) Brainstem activation specific to migraine headache. *Lancet* 357: 1016–17. http://dx.doi.org/10.1016/S0140-6736(00)04250-1

Bartsch T, Goadsby PJ (2001) Stimulation of the greater occipital nerve (GON) enhances responses of dural responsive convergent neurons in the trigemino-cervical complex in the rat. *Cephalalgia* 21: 401–2.

Bartsch T, Goadsby PJ (2002) Stimulation of the greater occipital nerve induces increased central excitability of dural afferent input. *Brain* 125: 1496–509. http://dx.doi.org/10.1093/brain/awf166

Bartsch T, Goadsby PJ (2005) Anatomy and physiology of pain referral in primary and cervicogenic headache disorders. *Headache Curr* 2: 42–8. http://dx.doi.org/10.1111/j.1743-5013.2005.20201.x

Bernard JF, Huang GF, Besson JM (1992) Nucleus centralis of the amygdala and the globus pallidus ventralis: electrophysiological evidence for an involvement in pain processes. *J Neurophysiol* 68: 551–69.

Brain SD, Grant AD (2004) Vascular actions of calcitonin gene-related peptide and adrenomedullin. *Physiol Rev* 84: 903–34. http://dx.doi.org/10.1152/physrev.00037.2003

Burstein R, Yamamura H, Malick A, Strassman AM (1998) Chemical stimulation of the intracranial dura induces enhanced responses to facial stimulation in brain stem trigeminal neurons. *J Neurophysiol* 79: 964–82.

Buzzi MG, Moskowitz MA (1990) The antimigraine drug, sumatriptan (GR43175), selectively blocks neurogenic plasma extravasation from blood vessels in dura mater. *Br J Pharmacol* 99: 202–6. http://dx.doi.org/10.1111/j.1476-5381.1990.tb14679.x

Buzzi MG, Moskowitz MA (1991) Evidence for 5-HT$_{1B/1D}$ receptors mediating the antimigraine effect of sumatriptan and dihydroergotamine. *Cephalalgia* 11: 165–8. http://dx.doi.org/10.1046/j.1468-2982.1991.1104165.x

Buzzi MG, Sakas DE, Moskowitz MA (1989) Indomethacin and acetylsalicylic acid block neurogenic plasma protein extravasation in rat dura mater. *Eur J Pharmacol* 165: 251–8. http://dx.doi.org/10.1016/0014-2999(89)90719-X

Chen AC (1993) Human brain measures of clinical pain: a review. II. Tomographic imaging. *Pain* 54: 133–44. http://dx.doi.org/10.1016/0304-3959(93)90201-Y

Christiansen T, Bruun A, Knight YE, Goadsby PJ, Edvinsson L (2004) Immunoreactivity of NOS, CGRP, PACAP, SP and VIP in the trigeminal nucleus caudalis and in the cervical spinal cord C1 and C2 of the cat. *J Headache Pain* 4: 156–63.

Chudler EH, Dong WK (1995) The role of the basal ganglia in nociception and pain. *Pain* 60: 33–8. http://dx.doi.org/10.1016/0304-3959(94)00172-B

Connor HE, Bertin L, Gillies S, Beattie DT, Ward P, The GR205171 Clinical Study Group (1998) Clinical evaluation of a novel, potent, CNS penetrating NK$_1$ receptor antagonist in the acute treatment of migraine. *Cephalalgia* 18: 392.

Connor KM, Shapiro RE, Diener HC et al (2009) Randomized, controlled trial of telcagepant for the acute treatment of migraine. *Neurology* 73: 970–7. http://dx.doi.org/10.1212/WNL.0b013e3181b87942

Cumberbatch MJ, Hill RG, Hargreaves RJ (1997) Rizatriptan has central antinociceptive effects against durally evoked responses. *Eur J Pharmacol* 328: 37–40. http://dx.doi.org/10.1016/S0014-2999(97)83024-5

Cumberbatch MJ, Hill RG, Hargreaves RJ (1998) Differential effects of the 5HT$_{1B/1D}$ receptor agonist naratriptan on trigeminal versus spinal nociceptive responses. *Cephalalgia* 18: 659–64. http://dx.doi. org/10.1046/j.1468-2982.1998.1810659.x

Cushing H (1904) The sensory distribution of the fifth cranial nerve. *Bull Johns Hopkins Hosp* 15: 213–32.

Cutrer FM, Limmroth V, Waeber C, Yu X, Moskowitz MA (1997) New targets for antimigraine drug development. In: Goadsby PJ, Silberstein SD, editors. *Headache*. Philadelphia: Butterworth-Heinemann, pp. 59–72.

Data J, Britch K, Westergaard N et al (1998) A double-blind study of ganaxolone in the acute treatment of migraine headaches with or without an aura in premenopausal females. *Headache* 38: 380.

Denuelle M, Fabre N, Payoux P, Chollet F, Geraud G (2004) Brainstem and hypothalamic activation in spontaneous migraine attacks. *Cephalalgia* 24: 775–814.

Derbyshire SWG, Jones AKP, Gyulai F, Clark S, Townsend D, Firestone LL (1997) Pain processing during three levels of noxious stimulation produces differential patterns of central activity. *Pain* 73: 431–45. http://dx.doi.org/10.1016/S0304-3959(97)00138-3

Diener H-C, Barbanti P, Dahlof C, Reuter U, Habeck J, Podhorna J (2011) BI 44370 TA, an oral CGRP antagonist for the acute treatment of migraine attacks: results from a phase II study. *Cephalalgia* 31: 573–84. http://dx.doi.org/10.1177/0333102410388435

Diener H-C, The RPR100893 Study Group (2003) RPR100893, a substance-P antagonist, is not effective in the treatment of migraine attacks. *Cephalalgia* 23: 183–5. http://dx.doi.org/10.1046/j.1468-2982.2003.00496.x

Dieterich M, Brandt T (1999) Episodic vertigo related to migraine (90 cases): vestibular migraine? *J Neurol* 246: 883–92. http://dx.doi.org/10.1007/s004150050478

Dimitriadou V, Buzzi MG, Moskowitz MA, Theoharides TC (1991) Trigeminal sensory fiber stimulation induces morphological changes reflecting secretion in rat dura mater mast cells. *Neuroscience* 44: 97–112. http://dx.doi.org/10.1016/0306-4522(91)90253-K

Dimitriadou V, Buzzi MG, Theoharides TC, Moskowitz MA (1992) Ultrastructural evidence for neurogenically mediated changes in blood vessels of the rat dura mater and tongue following antidromic trigeminal stimulation. *Neuroscience* 48: 187–203. http://dx.doi.org/10.1016/0306-4522(92)90348-6

Dong WK, Hayashi T, Roberts VJ, Fusco BM, Chudler EH (1996) Behavioral outcome of posterior parietal cortex injury in the monkey. *Pain* 64: 579–87. http://dx.doi.org/10.1016/0304-3959(95)00215-4

Doods H, Hallermayer G, Wu D et al (2000) Pharmacological profile of BIBN4096BS, the first selective small molecule CGRP antagonist. *Br J Pharmacol* 129: 420–3. http://dx.doi.org/10.1038/sj.bjp.0703110

Drummond PD, Lance JW (1983) Extracranial vascular changes and the source of pain in migraine headache. *Ann Neurol* 13: 32–7. http://dx.doi.org/10.1002/ana.410130108

Earl NL, McDonald SA, Lowy MT, 4991W93 Investigator Group (1999) Efficacy and tolerability of the neurogenic inflammation inhibitor, 4991W93, in the acute treatment of migraine. *Cephalalgia* 19: 357.

Fanciullacci M, Alessandri M, Figini M, Geppetti P, Michelacci S (1995) Increase in plasma calcitonin gene-related peptide from extracerebral circulation during nitroglycerin-induced cluster headache attack. *Pain* 60: 119–23. http://dx.doi.org/10.1016/0304-3959(94)00097-X

Feindel W, Penfield W, McNaughton F (1960) The tentorial nerves and localization of intracranial pain in man. *Neurology* 10: 555–63. http://dx.doi.org/10.1212/WNL.10.6.555

Foote SL, Berridge CW, Adams LM, Pineda JA (1991) Electrophysiological evidence for the involvement of the locus coeruleus in alerting, orienting, and attending. *Prog Brain Res* 88: 521–32. http://dx.doi.org/10.1016/S0079-6123(08)63831-5

Friberg L, Olesen J, Iversen HK, Sperling B (1991) Migraine pain associated with middle cerebral artery dilatation: reversal by sumatriptan. *Lancet* 338: 13–17. http://dx.doi.org/10.1016/0140-6736(91)90005-A

Fumal A, Laureys S, Di Clemente L et al (2006) Orbitofrontal cortex involvement in chronic analgesic-overuse headache evolving from episodic migraine. *Brain* 129: 543–50. http://dx.doi.org/10.1093/brain/awh691

Fureman BE, Hess EJ (2005) Noradrenergic blockade prevents attacks in a model of episodic dysfunction caused by a channelopathy. *Neurobiol Dis* 20: 227–32. http://dx.doi.org/10.1016/j.nbd.2005.03.004

Gallai V, Sarchielli P, Floridi A et al (1995) Vasoactive peptides levels in the plasma of young migraine patients with and without aura assessed both interictally and ictally. *Cephalalgia* 15: 384–90.

Gelfand AA, Thomas KC, Goadsby PJ (2012a) Before the headache: infant colic as an early life expression of migraine. *Neurology* 79: 1392–6. http://dx.doi.org/10.1212/WNL.78.1_MeetingAbstracts.S36.005

Gelfand AA, Thomas KC, Goadsby PJ (2012b) Infantile colic and migraine- how early does it all start? *Headache* in press.

Giffin NJ, Benton S, Goadsby PJ (2002) Benign paroxysmal torticollis of infancy: 4 new cases and linkage to CACNA1A. *Dev Child Neurol* 44: 490–3. http://dx.doi.org/10.1111/j.1469-8749.2002.tb00311.x

Goadsby PJ (2000) The pharmacology of headache. *Prog Neurobiol* 62: 509–25. http://dx.doi.org/10.1016/S0301-0082(00)00010-1

Goadsby PJ (2002) Neurovascular headache and a midbrain vascular malformation – evidence for a role of the brainstem in chronic migraine. *Cephalalgia* 22: 107–11. http://dx.doi.org/10.1046/j.1468-2982.2002.00323.x

Goadsby PJ, Duckworth JW (1987) Effect of stimulation of trigeminal ganglion on regional cerebral blood flow in cats. *Am J Physiol* 253: R270–4.

Goadsby PJ, Duckworth JW (1989) Low frequency stimulation of the locus coeruleus reduces regional cerebral blood flow in the spinalized cat. *Brain Res* 476: 71–7. http://dx.doi.org/10.1016/0006-8993(89)91537-0

Goadsby PJ, Edvinsson L (1994) Human *in vivo* evidence for trigeminovascular activation in cluster headache. *Brain* 117: 427–34. http://dx.doi.org/10.1093/brain/117.3.427

Goadsby PJ, Edvinsson L (1996) Neuropeptide changes in a case of chronic paroxysmal hemicrania- evidence for trigemino-parasympathetic activation. *Cephalalgia* 16: 448–50. http://dx.doi.org/10.1046/j.1468-2982.1996.1606448.x

Goadsby PJ, Hoskin KL (1996) Inhibition of trigeminal neurons by intravenous administration of the serotonin (5HT)$_{1B/D}$ receptor agonist zolmitriptan (311C90): are brain stem sites a therapeutic target in migraine? *Pain* 67: 355–9. http://dx.doi.org/10.1016/0304-3959(96)03118-1

Goadsby PJ, Hoskin KL (1997) The distribution of trigeminovascular afferents in the nonhuman primate brain *Macaca nemestrina*: a c-fos immunocytochemical study. *J Anat* 190: 367–75. http://dx.doi.org/10.1046/j.1469-7580.1997.19030367.x

Goadsby PJ, Hoskin KL (1999) Differential effects of low dose CP122,288 and eletriptan on fos expression due to stimulation of the superior sagittal sinus in cat. *Pain* 82: 15–22. http://dx.doi.org/10.1016/S0304-3959(99)00025-1

Goadsby PJ, Knight YE (1997) Inhibition of trigeminal neurons after intravenous administration of naratriptan through an action at the serotonin (5HT$_{1B/1D}$) receptors. *Br J Pharmacol* 122: 918–22. http://dx.doi.org/10.1038/sj.bjp.0701456

Goadsby PJ, Macdonald GJ (1985) Extracranial vasodilatation mediated by VIP (vasoactive intestinal polypeptide). *Brain Res* 329: 285–8. http://dx.doi.org/10.1016/0006-8993(85)90535-9

Goadsby PJ, Zagami AS (1991) Stimulation of the superior sagittal sinus increases metabolic activity and blood flow in certain regions of the brainstem and upper cervical spinal cord of the cat. *Brain* 114: 1001–11. http://dx.doi.org/10.1093/brain/114.2.1001

Goadsby PJ, Lambert GA, Lance JW (1982) Differential effects on the internal and external carotid circulation of the monkey evoked by locus coeruleus stimulation. *Brain Res* 249: 247–54. http://dx.doi.org/10.1016/0006-8993(82)90058-0

Goadsby PJ, Lambert GA, Lance JW (1985) The mechanism of cerebrovascular vasoconstriction in response to locus coeruleus stimulation. *Brain Res* 326: 213–17. http://dx.doi.org/10.1016/0006-8993(85)90030-7

Goadsby PJ, Edvinsson L, Ekman R (1988) Release of vasoactive peptides in the extracerebral circulation of man and the cat during activation of the trigeminovascular system. *Ann Neurol* 23: 193–6. http://dx.doi.org/10.1002/ana.410230214

Goadsby PJ, Edvinsson L, Ekman R (1990) Vasoactive peptide release in the extracerebral circulation of humans during migraine headache. *Ann Neurol* 28: 183–7. http://dx.doi.org/10.1002/ana.410280213

Goadsby PJ, Zagami AS, Lambert GA (1991) Neural processing of craniovascular pain: a synthesis of the central structures involved in migraine. *Headache* 31: 365–71. http://dx.doi.org/10.1111/j.1526-4610.1991.hed3106365.x

Goadsby PJ, Knight YE, Hoskin KL, Butler P (1997) Stimulation of an intracranial trigeminally-innervated structure selectively increases cerebral blood flow. *Brain Res* 751: 247–52. http://dx.doi.org/10.1016/S0006-8993(96)01344-3

Goadsby PJ, Dodick D, Silberstein SD (2005) *Chronic Daily Headache for Clinicians*. Hamilton, Canada: BC Decker Inc.

Goldstein DJ, Wang O, Saper JR, Stoltz R, Silberstein SD, Mathew NT (1997) Ineffectiveness of neurokinin-1 antagonist in acute migraine: a crossover study. *Cephalalgia* 17: 785–90. http://dx.doi.org/10.1046/j.1468-2982.1997.1707785.x

Goldstein DJ, Offen WW, Klein EG et al (2001) Lanepitant, an NK-1 antagonist, in migraine prevention. *Cephalalgia* 21: 102–6. http://dx.doi.org/10.1046/j.1468-2982.2001.00161.x

Grant AD, Tam CW, Lazar Z, Shih MK, Brain SD (2004) The calcitonin gene-related peptide (CGRP) receptor antagonist BIBN4096BS blocks CGRP and adrenomedullin vasoactive responses in the microvasculature. *Br J Pharmacol* 142: 1091–8. http://dx.doi.org/10.1038/sj.bjp.0705824

Grant AD, Pinter E, Salmon AM, Brain SD (2005) An examination of neurogenic mechanisms involved in mustard oil-induced inflammation in the mouse. *Eur J Pharmacol* 507: 273–80. http://dx.doi.org/10.1016/j.ejphar.2004.11.026

Guidetti V, Ottaviano S, Pagliarini M (1984) Childhood headache risk: warning signs and symptoms present during the first six months of life. *Cephalalgia* 4: 237–42. http://dx.doi.org/10.1046/j.1468-2982.1984.0404237.x

Haas DC, Kent PF, Friedman DI (1993) Headache caused by a single lesion of multiple sclerosis in the periaqueductal gray area. *Headache* 33: 452–55. http://dx.doi.org/10.1111/j.1526-4610.1993.hed3308452.x

Hansen JM, Sitarz J, Birk S et al (2006) Vasoactive intestinal polypeptide evokes only a minimal headache in healthy volunteers. *Cephalalgia* 26: 992–1003. http://dx.doi.org/10.1111/j.1468-2982.2006.01149.x

Harmar AJ, Fahrenkrug J, Gozes I et al (2012) IUPHAR reviews 1: pharmacology and functions of receptors for vasoactive intestinal peptide and pituitary adenylate cyclase-activating polypeptide. *Br J Pharmacol* 166: 4–17.

Hewitt DJ, Aurora SK, Dodick DW et al (2011) Randomized controlled trial of the CGRP receptor antagonist, MK-3207, in the acute treatment of migraine. *Cephalalgia* 31: 712–22. http://dx.doi.org/10.1177/0333102411398399

Ho TW, Ferrari MD, Dodick DW et al (2008) Efficacy and tolerability of MK-0974 (telcagepant), a new oral antagonist of calcitonin gene-related peptide receptor, compared with zolmitriptan for acute migraine: a randomised, placebo-controlled, parallel-treatment trial. *Lancet* 372: 2115–23. http://dx.doi.org/10.1016/S0140-6736(08)61626-8

Hoskin KL, Kaube H, Goadsby PJ (1996) Central activation of the trigeminovascular pathway in the cat is inhibited by dihydroergotamine. A c-Fos and electrophysiology study. *Brain* 119: 249–56. http://dx.doi.org/10.1093/brain/119.1.249

Hoskin KL, Zagami A, Goadsby PJ (1999) Stimulation of the middle meningeal artery leads to Fos expression in the trigeminocervical nucleus: a comparative study of monkey and cat. *J Anat* 194: 579–88. http://dx.doi.org/10.1046/j.1469-7580.1999.19440579.x

Hoskin KL, Bulmer DCE, Lasalandra M, Jonkman A, Goadsby PJ (2001) Fos expression in the midbrain periaqueductal grey after trigeminovascular stimulation. *J Anat* 197: 29–35. http://dx.doi.org/10.1046/j.1469-7580.2001.19810029.x

Hsieh JC, Stahle-Backdahl M, Hagermark O, Stone-Elander S, Rosenquist G, Ingvar M (1996) Traumatic nociceptive pain activates the hypothalamus and the periaqueductal gray: a positron emission tomography study. *Pain* 64: 303–14. http://dx.doi.org/10.1016/0304-3959(95)00129-8

Jones AK, Brown WD, Friston KJ, Qi LY, Frackowiak RSJ (1991a) Cortical and subcortical localization of response to pain in man using positron emission tomography. *Proc R Soc B* 244: 39–44. http://dx.doi.org/10.1098/rspb.1991.0048

Jones AK, Qi LY, Fujirawa T et al (1991b) *In vivo* distribution of opioid receptors in man in relation to the cortical projections of the medial and lateral pain systems measured with positron emission tomography. *Neurosci Lett* 126: 25–8. http://dx.doi.org/10.1016/0304-3940(91)90362-W

Kandere-Grzybowska K, Gheorghe D, Priller J et al (2003) Stress-induced dura vascular permeability does not develop in mast cell-deficient and neurokinin-1 receptor knockout mice. *Brain Res* 980: 213–20. http://dx.doi.org/10.1016/S0006-8993(03)02975-5

Kaube H, Hoskin KL, Goadsby PJ (1993a) Inhibition by sumatriptan of central trigeminal neurones only after blood–brain barrier disruption. *Br J Pharmacol* 109: 788–92. http://dx.doi.org/10.1111/j.1476-5381.1993.tb13643.x

Kaube H, Hoskin KL, Goadsby PJ (1993b) Intravenous acetylsalicylic acid inhibits central trigeminal neurons in the dorsal horn of the upper cervical spinal cord in the cat. *Headache* 33: 541–50. http://dx.doi.org/10.1111/j.1526-4610.1993.hed3310541.x

Kaube H, Keay KA, Hoskin KL, Bandler R, Goadsby PJ (1993c) Expression of c-*Fos*-like immunoreactivity in the caudal medulla and upper cervical cord following stimulation of the superior sagittal sinus in the cat. *Brain Res* 629: 95–102. http://dx.doi.org/10.1016/0006-8993(93)90486-7

Kerr FWL (1961) A mechanism to account for frontal headache in cases of posterior fossa tumous. *J Neurosurg* 18: 605–9. http://dx.doi.org/10.3171/jns.1961.18.5.0605

Kerr FWL, Olafson RA (1961) Trigeminal and cervical volleys. *Arch Neurol* 5: 69–76. http://dx.doi.org/10.1001/archneur.1961.00450140053005

Knight YE, Goadsby PJ (1999) Brainstem stimulation inhibits trigeminal neurons in the cat. *Cephalalgia* 19: 315.

Knight YE, Edvinsson L, Goadsby PJ (1999) Blockade of CGRP release after superior sagittal sinus stimula-tion in cat: a comparison of avitriptan and CP122,288. *Neuropeptides* 33: 41–6. http://dx.doi.org/10.1054/npep.1999.0009

Knight YE, Edvinsson L, Goadsby PJ (2001) 4991W93 inhibits release of calcitonin gene-related peptide in the cat but only at doses with $5HT_{1B/1D}$ receptor agonist activity. *Neuropharmacology* 40: 520–5.

Knight YE, Classey JD, Lasalandra MP et al. (2005) Patterns of fos expression in the rostral medulla and caudal pons evoked by noxious craniovascular stimulation and periaqueductal gray stimulation in the cat. *Brain Res* 10145: 1–11.

Kurth T, Mohamed S, Maillard P et al (2011) Headache, migraine, and structural brain lesions and function: population based Epidemiology of Vascular Ageing-MRI study. *BMJ* 342: c7357. http://dx.doi.org/10.1136/bmj.c7357

Lambert GA, Bogduk N, Goadsby PJ, Duckworth JW, Lance JW (1984) Decreased carotid arterial resis-tance in cats in response to trigeminal stimulation. *J Neurosurg* 61: 307–15. http://dx.doi.org/10.3171/jns.1984.61.2.0307

Lance JW, Goadsby PJ (2005) *Mechanism and Management of Headache*. New York: Elsevier.

Lipton RB, Bigal M (2006) *Migraine and Other Headache Disorders*. New York: Marcel Dekker, Taylor & Francis Books, Inc.

McNaughton FL (1966) The innervation of the intracranial blood vessels and the dural sinuses. In: Cobb S, Frantz AM, Penfield W, Riley HA, editors. *The Circulation of the Brain and Spinal Cord*. New York: Hafner Publishing Co. Inc., pp. 178–200.

McNaughton FL, Feindel WH (1977) Innervation of intracranial structures: a reappraisal. In: Rose FC, edi-tor. *Physiological Aspects of Clinical Neurology*. Oxford: Blackwell Scientific Publications, pp. 279–93.

Maltos KL, Menezes GB, Caliari MV et al (2004) Vascular and cellular responses to pro-inflammatory stimuli in rat dental pulp. *Arch Oral Biol* 49: 443–50. http://dx.doi.org/10.1016/j.archoralbio.2004.01.004

Markowitz S, Saito K, Moskowitz MA (1987) Neurogenically mediated leakage of plasma proteins occurs from blood vessels in dura mater but not brain. *J Neurosci* 7: 4129–36.

Martins IP, Baeta E, Paiva T, Campo T, Gomes L (1993) Headaches during intracranial endovascular procedures: a possible model of vascular headache. *Headache* 33: 227–33. http://dx.doi.org/10.1111/j.1526-4610.1993.hed3305227.x

Matsuyama T, Shiosaka S, Matsumoto M et al (1983) Overall distribution of vasoactive intestinal polypeptide-containing nerves on the wall of the cerebral arteries: an immunohistochemical study using whole-mounts. *Neuroscience* 10: 89–96. http://dx.doi.org/10.1016/0306-4522(83)90083-0

May A, Gijsman HJ, Wallnoefer A, Jones R, Diener HC, Ferrari MD (1996) Endothelin antagonist bosentan blocks neurogenic inflammation, but is not effective in aborting migraine attacks. *Pain* 67: 375–8. http://dx.doi.org/10.1016/0304-3959(96)03137-5

May A, Bahra A, Buchel C, Frackowiak RS, Goadsby PJ (1998a) Hypothalamic activation in cluster headache attacks. *Lancet* 352: 275–8. http://dx.doi.org/10.1016/S0140-6736(98)02470-2

May A, Shepheard S, Wessing A, Hargreaves RJ, Goadsby PJ, Diener HC (1998b) Retinal plasma extravasa-tion can be evoked by trigeminal stimulation in rat but does not occur during migraine attacks. *Brain* 121: 1231–7. http://dx.doi.org/10.1093/brain/121.7.1231

May A, Bahra A, Buchel C, Turner R, Goadsby PJ (1999) Functional MRI in spontaneous attacks of SUNCT: short-lasting neuralgiform headache with conjunctival injection and tearing. *Ann Neurol* 46: 791–3. http://dx.doi.org/10.1002/1531-8249(199911)46:5<791::AID-ANA18>3.0.CO;2-8

Melzack R, Casey KL (1968) Sensory, motivational and central control determinants of pain. In: Kenshalo DR, editor. *The Skin Senses*. Springfield, IL: C.C. Thomas, pp. 423–39.

Miller P, Barwell J, Poyner DR, Wigglesworth MJ, Garland SL, Donnelly D (2010) Non-peptidic antagonists of the CGRP receptor, BIBN4096BS and MK-0974, interact with the calcitonin receptor-like receptor via methionine-42 and RAMP1 via tryptophan-74. *Biochem Biophys Res Commun* 391: 437–42. http://dx.doi.org/10.1016/j.bbrc.2009.11.076

Moskowitz MA (1990) Basic mechanisms in vascular headache. *Neurol Clin* 8: 801–15.

Nichols FT, Mawad M, Mohr JP, Hilal S, Stein B, Michelson J (1990) Focal headache during balloon infla-tion in the internal carotid and middle cerebral arteries. *Stroke* 21: 555–9. http://dx.doi.org/10.1161/01.STR.21.4.555

Nichols FT, Mawad M, Mohr JP, Hilal S, Adams RJ (1993) Focal headache during balloon inflation in the ver-tebral and basilar arteries. *Headache* 33: 87–9. http://dx.doi.org/10.1111/j.1526-4610.1993.hed3302087.x

Norman B, Panebianco D, Block GA (1998) A placebo-controlled, in-clinic study to explore the preliminary safety and efficacy of intravenous L-758,298 (a prodrug of the NK1 receptor antagonist L-754,030) in the acute treatment of migraine. *Cephalalgia* 18: 407.

Nozaki K, Boccalini P, Moskowitz MA (1992) Expression of c-fos-like immunoreactivity in brainstem after meningeal irritation by blood in the subarachnoid space. *Neuroscience* 49: 669–80. http://dx.doi.org/10.1016/0306-4522(92)90235-T

Olesen J, Diener HC, Husstedt IW et al (2004) Calcitonin gene-related peptide receptor antagonist BIBN 4096 BS for the acute treatment of migraine. *N Engl J Med* 350: 1104–10. http://dx.doi.org/10.1056/NEJMoa030505

Olesen J, Tfelt-Hansen P, Ramadan N, Goadsby PJ, Welch KMA (2005) *The Headaches*. Philadelphia: Lippincott, Williams & Wilkins.

Olesen J, Bousser MG, Diener HC et al (2006) New appendix criteria open for a broader concept of chronic migraine. *Cephalalgia* 26: 742–6. http://dx.doi.org/10.1111/j.1468-2982.2006.01172.x

Ophoff RA, Terwindt GM, Vergouwe MN et al (1996) Familial hemiplegic migraine and episodic ataxia type-2 are caused by mutations in the Ca^{2+} channel gene CACNL1A4. *Cell* 87: 543–52. http://dx.doi.org/10.1016/S0092-8674(00)81373-2

Peroutka SJ (2005) Neurogenic inflammation and migraine: implications for therapeutics. *Mol Interv* 5: 306–13. http://dx.doi.org/10.1124/mi.5.5.10

Petersen KA, Birk S, Doods H, Edvinsson L, Olesen J (2004) Inhibitory effect of BIBN4096BS on cephalic vasodilatation induced by CGRP or transcranial electrical stimulation in the rat. *Br J Pharmacol* 143: 697–704. http://dx.doi.org/10.1038/sj.bjp.0705966

Petersen KA, Birk S, Lassen LH et al (2005) The CGRP-antagonist, BIBN4096BS does not affect cerebral or systemic haemodynamics in healthy volunteers. *Cephalalgia* 25: 139–47. http://dx.doi.org/10.1111/j.1468-2982.2004.00830.x

Piovesan EJ, Kowacs PA, Tatsui CE, Lange MC, Ribas LC, Werneck LC (2001) Referred pain after painful stmulation of the greater occipital nerve in humans: evidence of convergence of cervical afferents on trigeminal nuclei. *Cephalalgia* 21: 107–9. http://dx.doi.org/10.1046/j.1468-2982.2001.00166.x

Rahmann A, Wienecke T, Hansen JM, Fahrenkrug J, Olesen J, Ashina M (2008) Vasoactive intestinal peptide causes marked cephalic vasodilatation but does not induce migraine. *Cephalalgia* 28: 226–36. http://dx.doi.org/10.1111/j.1468-2982.2007.01497.x

Raskin NH, Hosobuchi Y, Lamb S (1987) Headache may arise from perturbation of brain. *Headache* 27: 416–20. http://dx.doi.org/10.1111/j.1526-4610.1987.hed2708416.x

Roon K, Olesen J, Diener HC et al (2000) No acute antimigraine efficacy of CP-122,288, a highly potent inhibitor of neurogenic inflammation: results of two randomized double-blind placebo-controlled clinical trials. *Ann Neurol* 47: 238–41.

Schytz HW, Birk S, Wienecke T, Kruuse C, Olesen J, Ashina M (2009) PACAP38 induces migraine-like attacks in patients with migraine without aura. *Brain* 132: 16–25. http://dx.doi.org/10.1093/brain/awn307

Shields KG, Goadsby PJ (2005) Propranolol modulates trigeminovascular responses in thalamic ventroposteromedial nucleus: a role in migraine? *Brain* 128: 86–97. http://dx.doi.org/10.1093/brain/awh298

Shields KG, Goadsby PJ (2006) Serotonin receptors modulate trigeminovascular responses in ventroposteromedial nucleus of thalamus: a migraine target? *Neurobiol Dis* 23: 491–501. http://dx.doi.org/10.1016/j.nbd.2006.04.003

Silberstein SD, Lipton RB, Goadsby PJ (2002) *Headache in Clinical Practice*. London: Martin Dunitz.

Sprenger T, Goadsby PJ (2010) What has functional neuroimaging done for primary headache... and for the clinical neurologist? *J Clin Neurosci* 17: 547–53. http://dx.doi.org/10.1016/j.jocn.2009.09.030

Sprenger T, Seifert CL, Valet M et al (2010) Abnormal interictal large-scale brain network connectivity in episodic migraine. *Headache* 50: 71.

Sprenger T, Maniyar FH, Monteith TS, Schankin C, Goadsby PJ (2012) Midbrain activation in the premonitory phase: a H215O-Positron emission tomography study. *Headache* 52: 863–4.

Steuer H, Jaworski A, Stoll D, Schlosshauer B (2004) In vitro model of the outer blood–retina barrier. *Brain Res Brain Res Protoc* 13: 26–36. http://dx.doi.org/10.1016/j.brainresprot.2003.12.002

Storer RJ, Akerman S, Goadsby PJ (2004) Calcitonin gene-related peptide (CGRP) modulates nociceptive trigeminovascular transmission in the cat. *Br J Pharmacol* 142: 1171–81. http://dx.doi.org/10.1038/sj.bjp.0705807

Strassman AM, Raymond SA, Burstein R (1996) Sensitization of meningeal sensory neurons and the origin of headaches. *Nature* 384: 560–3. http://dx.doi.org/10.1038/384560a0

Summ O, Charbit AR, Andreou AP, Goadsby PJ (2010) Modulation of nocioceptive transmission with calcitonin gene-related peptide receptor antagonists in the thalamus. *Brain* 133: 2540–8. http://dx.doi.org/10.1093/brain/awq224

Tam C, Brain SD (2004) The assessment of vasoactive properties of CGRP and adrenomedullin in the microvasculature: a study using in vivo and in vitro assays in the mouse. *J Mol Neurosci* 22: 117–24. http://dx.doi.org/10.1385/JMN:22:1-2:117

Tran-Dinh YR, Thurel C, Cunin G, Serrie A, Seylaz J (1992) Cerebral vasodilation after the thermocoagulation of the trigeminal ganglion in humans. *Neurosurgery* 31: 658–62. http://dx.doi.org/10.1227/00006123-199210000-00007

Tvedskov JF, Lipka K, Ashina M, Iversen HK, Schifter S, Olesen J (2005) No increase of calcitonin gene-related peptide in jugular blood during migraine. *Ann Neurol* 58: 561–8. http://dx.doi.org/10.1002/ana.20605

Uddman R, Edvinsson L, Ekman R, Kingman T, McCulloch J (1985) Innervation of the feline cerebral vasculature by nerve fibers containing calcitonin gene-related peptide: trigeminal origin and co-existence with substance P. *Neurosci Lett* 62: 131–6. http://dx.doi.org/10.1016/0304-3940(85)90296-4

Uddman R, Goadsby PJ, Jansen I, Edvinsson L (1993) PACAP, a VIP-like peptide, immunohistochemical localization and effect upon cat pial arteries and cerebral blood flow. *J Cereb Blood Flow Metab* 13: 291–7. http://dx.doi.org/10.1038/jcbfm.1993.36

Van der Schueren BJ, Blanchard R, Murphy MG et al (2011) The potent calcitonin gene-related peptide receptor antagonist, telcagepant, does not affect nitroglycerin-induced vasodilation in healthy men. *Br J Clin Pharmacol* 71: 708–17. http://dx.doi.org/10.1111/j.1365-2125.2010.03869.x

Veloso F, Kumar K, Toth C (1998) Headache secondary to deep brain implantation. *Headache* 38: 507–15. http://dx.doi.org/10.1046/j.1526-4610.1998.3807507.x

Weiller C, May A, Limmroth V et al (1995) Brain stem activation in spontaneous human migraine attacks. *Nat Med* 1: 658–60. http://dx.doi.org/10.1038/nm0795-658

Zagami AS, Goadsby PJ (1991) Stimulation of the superior sagittal sinus increases metabolic activity in cat thalamus. In: Rose FC, editor. *New Advances in Headache Research: 2*. London: Smith-Gordon and Co. Ltd, pp. 169–71.

Zagami AS, Lambert GA (1991) Craniovascular application of capsaicin activates nociceptive thalamic neurons in the cat. *Neurosci Lett* 121: 187–90. http://dx.doi.org/10.1016/0304-3940(91)90681-I

Zagami AS, Goadsby PJ, Edvinsson L (1990) Stimulation of the superior sagittal sinus in the cat causes release of vasoactive peptides. *Neuropeptides* 16: 69–75. http://dx.doi.org/10.1016/0143-4179(90)90114-E

Zagami AS, Edvinsson L, Hoskin KL, Goadsby PJ (1995) Stimulation of the superior sagittal sinus causes extracranial release of PACAP. *Cephalalgia* 15: 109.

4
HEREDITY AND GENETICS OF HEADACHE AND MIGRAINE

Michael Bjørn Russell

Introduction

Migraine, hemiplegic migraine, tension-type headache and cluster headache are paroxysmal disorders. This is also true for the chronic forms of migraine, tension-type headache and cluster headache, as the intensity of the headache varies and the vast majority of those with chronic headaches have hours, days or short periods without headache. This is important in relation to the genes responsible for hemiplegic migraine, and possibly also for the other types of headaches, although genes for these headache syndromes have not yet been identified.

Transmission of migraine from parents to children was reported as early as the seventeenth century (Willis 1682), almost 200 years before Gregor Mendel's famous theories of inheritance, written in 1866. However, Mendel's theories were forgotten for 34 years before they were rediscovered independently by Connens, de Vries and von Tscermak in 1900.

This promoted an enormous interest in heredity of migraine, whereas the interest in heredity of tension-type headache and cluster headache came later, i.e. in the 1990s. Tension-type headache was probably ignored because of the mild symptomatology and very high prevalence, whereas cluster headache was often classified as a subtype of migraine and not as a syndrome in its own right.

This chapter focuses on the heredity and genetics of different types of headache. The literature is based on adolescents and adults, as specific studies on children have not been conducted nor published to the knowledge of the author.

Co-occurrence of different types of headache

Migraine, hemiplegic migraine, tension-type headache and cluster headache are different headache syndromes and defined as such by the International Classification of Headache Disorders (Headache Classification Subcommittee of the International Headache Society 2004). The prevalence of co-occurrence of migraine without aura and migraine with aura is similar to the sum of the prevalences of each of the two types of migraine in the general population (Russell et al 1996a, 2002). This indicates that migraine without aura and migraine with aura are distinct syndromes. Co-occurrence of migraine without aura and migraine with aura is very frequent in the clinic population, but such data are biased by selection and the results are neither representative of nor generalisable to the general population. Hemiplegic migraine is distinct from migraine without aura and migraine with aura, but those with hemiplegic migraine have many abortive attacks of hemiplegic migraine that mimic typical migraine with aura (Thomsen et al 2003a,b). The prevalence and frequency of tension-type headache is higher in those with migraine than without migraine (Russell 2005). Thus, tension-type headache is a confounding factor in genetic studies of migraine and tension-type headache. The prevalence of migraine in those with cluster headache corresponds to the prevalence of migraine in the general population, indicating that migraine and cluster headache are distinct headache syndromes (Rasmussen et al 1991a, Russell 1997).

Family studies

GENERAL CONSIDERATIONS

A positive family history is imprecise, because it does not specify the number of affected individuals, family size or relation to the proband. For example, the lifetime prevalence of migraine is 16% in the general population (Rasmussen et al 1991a). This causes a positive family history simply by chance in more than 65% of families, if the proband has six first-degree relatives (parents, siblings and children), and one or both parents are affected in more than 30% of families. Furthermore, a positive family history does not include an interview of the relatives by a physician. Probands only identify about half of their affected first-degree relatives with migraine, which adds to the imprecision (Russell et al 1996b). A positive family history provides more information about heredity if the disorder is rare, as for instance with hemiplegic migraine or cluster headache.

Familial aggregation is a more precise estimation of the population relative risk, which is calculated by dividing the probability that a relative is affected by the probability that a random member of the general population is affected by the same condition (Weiss et al 1982).

As the prevalence of the different primary headaches depends on age and sex, the value of the denominator is adjusted according to the distribution of age and sex in the group of relatives studied. Hence, this standardised population relative risk is estimated by dividing the observed number of affected first-degree relatives by the expected number, according to the prevalence rates in the population. The expected number is calculated by adding the products of the current age- and sex-specific rates and the number of relatives within each cor-responding age–sex category. Some studies calculate the familial aggregation by comparing the families of probands with and without disease, a method that is less precise.

An increased familial risk can be caused by genetic as well as environmental factors. The risk among spouses can be used to evaluate this relationship, because probands and spouses in part share a common environment, but differ in genetic constitution.

MIGRAINE WITHOUT AURA AND MIGRAINE WITH AURA

Table 4.1 shows the population relative risk of migraine without aura and migraine with aura. All surveys except the American survey found that first-degree relatives of probands had a significantly increased risk of the proband's disorder as compared with the general population (Mochi et al 1993, Russell and Olesen 1995, Kalfakis et al 1996, Stewart et al 1997). The American survey is biased because family members were interviewed only about their most severe type of headache by lay interviewers (Stewart et al 1997). For an unerring diagnosis,

TABLE 4.1

Age- and sex-standardised risk of migraine without aura and migraine with aura

Disease in proband	Study population	Disease in first-degree relative	Number of affected relatives		Population relative risk (95% CI)
			Observed	Expected	
MO					
Mochi et al (1993)	Clinic	MO	64	17.7	3.6 (1.1–6.1)
Russell and Olesen (1995)	General	MO	102	54.8	1.9 (1.6–2.2)
		MA	42	29.2	1.4 (1.0–1.9)
Stewart et al (1997)	General	MO	30	21.0	1.4 (0.8–2.5)
		MA	10	4.2	2.4 (0.9–6.4)
MA					
Mochi et al (1993)	Clinic	MA	13	1.9	7.0 (3.2–10.8)
Russell and Olesen (1995)	General	MA	111	29.3	3.8 (3.2–4.4)
		MO	56	54.9	1.0 (0.8–1.3)
Stewart et al (1997)	General	MA	3	2.4	1.2 (0.3–5.5)
		MO	17	12.1	1.4 (0.7–2.8)
Kalfakis et al (1997)	Clinic	MA	58	4.9	11.9 (7.0–16.7)

The population relative risk is calculated using available data from papers by the author of this chapter (Russell 1997). CI, confidence interval; MO, migraine without aura; MA, migraine with aura.

interviews by physicians are preferred. Clinical populations are subject to selection bias. Thus, the Danish survey conducted by one physician who was blinded to the diagnosis of the probands is probably the most precise genetic epidemiological survey on migraine (Russell and Olesen 1995).

Spouses of probands with migraine without aura had a slightly increased risk of migraine without aura, while spouses of probands with migraine with aura had no increased risk of migraine with aura (Russell and Olesen 1995). All in all, the increased family risk indicates that both migraine without aura and migraine with aura are likely to be at least partly inherited. The family aggregation does not provide information about mode of inheritance. A classical segregation analysis analyses for Mendelian inheritance, i.e. autosomal dominant and recessive inheritance, and X-linked inheritance. However, a complex segregation analysis also analyses for multifactorial inheritance, as well as transmissible and non-transmissible environmental factors (Lalouel and Morton 1981). A complex segregation analysis of the Danish survey on migraine without aura suggested multifactorial inheritance, and the analysis of migraine with aura also suggested multifactorial inheritance (Russell et al 1995a).

TENSION-TYPE HEADACHE

Tension-type headache, with exception of its chronic form, is not suited for a genetic epidemiological survey owing to its high prevalence. A total of 122 consecutive probands with chronic tension-type headache from a Danish headache clinic were included in a family study (Østergaard et al 1997). The first-degree relatives of probands with chronic tension-type headache had a 3.1-fold increased risk of chronic tension-type headache as compared with the general population, whereas spouses of probands with chronic tension-type headache had no increased risk of chronic tension-type headache. This result indicates the importance of genetic factors. A complex segregation analysis suggested multifactorial inheritance (Russell et al 1998).

CLUSTER HEADACHE

Cluster headache was not considered to be inherited until the 1990s, as the family history was usually negative. However, as cluster headache is relatively rare, the positive family history of cluster headache among first-degree relatives (parents, siblings, children), found in 51 of 1406 families analysed in the literature up to 1995, strongly suggests heredity (Russell 1997, Russell et al 1994). Table 4.2 shows the population relative risk of four genetic epidemiological surveys conducted on two continents. The French survey is the most accurate, because all first-degree relatives were directly interviewed by a physician (El Amrani et al 2002). The Danish and Italian surveys probably underestimated the risk of cluster headache, as only those possibly affected were interviewed (Russell et al 1994, 1995b, Leone et al 2001). The American survey either under- or overestimated the risk of cluster headache, depending on the balance between underestimation and misclassification by the probands (Kudrow and Kudrow 1994). A diagnosis of cluster headache was confirmed in only 57%, while the remaining 43% had migraine in the Danish cluster headache survey (Russell et al 1995b). The increased familial risk of cluster headache among first- and second-degree relatives strongly suggests a genetic cause. Theoretically, a shared environment can produce relative risks of the magnitude observed for cluster headache only under extreme conditions (Khoury et al 1988). A complex segregation analysis of cluster headache suggested that an autosomal dominant

TABLE 4.2
Age- and sex-standardised risk of cluster headache

Disease in proband	Study population	Cluster headache in relatives	Number of affected relatives		Population relative risk (95% CI)
			Observed	Expected	
Russell et al (1994, 1995a,b)	Clinic	First degree	26	5	4.7 (3.1–6.9)
		Second degree	10	13.2	0.8 (0.4–1.4)
Kudrow and Kudrow (1994)	Clinic	First degree	41	2.7	15.2 (11.1–21.1)
De Simone et al (2003)	Clinic	First degree	39	2.97	13.1 (9.0–17.3)
		Second degree	18	6.69	2.7 (1.5–3.9)
El Amrani et al (2002)	Clinic	First degree	22	1.25	17.6 (10.2–24.9)

The population relative risk is calculated using available data from papers by the author of this chapter (Russell 1997). CI, confidence interval.

gene has a role in some families (Russell et al 1995c). An analysis of a single Italian pedigree suggested autosomal recessive inheritance in that particular family (De Simone et al 2003).

Twin studies

GENERAL CONSIDERATIONS

Studies of twin pairs is the classic method used to investigate the importance of genetic and environmental factors. Monozygotic twin pairs have identical genes, whereas dizygotic twin pairs share, on average, 50% of their genes, although the genes may be altered by epigenetic mechanisms, among others. Thus, if epigenetic and other mechanisms that can alter the genes are disregarded, monozygotic twin pairs should have 100% concordance if the condition is determined exclusively by genetic factors, whereas dizygotic twin pairs have a 50% or 25% concordance rate if the disorder has autosomal dominant or recessive inheritance. Lower concordance rates than mentioned above, in which monozygotic twin pairs have significantly higher concordance rates than dizygotic twin pairs, indicate multifactorial inheritance, i.e. the disorder is caused by a combination of genetic and environmental factors.

MIGRAINE

Diagnostic criteria, ascertainment methods and sampling sources have not been uniform in previous twin studies. The majority of twin studies are case reports or small series, whereas the larger series are based on questionnaires or non-evaluated lay interviews (Russell 1997). The validity of questionnaires may be questioned, as the diagnosis of migraine was not validated against the International Headache Society's criteria in a self-administered headache questionnaire (Rasmussen et al 1991b).

Unfortunately, most twin studies do not discriminate between migraine without aura and migraine with aura. The concordance is significantly higher in monozygotic than dizygotic twin pairs with unspecified migraine ($p<0.001$). The picture is less clear when analysing migraine without aura and migraine with aura. Thus, no firm conclusion can be drawn from early twin studies.

A large Danish survey based on a population-based twins registry, in which the twin pairs were blindly interviewed by physicians, was more precise than earlier studies (Gervil et al 1999a, Ulrich et al 1999a). Migraine without aura and migraine with aura were analysed separately. The probandwise concordance rate was significantly higher in monozygotic than same-sex dizygotic twin pairs in both migraine without aura (50% [95% confidence interval {CI} 38–62%] vs 21% [95% CI 12–30%]) and migraine with aura [40% (95% CI 33–48%) vs 28% (95% CI 23–33%)]. The following genetic analysis, estimated by means of structural equation modelling, found that the best fitting model implied that the liability to migraine with and without aura resulted from additive genetic effects [migraine without aura, 61% (95% CI 49–71%); migraine with aura, 65% (95% CI 49–78%)] and individual-specific environmental effects [migraine without aura, 39% (95% CI 29–51%); migraine with aura, 35% (95% CI 22–51%)] (Gervil et al 1999b, Ulrich et al 1999b). Thus, the results of the twin studies support the findings in family studies, i.e. both types of migraine are caused by a combination of genetic and environmental factors.

TENSION-TYPE HEADACHE

Migraine is a confounding factor of tension-type headache; for that reason it is important to exclude twin pairs with co-occurrence of migraine in a study of twin pair concordance.

Analysing no, infrequent, frequent and chronic tension-type headache separately, it seems that genetic factors play a role in no and frequent episodic tension-type headache, whereas infrequent episodic tension-type headache is caused primarily by environmental factors. The result regarding chronic tension-type headache was inconclusive owing to the small number of affected twin pairs (Russell et al 2006).

CLUSTER HEADACHE

Cluster headaches have been reported in five pairs of monozygotic twins (Russell 1997). All twin pairs were concordant for cluster headache, indicating the importance of genetic factors, although publication itself introduces selection bias (Motulsky 1978). A Swedish genetic epidemiological survey of twin pairs from the general population found that 2 of 12 monozygotic twin pairs, and 0 of 25 dizygotic twin pairs, were concordant for cluster headache (Ekbom et al 2006), i.e. the pairwise concordance rate was 17% in monozygotic and 0% in dizygotic twin pairs. The combined results are in favour of a combination of genetic and environmental factors being important in cluster headache.

Identification of headache genes

HEMIPLEGIC MIGRAINE

Sporadic and familial hemiplegic migraine are rare paroxysmal disorders characterised by motor aura (weakness) and headache (Headache Classification Subcommittee of the International Headache Society 2004). The diagnostic criterion differs with respect to familiarity, i.e. no affected versus at least one affected first- and/or second-degree relatives. Hemiplegic migraine was first described in 1910, and then again more than 40 years later (Clarke 1910, Whitty 1953, Chrást 1954, Blau and Whitty 1955). Since then, numerous publications have suggested that familial hemiplegic migraine has an autosomal dominant mode of inheritance (Russell and Ducros 2011). This led to an extensive search for the gene(s) responsible for familial hemiplegic migraine in the 1990s. The first major breakthrough was the identification of linkage to chromosome 19p (Joutel et al 1993). This discovery was soon to be followed by the identification of mutations in ion-channel genes *CACNA1A*, *ATP1A2* and *SCN1A*, all of which can cause familial hemiplegic migraine, i.e. genetic heterogeneity (Ophoff et al 1996, De Fusco et al 2003, Dichgans et al 2005).

Mutations in the *CACNA1A* gene can also cause episodic ataxia type 2 (*EA2*) or spinocerebellar ataxia type 6 (*SCA6*), whereas mutations in *SCN1A* genes can cause generalised epilepsy with febrile seizures and severe myoclonic epilepsy of infancy, i.e. allelic heterogeneity (Russell and Ducros 2011). Familial hemiplegic migraine with permanent cerebellar signs, i.e. nystagmus, ataxia and dysarthria, are experienced by 40% of the familial hemiplegic migraine families with mutations in the *CACNA1A* gene (Ducros et al 2001). Mutations in the *CACNA1A*, *ATP1A2* and *SCN1A* genes are identified in approximately 50%, 20% and 3%, respectively, of the large familial hemiplegic migraine families (calculated by the author of this paper) (Ducros et al 2001, Riant et al 2005, Vanmolkot et al 2007). Other gene mutations that can cause familial hemiplegic migraine with certainty await identification.

Sporadic hemiplegic migraine is sometimes caused by de novo mutations in known familial hemiplegic migraine genes.

MIGRAINE WITHOUT AURA, MIGRAINE WITH AURA, TENSION-TYPE HEADACHE AND CLUSTER HEADACHE

No genes have so far been identified with certainty for migraine without aura, migraine with aura, tension-type headache or cluster headache. However, several association studies have been conducted, especially in relation to migraine and cluster headache. Association studies for specific candidate genes are selected on the basis of their known (or, more often, hypothesised) biological functions relevant to the type of headache in question and have been done for many polymorphisms. Both linkage and association studies have been largely unsuccessful, for reasons that include small sample size, low sensitivity to detect moderate effects and the substantial locus heterogeneity that underlies the different types of headache.

Although studies with a smaller sample size find statistically significant results, they need to be confirmed in larger sample sizes in order to minimise the risk of type 1 and 2 errors. To overcome the power problem, a large sample size is necessary to locate common genetic factors of multifactorial disorders.

Future research

Familial hemiplegic migraine is the main model to study the molecular genetics of migraine. Future studies should focus on the identification of the genes implicated in pure familial hemiplegic migraine, followed by functional studies of the identified genes. Owing to intra-familial phenotypic variations, other genes are likely to have a modifying effect on the major autosomal dominant genes for familial hemiplegic migraine identified so far.

Identification and investigation of these genes will be important for elucidating the full story of hemiplegic migraine. Subsequently, the main challenge is to establish whether the research findings for hemiplegic migraine are also valid for the common types of migraine. It is anticipated that the challenges regarding tension-type headache and cluster headache will be at least of the magnitude of those of the typical types of migraine.

REFERENCES

Blau JN, Whitty CWM (1955) Familial hemiplegic migraine. *Lancet* 2: 1115–16. http://dx.doi.org/10.1016/S0140-6736(55)92952-4

Chrást B (1954) Migraena cerebellaris. *Lék List* 9: 271–6.

Clarke JM (1910) On recurrent motor paralysis in migraine. *Br Med J* 1: 1534–8. http://dx.doi.org/10.1136/bmj.1.2582.1534

De Fusco M, Marconi R, Silvestri L et al (2003) Haploinsufficiency of ATP1A2 encoding the Na$^+$/K$^+$ pump alpha2 subunit associated with familial hemiplegic migraine type 2. *Nat Genet* 33: 192–6. http://dx.doi.org/10.1038/ng1081

De Simone R, Fiorillo C, Bonuso S, Castaldo G (2003) A cluster headache family with possible autosomal recessive inheritance. *Neurology* 61: 578–9. http://dx.doi.org/10.1212/01.WNL.0000078698.05379.FF

Dichgans M, Freilinger T, Eckstein G et al (2005) Mutation in the neuronal voltage-gated sodium channel SCN1A in familial hemiplegic migraine. *Lancet* 366: 371–7. http://dx.doi.org/10.1016/S0140-6736(05)66786-4

Ducros A, Denier C, Joutel A et al (2001) The clinical spectrum of familial hemiplegic migraine associated with mutations in a neuronal calcium channel. *N Engl J Med* 345: 17–24. http://dx.doi.org/10.1056/NEJM200107053450103

Ekbom K, Svensson DA, Pedersen NL, Waldenlind E (2006) Lifetime prevalence and concordance risk of cluster headache in the Swedish twin population. *Neurology* 67: 798–803. http://dx.doi.org/10.1212/01.wnl.0000233786.72356.3e

El Amrani M, Ducros A, Boulan P et al (2002) Familial cluster headache: a series of 186 index patients. *Headache* 42: 974–7. http://dx.doi.org/10.1046/j.1526-4610.2002.02226.x

Gervil M, Ulrich V, Kyvik KO, Olesen J, Russell MB (1999a) Migraine without aura: a population based twin study. *Ann Neurol* 46: 606–11. http://dx.doi.org/10.1002/1531-8249(199910)46:4<606::AID-ANA8>3.0.CO;2-O

Gervil M, Ulrich V, Kaprio J, Olesen J, Russell MB (1999b) The relative role of genetic and environmental factors in migraine without aura. *Neurology* 53: 995–9. http://dx.doi.org/10.1212/WNL.53.5.995

Headache Classification Subcommittee of the International Headache Society (2004) The International Classification of Headache Disorders. *Cephalalgia* 24(Suppl 1): 9–160.

Joutel A, Bousser MG, Biousse V et al (1993) A gene for familial hemiplegic migraine maps to chromosome 19. *Nat Genet* 5: 40–5. http://dx.doi.org/10.1038/ng0993-40

Kalfakis N, Panas M, Vassilopoulos D, Malliara Loulakaki S (1996) Migraine with aura: segregation analysis and heritability estimation. *Headache* 36: 320–2. http://dx.doi.org/10.1046/j.1526-4610.1996.3605320.x

Khoury MJ, Beaty TH, Liang K-Y (1988) Can familial aggregation of diseases be explained by familial aggregation of environmental risk factors? *Am J Epidemiol* 127: 674–83.

Kudrow L, Kudrow DB (1994) Inheritance of cluster headache and its possible link to migraine. *Headache* 34: 400–7. http://dx.doi.org/10.1111/j.1526-4610.1994.hed3407400.x

Lalouel JM, Morton NE (1981) Complex segregation analysis with pointers. *Hum Hered* 31: 312–21. http://dx.doi.org/10.1159/000153231

Leone M, Russell MB, Rigamonti A et al (2001) Familial risk of cluster headache: a study of Italian families. *Neurology* 56: 1233–6. http://dx.doi.org/10.1212/WNL.56.9.1233

Mochi M, Sangiorgi S, Cortelli P et al (1993) Testing models for genetic determination in migraine. *Cephalalgia* 13: 389–94. http://dx.doi.org/10.1046/j.1468-2982.1993.1306389.x

Motulsky AG (1978) Biased ascertainment and the natural history of diseases. *N Engl J Med* 298: 1196–7. http://dx.doi.org/10.1056/NEJM197805252982111

Ophoff RA, Terwindt GM, Vergouwe MN et al (1996) Familial hemiplegic migraine and episodic ataxia type-2 are caused by mutations in the Ca2+ channel gene CACNL1A4. *Cell* 87: 543–52. http://dx.doi.org/10.1016/S0092-8674(00)81373-2

Østergaard S, Russell MB, Bendtsen L, Olesen J (1997) Comparison of first degree relatives and spouses of people with chronic tension type headache. *BMJ* 314: 1092–3. http://dx.doi.org/10.1136/bmj.314.7087.1092

Rasmussen BK, Jensen R, Schroll M, Olesen J (1991a) Epidemiology of headache in a general population – a prevalence study. *J Clin Epidemiol* 44: 1147–57. http://dx.doi.org/10.1016/0895-4356(91)90147-2

Rasmussen BK, Jensen R, Olesen J (1991b) Questionnaire versus clinical interview in the diagnosis of headache. *Headache* 31: 290–5. http://dx.doi.org/10.1111/j.1526-4610.1991.hed3105290.x

Riant F, De Fusco M, Aridon P et al (2005) ATP1A2 mutations in 11 families with familial hemiplegic migraine. *Hum Mutat* 26: 281. http://dx.doi.org/10.1002/humu.9361

Russell MB (1997) Genetic epidemiology of migraine and cluster headache. *Cephalalgia* 17: 683–701. http://dx.doi.org/10.1046/j.1468-2982.1997.1706683.x

Russell MB (2005) Tension-type headache in 40-year-olds: a Danish population-based sample of 4000. *J Headache Pain* 6: 441–7. http://dx.doi.org/10.1007/s10194-005-0253-3

Russell MB, Ducros A (2011) Sporadic and familial hemiplegic migraine: pathophysiological mechanisms, clinical characteristics, diagnosis, and management. *Lancet Neurol* 10: 457–70. http://dx.doi.org/10.1016/S1474-4422(11)70048-5

Russell MB, Olesen J (1995) Increased familial risk and evidence of genetic factor in migraine. *BMJ* 311: 541–4. http://dx.doi.org/10.1136/bmj.311.7004.541

Russell MB, Andersson PG, Thomsen LL (1994) Familial occurrence of cluster headache. *Genet Epidemiol* 11: 285–310.

Russell MB, Andersson PG, Thomsen LL (1995a) Familial occurrence of cluster headache. *J Neurol Neurosurg Psychiatry* 58: 341–3. http://dx.doi.org/10.1136/jnnp.58.3.341

Russell MB, Andersson PG, Thomsen LL, Iselius L (1995b) Cluster headache is an autosomal dominant inherited disorder in some families. A complex segregation analysis. *J Med Genet* 32: 954–6. http://dx.doi.org/10.1136/jmg.32.12.954

Russell MB, Iselius L, Olesen J (1995c) Investigation of inheritance of migraine by complex segregation analysis. *Hum Genet* 96: 726–30. http://dx.doi.org/10.1007/BF00210307

Russell MB, Rasmussen BK, Fenger K, Olesen J (1996a) Migraine without aura and migraine with aura are distinct clinical entities: a study of 484 male and female migraineurs from the general population. *Cephalalgia* 16: 239–45. http://dx.doi.org/10.1046/j.1468-2982.1996.1604239.x

Russell MB, Fenger K, Olesen J (1996b) Familial history of migraine. Direct versus indirect information. *Cephalalgia* 16: 156–60. http://dx.doi.org/10.1046/j.1468-2982.1996.1603156.x

Russell MB, Iselius L, Østergaard S, Olesen J (1998) A complex segregation analysis of chronic tension-type headache. *Hum Genet* 102: 138–40. http://dx.doi.org/10.1007/s004390050666

Russell MB, Ulrich V, Gervil M, Olesen J (2002) Migraine without aura and migraine with aura are distinct disorders. A population based twin survey. *Headache* 42: 332–6. http://dx.doi.org/10.1046/j.1526-4610.2002.02102.x

Russell MB, Saltyte-Benth J, Levi N (2006) Are infrequent episodic, frequent episodic and chronic tension-type headache inherited? A population-based study of 11 199 twin pairs. *J Headache Pain* 7: 119–26. http://dx.doi.org/10.1007/s10194-006-0299-x

Stewart WF, Staffa J, Lipton RB, Ottman R (1997) Familial risk of migraine: a population based study. *Ann Neurol* 41: 166–72. http://dx.doi.org/10.1002/ana.410410207

Thomsen LL, Ostergaard E, Romer SF et al (2003a) Evidence for a separate type of migraine with aura: sporadic hemiplegic migraine. *Neurology* 60: 595–601. http://dx.doi.org/10.1212/01.WNL.0000046524.25369.7D

Thomsen LL, Olesen J, Russell MB (2003b) Increased risk of migraine with typical aura in relatives of probands with familial hemiplegic migraine and their relatives *Eur J Neurol* 10: 421–7. http://dx.doi.org/10.1046/j.1468-1331.2003.00621.x

Ulrich V, Gervil M, Kyvik KO, Olesen J, Russell MB (1999a) Evidence of a genetic factor in migraine with aura: a population-based Danish twin study. *Ann Neurol* 45: 242–6. http://dx.doi.org/10.1002/1531-8249(199902)45:2<242::AID-ANA15>3.0.CO;2-1

Ulrich V, Gervil M, Kyvik KO, Olesen J, Russell MB (1999b) The inheritance of migraine with aura estimated by means of structural equation modelling. *J Med Gen* 36: 225–7.

Vanmolkot KR, Babini E, de Vries B et al (2007) The novel p.L1649Q mutation in the SCN1A epilepsy gene is associated with familial hemiplegic migraine: genetic and functional studies. *Hum Mutat* 28: 522. http://dx.doi.org/10.1002/humu.9486

Weiss KM, Chakraborty R, Majumder PP, Smouse PE (1982) Problems in the assessment of relative risk of affected individuals. *J Chronic Dis* 35: 539–51. http://dx.doi.org/10.1016/0021-9681(82)90073-X

Whitty CWM (1953) Familial hemiplegic migraine. *J Neurol Neurosurg Psychiat* 16: 172–7. http://dx.doi.org/10.1136/jnnp.16.3.172

Willis T (1682) *Opera Omnia*. Amstelaedami: Henricure Wetstenium, pp. 92–111.

5
CLASSIFICATION OF HEADACHE

Shashi S Seshia

Introduction

Classification schemes for clinical disorders are essential for standardising approaches to care and research, minimising inter- and intra-observer variability and ensuring uniformity of communication among professionals worldwide (American Psychiatric Association 2000, Seshia 2010). Olesen (2008) suggested that a set of medical disorders that lacked proper classification and diagnostic criteria was like a society without laws, the consequences being 'incoherence at best and chaos at worst'! Clinical assessment is still the foundation of diagnosis in headache disorders. In addition, in the absence of specific tests, clinical criteria form the basis for differentiating between the various primary headache types. Classifications based on the recommendations of a small group of experts are generally rated as low-level evidence. Ideally, clinical diagnostic criteria must aim for maximum specificity (Abu-Arafeh 2008). Clinicians must always be alert to the inevitable false-positive and false-negative diagnoses that occur when such criteria are used.

In 1962, an ad hoc committee tentatively presented an approach to the classification of headache (The Ad Hoc Committee on the Classification of Headache 1962). The first International Classification of Headache Disorders (ICHD-I) was published by the International Headache Society (IHS) in 1988 (Headache Classification Committee of the International Headache Society 1988), and began to be used by adult and paediatric headache specialists. The limitations of applying the adult-based ICHD-I criteria for migraine without aura to children (the term will be used to include adolescents) became quickly apparent, and suggestions for improvement followed (Mortimer et al 1992, Seshia et al 1994, Seshia and Wolstein 1995, Winner et al 1995, Wober-Bingol et al 1995). Attention was drawn to the shorter duration of migraine attacks in children, bilateral rather than unilateral location and the often limited information children were able to provide. A suggestion was also made to label the headache disorder as 'probable' when all criteria were not fulfilled (Seshia and Wolstein 1995). These issues were addressed in the subsequent, and still current, classification (ICHD-II) (Headache Classification Subcommittee of the International Headache Society 2004). A further revision, ICHD-III, is in progress (Olesen and Third International Headache Classification Committee of the International Headache Society 2011).

ICHD-II

Headache disorders, cranial neuralgias and central and primary facial pain are divided numerically into 14 major groups, separated into 'primary' and 'secondary'. Each group is further subdivided into types, subtypes and subforms (Appendix 5.1), giving a total of almost 200 conditions in which headache is a major feature, numerically coded to a three-digit level (Headache Classification Subcommittee of the International Headache Society 2004). The diagnostic criteria for each primary headache category include the proviso that

> History and physical and neurological examination do not suggest any of the disorders listed in groups 5–12 (*secondary headache*), or history and/or physical and/or neurological examination do suggest such disorder but is ruled out by appropriate investigations, or such disorder is present but attacks do not occur for the first time in close temporal relationship to the disorder [italics added].

Therefore, the challenges for clinicians lie in ensuring that a secondary cause is not masquerading as a primary headache. Clinical features that help in the differentiation have been discussed elsewhere in this book, including in Chapters 8 and 9.

A child may have more than one kind of headache disorder; each one has to be recognised for effective management, headache diaries being essential. When only some of the required criteria for diagnosis of a headache disorder are fulfilled, then the disorder should be classified as 'probable'.

As the classification is based on the work of a committee, it has the potential for being self-fulfilling, and sometimes inadequate. Also, it is not surprising that there is continuing debate about some entities, even among adult headache specialists. The challenges of applying ICHD-II in India have been discussed (Ravishankar 2010); observations that probably apply to much of the world's population.

A brief overview of the classification and the controversies follow, the perspective being paediatric. Arruda et al (2011) suggest that 113 of the 196 possible headache diagnoses in ICHD-II have been described in children. Hence, it is prudent to have some familiarity with these possibilities. An abbreviated ICHD-II classification considered most relevant for paediatric practice is presented in Appendix 5.1.

ICHD-II and childhood headache

As in adults, migraine without aura and tension-type headache are the most frequent headache types in children (Laurell et al 2004, Stovner et al 2007, Abu-Arafeh et al 2010, Alp et al 2010, Arruda et al 2010). Hence, the ICHD-II criteria for them have been well studied, but the criteria for many of the other 190-plus headache conditions have not been subject to critical review. These remarks apply in particular to secondary headache disorders (groups 5–12), for which the diagnostic criteria often do not reflect the protean clinical manifestations encountered in clinical practice. The IHS is subjecting secondary headache to further scrutiny (Olesen et al 2009).

Children can be unreliable historians, and parental accounts may be biased (Seshia et al 1994, Nakamura et al 2011); hence, it may not be possible to classify headaches with certainty, using ICHD criteria. In clinical practice, the classification of headache is often provisional at the first visit, and detailed diaries and follow-up reassessments are required for definite categorisation (see Chapter 8).

MIGRAINE

The ICHD-II criteria for migraine without aura for children (see Chapter 10) are applicable with a few provisos: children may use alternative terms for 'pulsating'; photophobia and phonophobia often have to be inferred from their behaviour; and, in the typical case, nausea is prominent, and vomiting occurs in over 75%. Children often go to sleep despite intense headache and wake up well, but the specificity and sensitivity of this feature has not been studied. Osmophobia, not yet a formal ICHD criteria, is considered to be relatively sensitive for migraine compared with tension-type headache (Zanchin et al 2007, Corletto et al 2008, De Carlo et al 2010, 2012). Nausea, vomiting and worsening with physical activity are not specific for migraine and can be seen with some secondary headache disorders; however, these are more characteristic of migraine than tension-type headache (Wober-Bingol et al 1995). Difficulty with thinking, light-headedness and fatigue have been suggested as additional features to improve sensitivity of migraine diagnosis (Hershey et al 2005). Family history of headache is not a useful discriminator, although at one time we thought it might be (Seshia and Wolstein 1995).

The diagnostic criteria for basilar-type migraine and childhood periodic syndromes, such as cyclical vomiting and abdominal migraine, appear satisfactory (Cuvellier and Lepine 2010), but to the author's knowledge have not been field tested. Some of these are discussed in detail elsewhere in this volume.

TENSION-TYPE HEADACHE

The criteria for infrequent episodic, frequent episodic and chronic tension-type headache (Table 5.1) are generally applicable to children (Rossi et al 2008, Seshia et al 2009). ICHD considers tension-type headache to be mild or moderate and migraine to be moderate or severe in intensity; however, children may describe tension-type headache as severe (Abu-Arafeh 2001), and be erroneously diagnosed as having migraine (Seshia et al 2009). Therefore, severity is *not a good discriminator* between migraine and tension-type headache. Tension-type headache is discussed in Chapter 18.

MIGRAINE WITHOUT AURA AND TENSION-TYPE HEADACHE

The co-occurrence of migraine without aura and tension-type headache is acknowledged in ICHD-II, and has been recognised in children for several years. Like many others, the author feels it may well represent an entity in its own right rather than a 'continuum' of migraine (Seshia et al 2009), although ICHD-II has not assigned the entity a distinct code. Recognition of both types is essential for management.

TABLE 5.1
Criteria for the diagnosis of tension-type headache

Diagnostic criteria	Infrequent episodic	Frequent episodic	Chronic
Frequency	<1d/mo, ≥10 episodes	1–15d/mo for ≥3mo	≥15d/mo for > 3mo
Duration	30min–7d	30min–7d	Hours – continuous
At least two of the following			
Intensity	Mild/moderate	Mild/moderate	Mild/moderate
Location	Bilateral	Bilateral	Bilateral
Quality	Pressing/tightening	Pressing/tightening	Pressing/tightening
Aggravated by activity	–	–	–
Both of the following			
Nausea or vomiting	–	–	Mild nausea ±
Photo- or phonophobia	+	+	+
Attributed to other disorder	–	–	–

Abbreviated version reproduced with permission of the International Headache Society (Headache Classification Subcommittee of the International Headache Society 2004) and the *Canadian Journal of Neurological Sciences* (Seshia et al 2009).

+, present; –, absent; ±, may be present or absent.

CLUSTER HEADACHE AND OTHER TRIGEMINAL AUTONOMIC CEPHALALGIAS

Cranial autonomic disturbances are the hallmark of the trigeminal autonomic cephalalgias (TACs), and by definition attacks often cluster (TACs are discussed in Chapter 19). Headaches occur unilaterally over the orbital, supraorbital and/or temporal region, are severe or very severe in intensity and may occur several times a day, for periods of several minutes to 3 hours. These conditions are uncommon in children (Pakalnis and Yonker 2010), and secondary causes must be excluded; thrashing about in bed may be the counterpart to restlessness and agitation in adults (Majumdar et al 2009). Attacks in paroxysmal hemicrania are shorter lasting than in cluster headache but occur more frequently; response to indometacin (indomethacin in North America) is diagnostic and a requisite feature of the disorder (Tarantino et al 2011). Autonomic symptoms are less common in hemicrania continua, another disorder for which indometacin responsivity is an essential diagnostic criterion. For this reason, it is common practice to consider a trial of indometacin when headache is unilateral. However, the IHS may need to reconsider the requirement for an absolute response to indometacin, as cases are described where all other criteria but this are fulfilled (Ji and Mack 2009, Marmura et al 2009).

OTHER PRIMARY HEADACHES

Primary exertional headache is not uncommon in children, headache being precipitated by any form of exercise. Headache occurs during or immediately after physical activity, and may be indometacin responsive (Moorjani and Rothner 2001). However, it is prudent to exclude

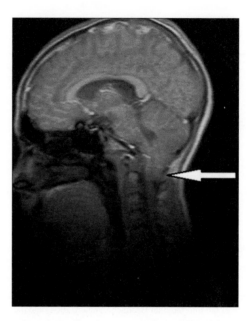

Fig. 5.1 Magnetic resonance imaging (sagittal T1 weighted) showing Chiari type 1 anomaly and congenitally narrow foramen magnum (craniocervical junction, arrow) in a 13-year-old male with occipital headache that occurred only with physical activity (see text).

secondary causes, such as type 1 Chiari malformation, when headache occurs during physical activity; type 1 Chiari malformation can be found incidentally in asymptomatic patients.

Case example

An athletically inclined 13-year-old male presented to the headache clinic with a 1-year history of occipital headache that occurred only during physical activity. Magnetic resonance imaging of the head and cervical spine (Fig. 5.1) showed a type 1 Chiari malformation and a developmentally narrow foramen magnum; findings that were confirmed at surgery. He was symptom free thereafter.

SECONDARY HEADACHE DISORDERS

Headaches attributed to high cerebrospinal fluid pressure, especially those due to idiopathic intracranial hypertension (IIH) and hydrocephalus, are particularly relevant for children, but their current diagnostic criteria (Headache Classification Subcommittee of the International Headache Society 2004) are unhelpful for clinical practice. ICHD-II recognises that IIH can occur without papilloedema. However, the occurrence of intracranial 'noises', tinnitus, transient visual obscuration and diplopia, which can be helpful in diagnosis, are not incorporated in the diagnostic criteria.

The criteria for headache attributed to hydrocephalus are similarly inadequate and need urgent modification to incorporate the shunt malfunction-related 'slit ventricle' syndrome

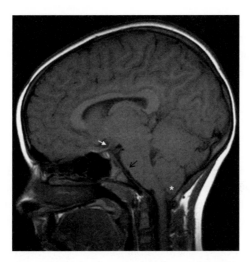

Fig. 5.2 Unenhanced sagittal T1-weighted magnetic resonance imaging of the brain, in a different child from Figure 5.1, with intracranial hypotension secondary to cerebrospinal fluid leak (see text). There is crowding of the posterior fossa structures with downward displacement of the cerebellar tonsils (*) below the level of the foramen magnum. There is 'slumping' of the brainstem with flattening of the ventral pons along the clivus (black arrow). The optic chiasm is draped over the dorsum sellae (white arrow). Reproduced with permission from the *Canadian Journal of Neurological Sciences* (Harder et al 2012).

(Seshia 1996, 2010); headache in this situation can mimic migraine without aura and tension-type headache (Seshia 1996).

Similarly, the criteria for 'headache attributed to spontaneous (or idiopathic) low cerebrospinal fluid pressure', a condition being recognised in children, especially those with inherited connective tissue disorders, need revision to reflect the protean clinical manifestations (Schievink et al 2011). Spontaneous spinal cerebrospinal fluid leaks are considered the most common cause, and can be from multiple sites. Figure 5.2 shows classic features of spontaneous intracranial hypotension in a child who presented with non-postural headache mimicking primary chronic daily headache (Harder et al 2012).

Case example of shunt malfunction masquerading as primary headache (Seshia 1996)
A 13-year-old male presented with a 3-year history of bouts of headache that at times fulfilled the criteria for migraine without aura and at others for probable tension-type headache. Previously, he had been diagnosed with hydrocephalus in infancy and had had a ventriculoperitoneal shunt placed, which had been revised on at least two occasions. Several computed tomograms taken over 6 years preceding the current visit had shown little or no serial change in ventricular size and were often reported as 'not showing convincing ventricular enlargement or evidence of shunt malfunction'. The most striking clinical feature was the aggravation of headache on lying down, prompting the suspicion of shunt malfunction with slit-ventricle syndrome. The diagnosis was confirmed on measuring the intracranial pressure, which exceeded 30cmH$_2$O.

Controversies in headache terminology and classification (ICHD-II)
The use of certain terms and definitions has provoked debate. Some of these have been discussed in several recent publications (Seshia 2010, 2012, Seshia et al 2010a,b). It is hoped that future revisions of ICHD will offer clear guidance.

DEFINITION OF 'CHRONIC'
The term 'chronic' is used inconsistently, which leads to confusion of usage. Chronic daily headache is conventionally defined as headache occurring at least 15 days a month for 3 months or more (see Chapter 20). However, 'chronic' is also used commonly in headache literature to describe headaches that occur over a period of at least 3 months regardless of attack frequency – chronic post-traumatic headache and recurrent headaches in migraine without aura or tension-type headache with attacks spread out over 3 months or more being examples in point. The situation would be clarified by limiting usage of 'chronic' to chronic daily headache.

CHRONIC DAILY HEADACHE
The IHS discouraged the use of chronic daily headache as a diagnostic entity, favouring 'chronic headache' as the umbrella term (Headache Classification Committee et al 2006), a view that was promptly challenged (Solomon 2007). Despite the injunction of the IHS, chronic daily headache remains the favoured term in both paediatric and adult literature, for its clinical utility (Welch and Goadsby 2002). Chronic daily headache is a useful descriptor for clinical research and practice. Chronic daily headache is also well understood by chronic daily headache sufferers and their families, the common expression being 'She is having headaches almost every day doctor; she should not be having headaches every day'. It is some comfort for them to know that there is indeed a simple name that clearly describes their experience.

It has been suggested that all subtypes of chronic daily headache be defined explicitly as headache occurring at least 15 days a month for at least 3 months, regardless of the duration of headache on any given day (Welch and Goadsby 2002, Seshia et al 2008, 2010a,b, Seshia 2010). Initially, an arbitrary average daily duration of more than 4 hours untreated was proposed (Siberstein et al 1994). Chronic daily headache is discussed in Chapter 20.

CHRONIC MIGRAINE
The revised definition for chronic migraine, requiring 'headache (tension-type and/or migraine) on at least 15 days per month for at least 3 months' (Headache Classification Committee et al 2006), is an implicit recognition of the existence of mixed chronic daily headache types. The incorporation of tension-type headache under chronic migraine has been questioned (Solomon 2007, Seshia et al 2008, 2010a,b, Manzoni and Torelli 2009, Seshia 2012). A more precise approach would be to classify chronic migraine as either (1) chronic migraine solely with migraine features or (2) chronic migraine with tension-type headache (Solomon 2007).

TRANSFORMED MIGRAINE
Transformed migraine was proposed as a subtype of chronic daily headache (Siberstein et al 1994). Originally, the term was used to reflect the evolution of episodic headache to chronic

daily headache (Mathew et al 1987). Unfortunately, transformed migraine implies that all cases of chronic migraine are transformed from episodic migraine, which is not the case. Chronic migraine can also be 'new daily persistent' from the outset.

NEW DAILY PERSISTENT HEADACHE

New daily persistent headache (NDPH) is discussed in Chapter 21. The current ICHD-II definition for NDPH and its inclusion under primary headache do not reflect clinical experience. As currently defined, the criteria for NDPH are similar to those for chronic tension-type headache with the exception of the onset, which is abrupt. However, migraine features are common in adults and children with NDPH (Kung et al 2009, Young 2011), and the onset may coincide with systemic illness or minor head injury, suggesting secondary headache (Mack 2004, Manzoni and Torelli 2011). NDPH and transformed migraine reflect the opposite ends of onset, and the classification of headache disorders on the basis of mode of onset is not desirable. For these reasons, the current definition of NDPH and its inclusion exclusively as a primary headache disorder need reconsideration.

MEDICATION OVERUSE HEADACHE

Medication overuse is not a major issue in most paediatric case series (Seshia et al 2010a). The criteria for medication overuse in ICHD-II are adult oriented and do not apply to children. Criteria should be based not only on duration of use and the nature of the drug but also on doses and age. The incorporation of medication overuse headache as a distinct headache type has confounded the diagnosis of chronic migraine (Manack et al 2009, Sun-Edelstein et al 2009, Manzoni and Torelli 2010). Data have been reviewed elsewhere to show that medication overuse (in the context of headache) invariably occurs on the background of a primary headache disorder, is a major risk for chronification, in some cases reflects addictive behaviour (Radat and Lanteri-Minet 2011) and may be subject to genetic influences (Hershey et al 2011).

In paediatric practice, an arbitrary definition of analgesia overuse, the most common potentially overused drug in children with headache, could be the use of analgesics at least once daily, 5 days or more a week, for more than 2 weeks – the reason being that usage beyond this period may cause transformation to chronic daily headache, an opinion for which there is no evidence. Clearly, there is urgent need to have a universal definition for medication overuse for children.

Multiaxial classification for headache disorders

A number of factors contribute to or are associated with primary headache disorders, especially primary chronic daily headache, associated psychiatric disorders being common. Hence, a multiaxial scheme, pioneered in psychiatry (American Psychiatric Association 2000), would help to capture all information relevant for clinical practice and research in a time-efficient and consistent manner (Seshia et al 2008, 2010a,b, Seshia 2010). Comorbidities to primary headache disorders would have been readily identified in earlier studies, had a multiaxial approach been adopted. A tentative classification, initially proposed for chronic daily headache, is outlined in Table 5.2.

TABLE 5.2
Multiaxial classification for headache

Axis I	Aetiological classification (primary or secondary)
Axis II	Types, subtypes and subforms (ICHD codes)
Axis III	Associated medical conditions (e.g. psychiatric disorders such as anxiety or depressive disorders, other pain syndromes, obesity, sleep disorders, etc.)
Axis IV	Contributory factors (e.g. adverse life events, concussion, analgesia overuse, other substance abuse, caffeine, poor sleep habits, infections, etc.)
Axis V	Functional impairment (specify sphere of activity)
Axis VI	Pain severity

(Seshia et al 2008) Reproduced with permission of John Wiley and Sons Ltd. ICHD, International Classification of Headache Disorders.

ICHD in paediatric practice

Clinical researchers will continue to use ICHD and strive to make it more relevant for childhood headache. ICHD-II is cumbersome for routine clinical use, and has three possible limitations: (1) with a few exceptions, many of the entities are not usually encountered in paediatric practice; (2) the criteria for most of the nearly 150 secondary headache disorders are clinically inadequate, and therefore potentially misleading; and (3) chronic daily headache, a frequently encountered, often primary headache syndrome, is not included.

In clinical practice, clinicians should try to classify headache disorders to the first- or second-digit level (e.g. migraine with or without aura, tension-type headache or episodic tension-type headache), and neurologists and headache specialists would ideally attempt to classify to the third-digit level. ICHD has done us a service by reminding us that individuals may have more than one type of headache and each should be classified (Headache Classification Subcommittee of the International Headache Society 2004).

Clinicians should be familiar with the diagnostic criteria for (1) the various forms of migraine, (2) tension-type headache (as it is just as common as migraine but often underdiagnosed), recognising that the two often co-occur, and (3) chronic daily headache, as these are common in clinical practice. Cranial autonomic symptomatology should always be sought for and along with unilateral orbital, supraorbital or temporal location of pain, would suggest a trigeminal autonomic cephalalgia or hemicrania continua. Clinicians must be familiar with red flags that will help them to recognise a secondary headache disorder presenting under the guise of a primary headache, and to features that suggest maltreatment, significant stressors or psychiatric disorders.

Conclusion

The ICHD has resulted in a consistency of approach in the diagnosis of headaches in children and adults. The diagnostic criteria for primary headache disorders are becoming increasingly robust. However, diagnostic criteria for most of the secondary headache disorders are inadequate for clinical practice or research. As the classification is based on expert opinion, continuing refinements, especially for children, will need to be made to ensure relevance. The ICHD classification can be readily incorporated into a broader multiaxial scheme, one that will also record additional information such as triggers, precipitating factors and comorbid conditions, crucial not only for biopsychosocial management, but also for epidemiological and clinic-based research. Many of the headache diagnoses in ICHD are not relevant for children, and the diagnostic criteria for those that are could be made more child-specific. There is a clear need for a separate user-friendly ICHD for children.

REFERENCES

Abu-Arafeh I (2001) Chronic tension-type headache in children and adolescents. *Cephalalgia* 21: 830–6. http://dx.doi.org/10.1046/j.0333-1024.2001.00275.x

Abu-Arafeh I (2008) Classification of headache. *Dev Med Child Neurol* 50: 246. http://dx.doi.org/10.1111/j.1469-8749.2008.00246.x

Abu-Arafeh I, Razak S, Sivaraman B, Graham C (2010) Prevalence of headache and migraine in children and adolescents: a systematic review of population-based studies. *Dev Med Child Neurol* 52: 1088–97. http://dx.doi.org/10.1111/j.1469-8749.2010.03793.x

Alp R, Alp SI, Palanci Y et al (2010) Use of the International Classification of Headache Disorders, 2nd edn, criteria in the diagnosis of primary headache in schoolchildren: epidemiology study from eastern Turkey. *Cephalalgia* 30: 868–77.

American Psychiatric Association (2000) *Diagnostic and Statistical Manual of Mental Disorders DSM-IV-TR*. Washington, DC: American Psychiatric Association.

Arruda MA, Albuquerque RC, Bigal ME (2011) Uncommon headache syndromes in the pediatric population. *Curr Pain Headache Rep* 15: 280–8. http://dx.doi.org/10.1007/s11916-011-0192-4

Arruda MA, Guidetti V, Galli F, Albuquerque RC, Bigal ME (2010) Primary headaches in childhood – a population-based study. *Cephalalgia* 30: 1056–64. http://dx.doi.org/10.1177/0333102409361214

Corletto E, Dal Zotto L, Resos A et al (2008) Osmophobia in juvenile primary headaches. *Cephalalgia* 28: 825–31. http://dx.doi.org/10.1111/j.1468-2982.2008.01589.x

Cuvellier JC, Lepine A (2010) Childhood periodic syndromes. *Pediatric Neurol* 42: 1–11. http://dx.doi.org/10.1016/j.pediatrneurol.2009.07.001

De Carlo D, Dal Zotto L, Perissinotto E et al (2010) Osmophobia in migraine classification: a multicentre study in juvenile patients. *Cephalalgia* 30: 1486–94. http://dx.doi.org/10.1177/0333102410362928

De Carlo D, Toldo I, Dal Zotto L et al (2012) Osmophobia as an early marker of migraine: a follow-up study in juvenile patients. *Cephalalgia* 32: 401–6. http://dx.doi.org/10.1177/0333102412438975

Harder S, Griebel RW, Lemire EG, Kriegler S, Gotlin J, Seshia SS (2012) Spinal CSF leaks: mimicker of primary headache disorder in a child. *Can J Neurol Sci* 39: 388–92.

Headache Classification Committee of the International Headache Society (1988) Classification and diagnostic criteria for headache disorders, cranial neuralgias and facial pain. *Cephalalgia* 8(Suppl 7): 1–96.

Headache Classification Committee, Olesen J, Bousser MG et al (2006) New appendix criteria open for a broader concept of chronic migraine. *Cephalagia* 26: 742–6. http://dx.doi.org/10.1111/j.1468-2982.2006.01172.x

Headache Classification Subcommittee of the International Headache Society (2004) The International Classification of Headache Disorders: 2nd edition. *Cephalalgia* 24(Suppl 1): 9–160.

Hershey AD, Winner P, Kabbouche MA et al (2005) Use of the ICHD-II criteria in the diagnosis of pediatric migraine. *Headache* 45: 1288–97. http://dx.doi.org/10.1111/j.1526-4610.2005.00260.x

Hershey AD, Burdine D, Kabbouche MA, Power SW (2011) Genomic expression patterns in medication overuse headaches. *Cephalalgia* 31: 161–71. http://dx.doi.org/10.1177/0333102410373155

Ji T, Mack KJ (2009) Unilateral chronic daily headache in children. *Headache* 49: 1062–5. http://dx.doi.org/10.1111/j.1526-4610.2009.01455.x

Kung E, Tepper SJ, Rapoport AM, Sheftell FD, Bigal ME (2009) New daily persistent headache in the paediatric population. *Cephalalgia* 29: 17–22. http://dx.doi.org/10.1111/j.1468-2982.2008.01647.x

Laurell K, Larsson B, Eeg-Olofsson O (2004) Prevalence of headache in Swedish schoolchildren, with a focus on tension-type headache. *Cephalalgia* 24: 380–8. http://dx.doi.org/10.1111/j.1468-2982.2004.00681.x

Mack KJ (2004) What incites new daily persistent headache in children? *Pediatr Neurol* 31: 122–5. http://dx.doi.org/10.1016/j.pediatrneurol.2004.02.006

Majumdar A, Ahmed MA, Benton S (2009) Cluster headache in children--experience from a specialist headache clinic. *Eur J Paediatr Neurol* 13: 524–9. http://dx.doi.org/10.1016/j.ejpn.2008.11.002

Manack A, Turkel C, Silberstein S (2009) The evolution of chronic migraine: classification and nomenclature. *Headache* 49: 1206–13. http://dx.doi.org/10.1111/j.1526-4610.2009.01432.x

Manzoni GC, Torelli P (2009) Chronic migraine and chronic tension-type headache: are they the same or different? *Neurol Sci* 30 (Suppl 1): S81–4. http://dx.doi.org/10.1007/s10072-009-0078-y

Manzoni GC, Torelli P (2011) Does NDPH exist? Some clinical considerations. *Neurol Sci* 32(Suppl 1): S45–9. http://dx.doi.org/10.1007/s10072-011-0534-3

Manzoni GC, Torelli P (2010) Proposal for a new classification of chronic headache. *Neurol Sci* 31(Suppl 1): S9–13. http://dx.doi.org/10.1007/s10072-010-0265-x

Marmura MJ, Silberstein SD, Gupta M (2009) Hemicrania continua: who responds to indomethacin? *Cephalalgia* 29: 300–7. http://dx.doi.org/10.1111/j.1468-2982.2008.01719.x

Mathew NT, Reuveni U, Perez F (1987) Transformed or evolutive migraine. *Headache* 27: 102–6. http://dx.doi.org/10.1111/j.1526-4610.1987.hed2702102.x

Moorjani BI, Rothner AD (2001) Indomethacin-responsive headaches in children and adolescents. *Sem Pediatr Neurol* 8: 40–5. http://dx.doi.org/10.1053/spen.2001.23328

Mortimer MJ, Kay J, Jaron A (1992) Epidemiology of headache and childhood migraine in an urban general practice using Ad Hoc, Vahlquist and IHS criteria. *Dev Med Child Neurol* 34: 1095–101. http://dx.doi.org/10.1111/j.1469-8749.1992.tb11423.x

Nakamura EF, Cui L, Lateef T, Nelson KB, Merikangas KR (2011) Parent-child agreement in the reporting of headaches in a national sample of adolescents. *J Child Neurol* 27: 61–7. http://dx.doi.org/10.1177/0883073811413580

Olesen J (2008) The International Classification of Headache Disorders. *Headache* 48: 691–3. http://dx.doi.org/10.1111/j.1526-4610.2008.01121.x

Olesen J, Steiner T, Bousser MG et al (2009) Proposals for new standardized general diagnostic criteria for the secondary headaches. *Cephalalgia* 29: 1331–6. http://dx.doi.org/10.1111/j.1468-2982.2009.01965.x

Olesen J, Third International Headache Classification Committee of the International Headache Society (2011) New plans for headache classification: ICHD-3. *Cephalalgia* 31: 4–5. http://dx.doi.org/10.1177/0333102410375628

Pakalnis A, Yonker M (2010) 'Other' headache syndromes in children. *Pediatr Ann* 39: 440–6. http://dx.doi.org/10.3928/00904481-20100623-08

Radat F, Lanteri-Minet M (2011) Addictive behaviour in medication overuse headache: A review of recent data. *Rev Neurol (Paris)* 167: 568–78. http://dx.doi.org/10.1016/j.neurol.2011.02.036

Ravishankar K (2010) The "IHS" Classification (1988, 2004) – contributions, limitations and suggestions. *J Assoc Physicians India* 58(Suppl): 7–9.

Rossi L N, Vajani S, Cortinovis I, Spreafico F, Menegazzo L (2008) Analysis of the International Classification of Headache Disorders for diagnosis of migraine and tension-type headache in children. *Dev Med Child Neurol* 50: 305–10. http://dx.doi.org/10.1111/j.1469-8749.2008.02041.x

Schievink WI, Dodick DW, Mokri B, Silberstein S, Bousser MG, Goadsby PJ (2011) Diagnostic criteria for headache due to spontaneous intracranial hypotension: a perspective. *Headache* 51: 1442–4. http://dx.doi.org/10.1111/j.1526-4610.2011.01911.x

Seshia SS (1996) Specificity of IHS criteria in childhood headache. *Headache* 36: 295–9. http://dx.doi.org/10.1046/j.1526-4610.1996.3605295.x

Seshia SS (2010) The classification of headache: room for improvement. In: Chowdhury D, Gupta M, Balta A, editors. *Headache and Related Disorders*. New Delhi: GB Pant Hospital, pp. 2–4.

Seshia SS (2012) Chronic daily headache in children and adolescents. *Curr Pain Headache Rep* 16: 60–72. http://dx.doi.org/10.1007/s11916-011-0228-9

Seshia SS, Wolstein JR (1995) International Headache Society classification and diagnostic criteria in children: a proposal for revision. *Dev Med Child Neurol* 37: 879–82. http://dx.doi.org/10.1111/j.1469-8749.1995.tb11940.x

Seshia SS, Wolstein JR, Adams C, Booth FA, Reggin JD (1994) International headache society criteria and childhood headache. *Dev Med Child Neurol* 36: 419–28. http://dx.doi.org/10.1111/j.1469-8749.1994.tb11868.x

Seshia SS, Phillips DF, Von Baeyer CL (2008) Childhood chronic daily headache: a biopsychosocial perspective. *Dev Med Child Neurol* 50: 541–5. http://dx.doi.org/10.1111/j.1469-8749.2008.03013.x

Seshia SS, Abu-Arafeh I, Hershey AD (2009) Tension-type headache in children: the Cinderella of headache disorders! *Can J Neurol Sci* 36: 687–95.

Seshia SS, Wang S, Abu-Arafeh I et al (2010a) Chronic daily headache in children and adolescents: a multifaceted syndrome. *Can J Neurol Sci* 37: 769–82.

Seshia SS, Wober-Bingol C, Guidetti V (2010b) The classification of chronic headache: room for further improvement? *Cephalalgia* 30: 1268–70. http://dx.doi.org/10.1177/0333102410374143

Siberstein SD, Lipton RB, Solomon S, Mathew NT (1994) Classification of daily and near-daily headaches: proposed revisions to the IHS criteria. *Headache* 34: 1–7. http://dx.doi.org/10.1111/j.1526-4610.1994.hed3401001.x

Solomon S (2007) New appendix criteria open for a broader concept of chronic migraine. *Cephalalgia* 27: 469; author reply 469–70. http://dx.doi.org/10.1111/j.1468-2982.2007.01292_1.x

Stovner L, Hagen K, Jensen R et al (2007) The global burden of headache: a documentation of headache prevalence and disability worldwide. *Cephalalgia* 27: 193–210. http://dx.doi.org/10.1111/j.1468-2982.2007.01288.x

Sun-Edelstein C, Bigal ME, Rapoport AM (2009) Chronic migraine and medication overuse headache: clarifying the current International Headache Society classification criteria. *Cephalalgia* 29: 445–2. http://dx.doi.org/10.1111/j.1468-2982.2008.01753.x

Tarantino S, Vollono C, Capuano A, Vigevano F, Valeriani M (2011) Chronic paroxysmal hemicrania in paediatric age: report of two cases. *J Headache Pain* 12: 263–7. http://dx.doi.org/10.1007/s10194-011-0315-7

The Ad Hoc Committee On The Classification Of Headache (1962) Classification of headache. *Arch Neurol* 6: 173–6. http://dx.doi.org/10.1001/archneur.1962.00450210001001

Welch KM, Goadsby PJ (2002) Chronic daily headache: nosology and pathophysiology. *Curr Opin Neurol* 15: 287–95. http://dx.doi.org/10.1097/00019052-200206000-00011

Winner P, Martinez W, Mate L, Bello L (1995) Classification of pediatric migraine: proposed revisions to the IHS criteria. *Headache* 35: 407–10. http://dx.doi.org/10.1111/j.1526-4610.1995.hed3507407.x

Wober-Bingol C, Wober C, Karwautz A et al (1995) Diagnosis of headache in childhood and adolescence: a study in 437 patients. *Cephalalgia* 15: 13–21. http://dx.doi.org/10.1046/j.1468-2982.1995.1501013.x

Young WB (2011) New daily persistent headache: controversy in the diagnostic criteria. *Curr Pain Headache Rep* 15: 47–50. http://dx.doi.org/10.1007/s11916-010-0160-4

Zanchin G, Dainese F, Trucco M, Mainardi F, Mampreso E, Maggioni F (2007) Osmophobia in migraine and tension-type headache and its clinical features in patients with migraine. *Cephalalgia* 27: 1061–8. http://dx.doi.org/10.1111/j.1468-2982.2007.01421.x

Appendix 5.1 Headache disorders most relevant for paediatric practice – abbreviated version of ICHD-II

PART 1: The primary headaches: *Most important category for clinicians*	Comments
1. Migraine	
1.1 Migraine without aura	*Most common type of migraine*
1.2 Migraine with aura	
1.2.1 Typical aura with migraine headache	
1.2.4 Familial hemiplegic migraine (FHM)	
1.2.5 Sporadic hemiplegic migraine	
1.2.6 Basilar-type migraine	
1.3 Childhood periodic syndromes precursors of migraine	
1.3.1 Cyclical vomiting	
1.3.2 Abdominal migraine	
1.3.3 Benign paroxysmal vertigo of childhood	
1.5 Complication of migraine	
1.5.1 Chronic migraine	*A type of chronic daily headache*
1.6 Probable migraine	
2. Tension-type headache	*A very common type*
2.1 Infrequent tension-type headache	
2.2 Frequent tension-type headache	
2.3 Chronic tension-type headache	
2.4 Probable tension-type headache	

A combination of 1 and 2 *(is very common in clinical practice, but has no code in ICHD-II)* may include 1.1 (migraine without aura) and 2.1 (infrequent) or 2.2 (frequent tension-type headache), and 1.5.1 and 2.3 (chronic migraine with chronic tension-type headache)

3. Cluster headache and other trigeminal autonomic cephalalgias	*Cluster headache is rare in children; exclude secondary causes*
3.1 Cluster headache	
3.1.1 Episodic cluster headache	
3.1.2 Chronic cluster headache	
3.2 Paroxysmal hemicranias	
3.2.1 Episodic paroxysmal hemicranias	
3.2.2 Chronic paroxysmal hemicranias (CPH)	
3.3 Short-lasting unilateral neuralgiform headache attacks with conjunctival injection and tearing (SUNCT)	
3.4 Probable trigeminal autonomic cephalalgia	
4. Other primary headaches	
4.1 Primary stabbing headache (ice-pick headache, jabs and jolts, etc.)	
4.2 Primary cough headache	
4.3 Primary exertional headache	
4.6 Primary thunderclap headache (high intensity of abrupt onset)	
4.7 Hemicrania continua (HC)	*Response to indometacin is currently required for diagnosis of HC*
4.8 New daily persistent headache (NDPH)	*See text*

PART 2: The secondary headaches: *ICHD criteria unlikely to be helpful in clinical practice; see text*

5. Headache attributed to head and/or neck trauma
    5.1 Acute post-traumatic headache
    5.2 Chronic post-traumatic headache
    5.3 Acute headache attributed to whiplash injury
    5.4 Chronic headache attributed to whiplash injury
    5.5 Traumatic intracranial haematoma

6. Headache attributed to cranial or cervical vascular disorder
    6.1 Ischemic stroke or transient ischemic attack
    6.2 Non-traumatic intracranial haemorrhage
    6.3 Unruptured vascular malformation
    6.4 Arteritis
    6.5 Carotid or vertebral artery pain
      6.5.1 Attributed to dissection
    6.6 Attributed to cerebral venous thrombosis (CVT)
    6.7 Other intracranial vascular disorder
      6.7.1 Cerebral autosomal dominant arteriopathy with subcortical infarcts and leukoencephalopathy (CADASIL)

      6.7.2. Mitochondrial encephalopathy, lactic acidosis and stroke-like episodes (MELAS)

Strokes are recognised in childhood; some populations are at high risk

6.3 may mimic migraine with aura or primary chronic daily headache; Moya Moya disease should be included; can present in childhood

6.7.1 migraine with aura, dementia, ischemic strokes, abnormal white matter on MRI; mutation of Notch 3 gene; childhood case described

6.7.2 not a vascular disorder; may present in children/adolescents

7. Headache attributed to non-vascular intracranial disorder
    7.1 High cerebrospinal fluid (CSF) pressure
      7.1.1 Idiopathic intracranial hypertension (IIH)
      7.1.3 Intracranial hypertension due to hydrocephalus
    7.2 Headache attributed to low CSF pressure
      7.2.2 Post dural puncture headache
      7.2.3 CSF fistula headache
      7.2.3 Spontaneous (or idiopathic) low CSF pressure
    7.4 Headache attributed to intracranial neoplasm
    7.7 Headache attributed to Chiari malformation type I

7.1 extremely important in children; see text

7.2 important in children with connective tissue disorders; usually due to a leak

7.7 occipital headache brought on or worsened with physical activity

8. Headache attributed to a substance or its withdrawal
    8.1 Headache induced by acute substance use or exposure
      8.1.5 Induced by food components and additives
    8.2 Medication overuse headache
      8.2.1 Ergotamine overuse headache
      8.2.2 Triptan overuse headache
      8.2.3 Analgesic overuse headache
      8.2.4 Opioid overuse
      8.2.5 Combination medication overuse headache
      8.2.6 Headache attributed to other medication overuse
      8.2.7 Probable medication overuse headache

See text for discussion; prevalence is not well established but in most centres considered uncommon

Ergotamine is not relevant, triptan may be relevant and analgesia is most relevant for children

Exposure to a low level of carbon monoxide, from defects in furnaces used to heat homes, may be associated with frequent or chronic daily headache (code 8.1.3)

9. Headache attributed to infection	
9.1. Headache attributed to intracranial infection	
9.2. Headache attributed to systemic infection	
9.3. Headache attributed to HIV/AIDS	
9.4. Chronic post infectious headache	
10. Headache attributed to disorder of homoeostasis	
11. Attributed to disorder of cranium, neck, eyes, ears, nose, sinuses, teeth, mouth or other facial or cranial structures	*Rare in children*
11.2 Attributed to disorders of the neck	
11.2.1 Cervicogenic headache	
11.3 Attributed to disorders of eyes	*Eyes disorders are an important, but often missed, cause*
11.5 Attributed to rhinosinusitis	*Sinusitis, an incidental finding on MRI, often confounds diagnosis of child's headache*
11.6 Disorder of teeth, jaws or related structures	
11.7 Temporomandibular joint (TM) disorder	
12. Headache attributed to psychiatric disorder	

Comments: *Better termed psychiatric disorders associated with headache; there is increasing evidence for the association of psychiatric disorders, particularly mood – especially depressive – and anxiety disorders with a number of specific headache disorders including migraine, tension-type headache and chronic daily headache; note that post-traumatic stress disorder is classified under anxiety disorders in DSM-IV; recognition of psychiatric and psychological disorders in those with headache is extremely important in clinical practice*

PART 3: Cranial neuralgias, central and primary facial pain and other headaches

13. Cranial neuralgias and central causes of facial pain	*Uncommon in children; secondary causes must always be excluded*
13.1 Trigeminal neuralgia	
13.2 to 13.8 A variety of other neuralgias	
13.11 Cold-stimulus headache	
13.12 Ingestion or inhalation of cold stimulus	*13.12 also called ice cream headache!*
13.16 Tolosa–Hunt syndrome	*13.16 interesting entity; extremely rare*
13.17 Ophthalmoplegic 'migraine'	*13.17 considered by ICHD-II as unlikely to be a variant of migraine, but secondary causes being common*

Comments in italics represent personal observations. Some conditions, including those discussed in the Appendix to ICHD-II, are not included. These include alternating hemiplegia of childhood and benign paroxysmal torticollis, often linked to benign paroxysmal vertigo of childhood and other forms of migraine. Posterior fossa and high cervical intra- and extramedullary cord lesions must always be excluded in those with paroxysmal torticollis.

Abbreviated version reproduced with permission of the International Headache Society (Headache Classification Subcommittee of the International Headache Society 2004).

6
EPIDEMIOLOGY OF HEADACHE AND MIGRAINE

Ishaq Abu-Arafeh

Introduction

Headache is a common complaint in people of all ages, including children. Primary headache, mainly tension-type headache (TTH) and migraine, has been reported from communities all over the world of diverse backgrounds, regardless of race, ethnic origin or socio-economic status. Apart from small geographical variations in the prevalence of headache and migraine, the overall trend in occurrence is similar worldwide.

It is conceivable that young children and even infants may suffer from headache, despite their inability to describe the pain or its location. It may be easier to understand the infant with head pain secondary to trauma or the newborn infant with tense cephalhaematoma after a difficult birth. It is also possible to understand the head pain in infants with scalp or periorbital cellulitis or intracranial infection. However, primary headache and most commonly migraine, which may have its first attack during infancy, cannot be easily recognised and diagnosed in a timely manner. In children with early-onset primary headache, the diagnosis may become apparent at a later age when the child can describe head pain during the discrete episodes of distress, crying, pallor, vomiting and lethargy that last a few hours to a day and may have been occurring from an early age. Many case reports describing such a pattern of headache in infants have been documented (Vahlquist and Hackzell 1949, Bille 1962, Woody and Blaw 1986, Elser and Woody 1990). Migraine was presumed to have started in an infant at the age of 2 weeks, who manifested episodes typical of cyclical vomiting syndrome (Chapter 14) that evolved in late childhood into episodes of migraine (Russell 1903). However, in early childhood, secondary headache is probably more common than primary headache (Vahlquist and Hackzell 1949, Barlow 1984).

Many population-based studies on the epidemiology of headache in children and adolescents have been published from many parts of the world over the past 30 years. The heightened interest in the study of headache epidemiology was influenced by several factors, including the introduction of the International Headache Society's Classification and Diagnostic Criteria of Headache Disorders (Classification Committee of the International Headache Society 1988), the increased awareness of the adverse impact of headache on quality of life and also the increased number of effective medications to treat acute attacks of migraine in the early 1990s. The treatment of headache in children has consequently benefited from the advances in the understanding and management of headache in adults.

Epidemiology of headache

For a long period of time, headache was considered a problem for adults, and many lay people and some healthcare professionals denied its existence in children. It was not unusual for a referral letter from primary to secondary specialist care to state 'if he/she was not a child, I would have no hesitation in making a diagnosis of migraine, but because of his/her young age I would like to seek your specialist opinion.'

Headache is not common in young preschool children, but the prevalence increases steadily and reaches the adult population prevalence during adolescence. The observed steady increase is probably multifactorial including, as well as age, several biological, physical and psychosocial factors that influence the prevalence and symptoms of headache.

HEADACHE IN PRESCHOOL-AGE CHILDREN

Most studies of headache in young children are based on clinic populations and case reports. Data from population-based studies of headache in young children under 5 years of age would be ideal to analyse the causes and clinical features of headache disorders. Unfortunately, such data are hard to obtain for many reasons, including the fact that preschool nursery education is seldom universal in any society, the ascertainment of a study population cannot be guaranteed and also headache is relatively less common in preschool children than in schoolchildren. For these reasons, many reports on headache in young preschool-age children come from specialist clinics in which a selected group of patients who seek medical advice are described. These reports are likely to be biased towards the severe end of the headache spectrum or would reflect parents' attitudes to headache and pain in general. Studies on clinic populations would inevitably exclude patients who are treated at home by the parents or at primary care.

For the above reasons, it is not possible to estimate the prevalence of headache with any accuracy in infants under the age of 3 years, especially as the diagnosis of primary headache disorders can be extremely difficult, although it may become clearer as the child grows older and is better able to describe symptoms. In many cases, pain in young children can be recognised by the associated behavioural (refusal to feed, crying, distress and poor sleep) and physiological (tachycardia, pallor and sweating) manifestations, but unfortunately they are non-specific. However, if symptoms occur in the context of recurrent attacks of pain, headache should be considered as a possible source of pain and treated accordingly (Beyer and Wells 1989, Bhatt-Mehta 1996). Headache in infancy is commonly secondary to organic diseases such as upper respiratory tract infections, otitis media or hydrocephalus or as a precursor for migraine.

The prevalence of headache increases with age from around 20% in preschool age to around 80% during adolescence and early adulthood (Abu-Arafeh and Russell 1994, Pothmann et al 1994). A follow-up study of a cohort of infants born in the early 1980s in Finland provided valuable data on the occurrence of headache in young children. At the age of 5 years, 4402 children were assessed for headache. Recurrent headache was reported by 861 children (19.5%) and was described as highly frequent in 0.2%, fairly frequent in 0.5%, less frequent in 4.3% and infrequent in 14.5% (Sillanpää et al 1991). Increased risk of headache was associated with a birthweight over 4.0kg and preterm birth (birth before 37 completed weeks of gestation).

A large study of 4825 children at age 7 years also in Finland showed that 1596 children (37.7%) had recurrent headache. Headache frequency was 2 to 11 times per year in 46% of children, 1 to 3 times per month in 18%, 1 to 6 times per week in 5.4% and daily in 1.3% (Sillanpää 1976).

HEADACHE IN SCHOOLCHILDREN AND ADOLESCENTS

A recent systematic review of published population-based studies of the prevalence of head-ache in children and adolescents between 5 and 20 years of age has shown a wide variation of reported prevalence across the world (Abu-Arafeh et al 2010). The reported prevalence of headache and the calculated 95% confidence intervals in all studies are shown in Figure 6.1 and demonstrate the variability in prevalence among studies. Such variation in prevalence is likely to be due to the variations in methodology of the published studies rather than a varia-tion in reporting or population predisposition to headache. The overall estimated prevalence of headache in children and adolescents (a total combined population of 80 876 children) was 58.4% [95% confidence interval (CI) 58.1–58.8%]. Females are more likely to have headache than males (odds ratio 1.53; 95% CI 1.48–1.60%), and this is also shown in Figure 6.2.

During the first primary school year (age 5–6 y) a small prevalence peak of 40% to 50% is noted (Sillanpää and Anttila 1996). It is very likely that the high prevalence of headache at the age of school entry is related to the fact that starting school is a major life event for the child and the family (Abu-Arafeh and Russell 1994).

Further increases in the prevalence of headache are seen during subsequent school years (Bille 1995). Interestingly, a second prevalence peak at the age of 12 to 14 years, followed by a temporary decrease in the prevalence, has been noted (Sillanpää 1983a,b, Abu-Arafeh and Russell 1994, Pothmann et al 1994, Raieli et al 1995, Bener et al 2000). Stressful events related to moving to secondary schools (Andrasik et al 1980), sitting examinations or other changes in the school systems in different countries might, in part, explain the peak. Puberty may also have a part to play in the second peak. Eighty-nine per cent of females between 13 and 15 years of age who had started menstruation had a significantly higher migraine preva-lence than those who had not (Lu et al 2000).

Bille's work on headache in 8993 schoolchildren from the city of Uppsala (Sweden) was extensive, representative and carefully performed. It showed that the prevalence of headache increased in males and females in equal proportions up to 10 to 12 years of age, but thereaf-ter more so in females. This trend has since been confirmed by many studies (Holguin and Fenichel 1967, Prensky and Sommer 1979, Sillanpää 1983a, Abu-Arafeh and Russell 1994, Aromaa et al 2000).

Epidemiology of migraine

MIGRAINE IN PRESCHOOL-AGE CHILDREN

The prevalence of headache in 7-year-old children was studied twice, using virtually identical study designs and circumstances in 1974 and 1992 in Finland. Highly significant increases in the prevalence of overall headache (from 23.4% to 71.1%) and migraine (from 1.9% to 5.7%) were demonstrated. The increase was more marked in males than in females (4.4% vs

Author	Total	Headache n	%
King and Sharpley	900	513	57
Mortimer et al	1083	409	38
Kristjánsdóttir and Wahlberg	1016	533	53
Kristjánsdóttir and Wahlberg	1124	567	50
Abu-Arafeh and Russell	1754	1166	67
Pothmann et al	4835	4297	89
Raieli et al	1445	345	24
Barea et al	538	446	83
Carlsson	1144	281	25
Antoniuk et al	460	414	90
Aaromaa et al	968	204	21
Bener et al	1159	428	37
Metsahonkala et al	3580	1306	37
Anttila et al	1290	725	56
Krasnik	2353	1759	75
Bendel-Hockstra et al	2358	2145	91
Al Jumah et al	1181	588	50
Fichtel and Larsson	792	258	33
Ho and Ong	205	174	85
Shivpuri et al	1305	255	20
Laurel et al	1371	614	45
Zwart et al	5847	4535	78
Bessisso et al	851	706	83
Bugdayci et al	5562	2739	49
Roth-Isgkeit et al	749	453	61
Alawneh and Bataineh	1120	269	24
Ayotalahi and Khorsavi	2226	691	31
Karli et al	2387	1245	52
Lundqvist et al	2126	1225	58
Siddiqui et al	1211	1035	86
Van Dijk et al	495	386	78
Aykol et al	7721	6431	83
Brun Sundblad et al	1903	1122	59
Kroner-Herwig et al	5474	2927	54
Isik et al	2228	700	31
Milovanovic	1259	413	33
Unalp et al	2384	1090	46
Ando et al	6472	3872	60
Total	80876	47266	58

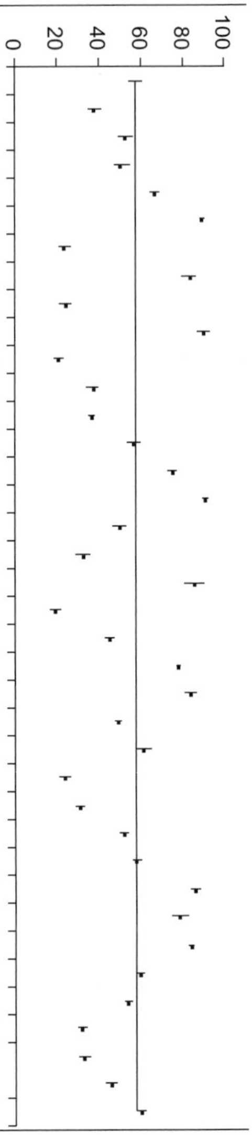

Fig. 6.1 Prevalence of headache (Abu-Arafeh et al 2010).

3%) (Sillanpää and Anttila 1996). The authors were able to confirm that 'the study design and methodology of collecting headache and other data were as identical as possible in the two measurements' and 'the correctness of the questionnaire data was ascertained by face-to-face interview. In addition, a clinical examination was performed to detect, among other things, possible causes of secondary headache' (Sillanpää and Anttila 1996). The authors were unable to detect 'reporting bias' between the two cohorts and suggested that 'even if it was present, it could not be the entire explanation of the increased prevalence'.

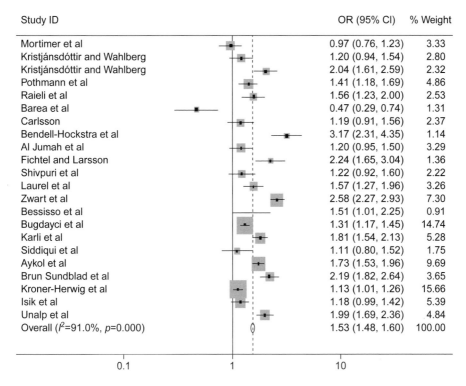

Study ID		OR (95% CI)	% Weight
Mortimer et al		0.97 (0.76, 1.23)	3.33
Kristjánsdóttir and Wahlberg		1.20 (0.94, 1.54)	2.80
Kristjánsdóttir and Wahlberg		2.04 (1.61, 2.59)	2.32
Pothmann et al		1.41 (1.18, 1.69)	4.86
Raieli et al		1.56 (1.23, 2.00)	2.53
Barea et al		0.47 (0.29, 0.74)	1.31
Carlsson		1.19 (0.91, 1.56)	2.37
Bendell-Hockstra et al		3.17 (2.31, 4.35)	1.14
Al Jumah et al		1.20 (0.95, 1.50)	3.29
Fichtel and Larsson		2.24 (1.65, 3.04)	1.36
Shivpuri et al		1.22 (0.92, 1.60)	2.22
Laurel et al		1.57 (1.27, 1.96)	3.26
Zwart et al		2.58 (2.27, 2.93)	7.30
Bessisso et al		1.51 (1.01, 2.25)	0.91
Bugdayci et al		1.31 (1.17, 1.45)	14.74
Karli et al		1.81 (1.54, 2.13)	5.28
Siddiqui et al		1.11 (0.80, 1.52)	1.75
Aykol et al		1.73 (1.53, 1.96)	9.69
Brun Sundblad et al		2.19 (1.82, 2.64)	3.65
Kroner-Herwig et al		1.13 (1.01, 1.26)	15.66
Isik et al		1.18 (0.99, 1.42)	5.39
Unalp et al		1.99 (1.69, 2.36)	4.84
Overall (I^2=91.0%, p=0.000)		1.53 (1.48, 1.60)	100.00

0.1   1   10

Fig. 6.2 Female predominance of headache prevalence (Abu-Arafeh et al 2010).

The same authors studied, for the third time, the incidence of migraine among 7-year-old children in the same Finnish population in 2002 and were able to show that migraine incidence had increased over the three decades (1974–2002) from 19.7 to 133.2 per 1000 persons-year, representing an increase in prevalence from 1.5% to 8% over the 30-year period (Anttila et al 2006). The authors observed a similar increase in the incidence of other pain syndromes, such as abdominal pain, back pain and toothache, over that period in Finland.

The reasons for the increase are *not known* and only a speculative attempt can be made to define possible factors. Having excluded possible variations in study methods and case definition, the authors of the above studies suggested 'several reasons for the increase in headache in children: a general trend of decreasing sleep in Finnish schoolchildren, an increase in use of information technology and an increase in daily sedentary life-style, a two-fold increase in soft drink consumption among children and adolescents (6–17 years) between 1977 and 1998' (Anttila et al 2006). They also suggested, but were unable to provide evidence, that 'early onset headache in children may be partly associated with the stressful lifestyle starting earlier than before or changes in the social environment'.

In younger children the diagnosis of early-onset headache disorders can be delayed because of the non-specific nature of symptoms, as shown in a study of six young children (aged 5mo–3y and 6mo) who had a strong family history of migraine and prominent features including facial pallor, irritability, sleep disturbance or mood changes (Elser and Woody 1990). Awareness of these symptoms beginning in infancy is important for the recognition and diagnosis of migraine. Other specific types of migraine, such as basilar-type migraine, were reported in eight children with onset prior to 4 years of age (Golden and French 1975).

MIGRAINE IN SCHOOL-AGE CHILDREN
The prevalence of migraine in schoolchildren has also been shown to increase in epidemiological studies in the USA and Europe. In the USA, the incidence of migraine rose from 634.5 cases per 100 000 person-years in 1979 to 1981 to 986.4 in the 1989 to 1990 period (Rozen et al 1999). Two closely comparable population-based studies in Europe, more than 30 years apart, showed an increase in the prevalence of migraine from 3.7% to 10.6% in 5- to 15-year-old schoolchildren (Bille 1962, Abu-Arafeh and Russell 1994). Although the definition of migraine was slightly different in the two studies, it is very unlikely that these differences can account for the large difference in prevalence. Also, it is extremely unlikely that population genetics have changed. However, it is reasonable to say that over the past 40 years there have been marked social and economic changes that have impacted on children's family structures and family lifestyles. There have also been changes in children's leisure activities away from outdoor sports and towards sedentary indoor activities such as excessive television watching and playing electronic video games. These changes in lifestyle are associated with increased numbers of children with weight problems. These changes may have added stress factors that have unmasked a genetic predisposition for headache in general, and migraine in particular.

A systematic review of population-based studies provided data on the prevalence of migraine in people under the age of 20 years. The diagnosis of migraine was made on the application of the International Headache Society's criteria of 1988 or the second edition of the International Classification of Headache Disorders 2004 (Classification Committee of the International Headache Society 1988, Headache Classification Subcommittee of the International Headache Society 2004). Two of the studies used revised criteria. The reported prevalence figures of migraine (and 95% CI) are shown in Figure 6.3. The cumulative analysis showed the overall prevalence of migraine in children and adolescents to be 7.7% (95% CI 7.6–7.8%).

The overall prevalence of migraine in female children and adolescents was 9.7% (95% CI 9.4–9.9%) and in males 6.0% (95% CI 5.8–6.2%; difference=3.7%, 95% CI 3.4–3.9%, $p<0.001$, as seen in the systematic review of population-based studies) (Abu-Arafeh et al 2010). The odds ratio for prevalence of migraine in females, as shown in Figure 6.4, is 1.67 (95% CI 1.60 to 1.75). The male to female ratio of children with migraine is almost equal for those under the age of 12 years, but there is a definite shift towards a higher prevalence of migraine in females after the age of 12 by a ratio of 1.5:1. This has been shown in individual population-based studies and to a certain extent by systematic reviews of published studies. Puberty, female sex hormones, genetics and other factors may be responsible for the increased prevalence of migraine in females.

The introduction of the second edition of the International Classification of Headache Disorders (Headache Classification Subcommittee of the International Headache Society 2004) allowed the criteria for the diagnosis of migraine in children to accept headache attacks

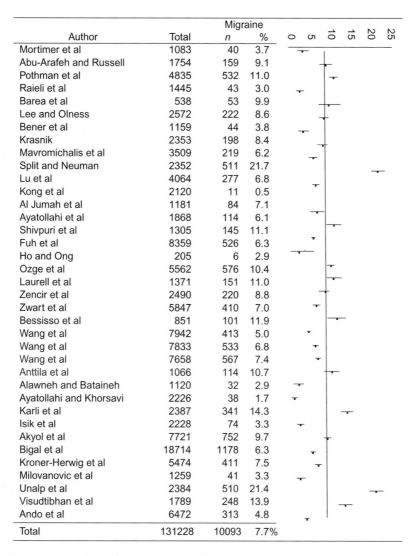

Author	Total	Migraine		0 5 10 15 20 25
		n	%	
Mortimer et al	1083	40	3.7	
Abu-Arafeh and Russell	1754	159	9.1	
Pothman et al	4835	532	11.0	
Raieli et al	1445	43	3.0	
Barea et al	538	53	9.9	
Lee and Olness	2572	222	8.6	
Bener et al	1159	44	3.8	
Krasnik	2353	198	8.4	
Mavromichalis et al	3509	219	6.2	
Split and Neuman	2352	511	21.7	
Lu et al	4064	277	6.8	
Kong et al	2120	11	0.5	
Al Jumah et al	1181	84	7.1	
Ayatollahi et al	1868	114	6.1	
Shivpuri et al	1305	145	11.1	
Fuh et al	8359	526	6.3	
Ho and Ong	205	6	2.9	
Ozge et al	5562	576	10.4	
Laurell et al	1371	151	11.0	
Zencir et al	2490	220	8.8	
Zwart et al	5847	410	7.0	
Bessisso et al	851	101	11.9	
Wang et al	7942	413	5.0	
Wang et al	7833	533	6.8	
Wang et al	7658	567	7.4	
Anttila et al	1066	114	10.7	
Alawneh and Bataineh	1120	32	2.9	
Ayatollahi and Khorsavi	2226	38	1.7	
Karli et al	2387	341	14.3	
Isik et al	2228	74	3.3	
Akyol et al	7721	752	9.7	
Bigal et al	18714	1178	6.3	
Kroner-Herwig et al	5474	411	7.5	
Milovanovic et al	1259	41	3.3	
Unalp et al	2384	510	21.4	
Visudtibhan et al	1789	248	13.9	
Ando et al	6472	313	4.8	
Total	131228	10093	7.7%	

Fig. 6.3 Migraine prevalence (Abu-Arafeh et al 2010).

of 1-hour duration if supported by appropriate prospective diaries, rather than the compulsory 2 hours. This minor change did not result in any increase of the prevalence of migraine on analysis of data in the systematic review. There was almost an identical prevalence of migraine whether the criteria of 1988 (7.5%; 95% CI 7.3–7.7%) or those of 2004 (7.8%; 95% CI 7.6–8.0%) were used.

Minor variations in prevalence are noted in different parts of the world. However, it is not possible to attribute these variations in prevalence to racial or genetic reasons, as many studies did not specify the ethnic origin of the people surveyed and did not analyse data based on

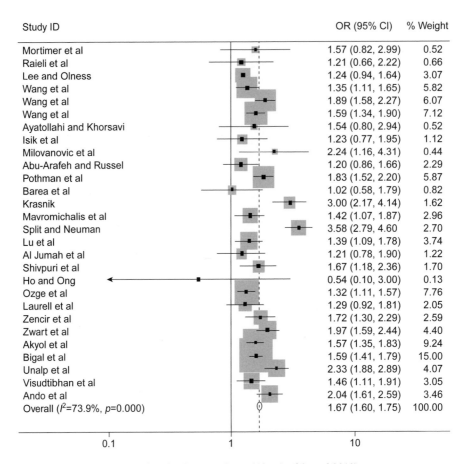

Study ID		OR (95% CI)	% Weight
Mortimer et al		1.57 (0.82, 2.99)	0.52
Raieli et al		1.21 (0.66, 2.22)	0.66
Lee and Olness		1.24 (0.94, 1.64)	3.07
Wang et al		1.35 (1.11, 1.65)	5.82
Wang et al		1.89 (1.58, 2.27)	6.07
Wang et al		1.59 (1.34, 1.90)	7.12
Ayatollahi and Khorsavi		1.54 (0.80, 2.94)	0.52
Isik et al		1.23 (0.77, 1.95)	1.12
Milovanovic et al		2.24 (1.16, 4.31)	0.44
Abu-Arafeh and Russel		1.20 (0.86, 1.66)	2.29
Pothman et al		1.83 (1.52, 2.20)	5.87
Barea et al		1.02 (0.58, 1.79)	0.82
Krasnik		3.00 (2.17, 4.14)	1.62
Mavromichalis et al		1.42 (1.07, 1.87)	2.96
Split and Neuman		3.58 (2.79, 4.60)	2.70
Lu et al		1.39 (1.09, 1.78)	3.74
Al Jumah et al		1.21 (0.78, 1.90)	1.22
Shivpuri et al		1.67 (1.18, 2.36)	1.70
Ho and Ong		0.54 (0.10, 3.00)	0.13
Ozge et al		1.32 (1.11, 1.57)	7.76
Laurell et al		1.29 (0.92, 1.81)	2.05
Zencir et al		1.72 (1.30, 2.29)	2.59
Zwart et al		1.97 (1.59, 2.44)	4.40
Akyol et al		1.57 (1.35, 1.83)	9.24
Bigal et al		1.59 (1.41, 1.79)	15.00
Unalp et al		2.33 (1.88, 2.89)	4.07
Visudtibhan et al		1.46 (1.11, 1.91)	3.05
Ando et al		2.04 (1.61, 2.59)	3.46
Overall (I^2=73.9%, p=0.000)		1.67 (1.60, 1.75)	100.00

0.1   1   10

Fig. 6.4 Female predominance in migraine prevalence (Abu-Arafeh et al 2010).

race. It would be reasonable to attribute the difference, as seen in Table 6.1, to geographical locations rather than race.

Migraine without aura is the most common type of migraine. In most population studies, between 75% and 80% of children with migraine have migraine without aura and between 15% and 20% have migraine with aura. It is not uncommon for some children to have mixed types of migraine and, in particular, episodes of migraine without aura as well as attacks of migraine with aura.

Basilar artery-type migraine is relatively rare (2.3–3.7% of all cases of migraine). Reliable data on population prevalence of basilar artery-type migraine are hard to find and often difficult to interpret owing to the use of less strict diagnostic criteria, which may include cases of migraine with aura (Watson and Steele 1974, Jay and Tomasi 1981). Ophthalmoplegic migraine was found in 0.2% of patients with migraine in a clinic series (Friedman et al 1962).

Chronic migraine in children is rare and the estimated prevalence from population-based studies in Italy is 1% (Arruda et al 2010).

TABLE 6.1
Geographical prevalence rates of migraine

Geographical region	Number of studies	Total population	Number with migraine	Prevalence	95% confidence interval
Europe	11	46 580	3888	8.35%	8.10–8.60
Middle East	15	38 829	3374	8.69%	8.41–8.97
Far East	6	39 486	2646	6.70%	6.45–6.95
USA	2	21 286	1400	6.58%	6.24–6.91

Adapted from Abu-Arafeh et al (2010).

PREVALENCE OF CHILDHOOD SYNDROMES RELATED TO MIGRAINE
Limited studies are available on the prevalence of these syndromes. The prevalence of abdominal migraine in Aberdeen (Scotland) schoolchildren of 5 to 15 years of age was 4.1% (Abu-Arafeh and Russell 1995a). In a study of 1083 children between 3 and 11 years of age, in a general practice in the UK, 26 children had abdominal migraine, a prevalence of 2.4%. One-third of the children had concomitant migraine headache (Mortimer et al 1993). In a recent study from Sri Lanka, the prevalence of abdominal migraine was estimated at 1%, but a further 4.4% of children suffered functional abdominal pain (Devanarayana et al 2011).

The prevalence of cyclical vomiting syndrome was 1.9% in Aberdeen schoolchildren and also in a population-based study in Turkey (Abu-Arafeh and Russell 1995b, Ertekin et al 2006). The prevalence of benign paroxysmal vertigo was 2.5% with a peak incidence at age 12 (Abu-Arafeh and Russell 1995c). Recurrent limb pain affected 2.6% of schoolchildren and with similar triggers as in vertigo and migraine (Abu-Arafeh and Russell 1996).

Epidemiology of tension-type headache
Until 2004, TTH was referred to as episodic TTH (ETTH) if it occurred on fewer than 15 days per month, or chronic TTH (CTTH) if it occurred on at least 15 days per month, and hence most published studied used this classification. Recent classification refers to TTH as infrequent (1 day per month), frequent (1–15 days per month) or chronic (more than 15 days per month).

Studies on the prevalence of ETTH are limited in number, probably because of the common perception that ETTH has a lower or minimal impact on patients as compared with migraine and CTTH. Also ETTH may co-exist or can easily be confused with mild attacks of migraine without aura.

Several studies on the epidemiology of TTH did not specify the frequency of headache attacks and were unable to differentiate between ETTH and CTTH. The prevalence of unspecified TTH varied between 12.1% in a study of 1868 children in Iran (Ayatollahi et al 2002), 12.5% for males and 23.2% for females in a study of 5847 children in Turkey (Zwart et al 2004) and 25.6% in a small study of 538 children in Brazil (Barea et al 1996).

The prevalence of ETTH, when specified, varied between 4.7% and 24.6%, as shown in Table 6.2.

TABLE 6.2
Prevalence of episodic tension-type headache (ETTH)

Author reference	Number	Prevalence of ETTH (%)	Infrequent ETTH (%)[a]	Frequent ETTH (%)[a]
Anttila et al (2002)	1135	12.2		
Özge et al (2003)	5562	23.2		
Laurell et al (2004)	1371	23.0		
Unlap et al (2007)	2384	4.7	1.9	2.8
Arruda et al (2012)	1994	24.6	23	1.6

[a]Headache Classification Subcommittee of the International Headache Society (2004) The International Classification of Headache Disorders. 2nd edn. *Cephalalgia* 24 (Suppl. 1): 1–52.

CTTH is relatively uncommon in children, and several studies have shown consistent findings of low prevalence between 0.1% and 1.6% (Abu-Arafeh and Russell 1994, Anttila et al 2002, Özge et al 2003, Laurell et al 2004, Unlap et al 2007, Arruda et al 2010). CTTH can also occur in the context of chronic daily headache, which may include other types of headache. Children with CTTH are more likely to seek medical advice than children with ETTH. Around 6% of children attending a general practice clinic because of headache, and around 20% of those attending specialist clinics, suffer from CTTH (van der Wouden et al 1999, Abu-Arafeh and MacLeod 2005).

Epidemiology of other types of headaches
Cluster headache, paroxysmal hemicrania, hemicrania continua, short-lasting unilateral neuralgiform headache attacks with conjunctival injection and tearing (SUNCT), other trigeminal autonomic cephalalgias and chronic post-traumatic headaches are rare, and no prevalence studies are available in children. These conditions will be discussed in appropriate chapters.

Headache comorbidities
Owing to its high prevalence in all communities, there have been many reports of an association between migraine and many diseases and health issues. A large study of 46 418 twins, residing in Denmark and born between 1931 and 1982, provided important data on the prevalence of many conditions in patients with migraine and those without migraine during adult life. Data have shown slight, but statistically significant, increases in the prevalence of low back pain (69.5% in people with migraine vs 56.3% in people without migraine), any atopic disease (24.8% vs 20.4%), asthma (10.6% vs 8.0%) and epilepsy (2.3% vs 1.5%) (Le et al 2011). The nature of these associations and comorbidities cannot be explained purely on the grounds of coincidence, but are probably due to a shared inflammatory pathway.

Non-specific Recurrent Pain Syndrome
Recurrent pains and aches are common in children and adolescents. Recurrent headache, as shown above, is very common and its association with recurrent abdominal pain and limb pain

has been well established over a long time. However, the causes and the pathophysiology of multiple pains in children are not well understood and may have psychological, familial or genetic predisposition.

The co-occurrence of recurrent pains at different body locations in children has been well demonstrated in a longitudinal population-based study of over 2000 children (aged 9–14y), who were surveyed on four occasions over a 4-year period (Van Gessel et al 2011). The prevalence of multiple pains (at least two recurrent pain locations, e.g. headache, abdominal pain or back pain) increased steadily from 45% at baseline to 54% after 4 years. Females were noted to be more likely to report recurrent pain than males by a factor of 1.5 to 3.0. Sex differences in prevalence of headache and abdominal pain were also noted in other studies.

In a study of 285 adolescents with frequent headache (at least once a week), 32% also reported back pain, 32% muscle pain, 25% abdominal pain, 23% joint pain, 7% earache and 4% toothache. One-third of the adolescents had one other frequent pain, and one-third had at least two other frequent pains (Fichtel and Larsson 2002).

Children with migraine seem to have a particularly strong tendency to have other associated recurrent pains such as abdominal pain, musculoskeletal limb pain and back pain (Abu-Arafeh and Russell 1996, Sillanpää and Aro 2000, Anttila et al 2001).

ATOPIC DISORDERS
Atopic disorders are common in children. About one in four children may have asthma, eczema and/or hay fever. Therefore, it is not unusual for children with migraine, which is also common, to have an atopic disorder. However, some studies have shown unexpectedly higher prevalence of atopic disorders in children with migraine and suggested a possible pathophysiological comorbidity.

The relationship between atopic diseases and migraine was recently studied in migraine patients who reported at least one atopic condition. Pulmonary function tests showed decreased pulmonary capacity, high eosinophil count and raised immunoglobulin E (IgE) levels during headache-free periods (Özge et al 2006). However, IgE tests and skin prick tests against common foods on 50 patients with migraine did not show any associations (Pradalier et al 1983).

IgG antibodies may provide another possible mechanism for food allergy in patients with migraine. From two double-blind, placebo-controlled trials of 30 patients in Turkey and 56 patients in Mexico, IgG antibodies were statistically more frequent in the migraine patients, who then improved on an elimination diet (Arroyave Hernandez et al 2007, Alpay et al 2010).

Studies of children have also shown atopic diseases to be more common in those with migraine than in comparison individuals. In a population-based study, bronchial asthma occurred more than expected in patients with migraine (14% of males and 4% of females) at any time between the ages of 7 and 22 years (Sillanpää and Aro 2000). Children born to mothers with migraine had a two-fold risk of bronchial asthma in another study (Chen and Leviton 1990).

Conclusions
Headache is a very common complaint across the world, affecting about 60% of children and adolescents. ETTH (prevalence of 20–25%) is the most common cause of primary headache,

followed by migraine (prevalence of 8%). The prevalence of migraine increases with children's age and reaches adult prevalence by late adolescence. Migraine without aura is three to four times more common than migraine with aura. Females and males under the age of 12 years are equally affected by migraine, but more females than males are affected by migraine after the age of 12 years.

REFERENCES

Abu-Arafeh I, MacLeod S (2005) Serious neurological disorders in children with chronic headache. *Arch Dis Child* 90: 937–40. http://dx.doi.org/10.1136/adc.2004.067256

Abu-Arafeh I, Russell G (1994) Prevalence of headache and migraine in schoolchildren. *BMJ* 309: 765–9. http://dx.doi.org/10.1136/bmj.309.6957.765

Abu-Arafeh I, Russell G (1995a) Prevalence and clinical features of abdominal migraine compared with those of migraine headache. *Arch Dis Child* 72: 413–17. http://dx.doi.org/10.1136/adc.72.5.413

Abu-Arafeh I, Russell G (1995b) Cyclical vomiting in children: a population-based study. *J Pediatr Gastroenterol Nutr* 21: 454–8. http://dx.doi.org/10.1097/00005176-199511000-00014

Abu-Arafeh I, Russell G (1995c) Paroxysmal vertigo as migraine equivalent in children. *Cephalalgia* 15: 22–5. http://dx.doi.org/10.1046/j.1468-2982.1995.1501022.x

Abu-Arafeh I, Russell G (1996) Recurrent limb pain in schoolchildren. *Arch Dis Child* 74: 336–9. http://dx.doi.org/10.1136/adc.74.4.336

Abu-Arafeh I, Razak S, Sivaraman B, Graham C (2010) Prevalence of headache and migraine in children and adolescents: A systematic review of population-based studies. *Dev Med Child Neurol* 52: 1088–97. http://dx.doi.org/10.1111/j.1469-8749.2010.03793.x

Alpay K, Ertas M, Orhan EK, Ustay DK, Lieners C, Baykan B (2010) Diet restriction in migraine, based on IgG against foods: a clinical double-blind, randomized, crossover trial. *Cephalalgia* 30: 829–37. http://dx.doi.org/10.1177/0333102410361404

Andrasik F, Holroyd KA, Abell T (1980) Prevalence of headache within a college student population: a preliminary analysis. *Headache* 19: 384–7. http://dx.doi.org/10.1111/j.1526-4610.1979.hed1907384.x

Aromaa M, Sillanpää M, Aro H (2000) A population-based follow-up study of headache from age 7 to 22 years. *J Headache Pain* 1: 11–15. http://dx.doi.org/10.1007/s101940050004

Anttila P, Metsähonkala L, Mikkelsson M, Helenius H, Sillanpää M (2001) Comorbidity of other pains in schoolchildren with migraine or nonmigrainous headache. *J Pediatr* 138: 176–80. http://dx.doi.org/10.1067/mpd.2001.112159

Anttila P, Metsahonkala L, Aromaa M et al (2002) Determinants of tension-type headache in children. *Cephalalgia* 22: 401–8. http://dx.doi.org/10.1046/j.1468-2982.2002.00381.x

Anttila P, Metsahonkala L, Sillanpaa M (2006) Long-term trends in the incidence of headache in Finnish schoolchildren. *Pediatrics* 117: e1197–201. http://dx.doi.org/10.1542/peds.2005-2274

Arroyave Hernandez CM, Echevarria Pinto M, Hernandez Montiel HL (2007) Food allergy mediated by IgG antibodies associated with migraine in adults. *Rev Alerg Mex* 54: 162–8.

Arruda MA, Guidetti V, Galli F, Albuquerque RCAP, Bigal ME (2010) Primary headaches in childhood – a population-based study. *Cephalalgia* 30: 1056–64. http://dx.doi.org/10.1177/0333102409361214

Ayatollahi SM, Moradi F, Ayatollahi SA (2002) Prevalences of migraine and tension-type headache in adolescent girls of Shiraz (Southern Iran). *Headache* 42: 287–90. http://dx.doi.org/10.1046/j.1526-4610.2002.02082.x

Barea LM, Tannhauser M, Rotta NT (1996) An epidmeiologic study of headache among children and adolescents of southern Brazil. *Cephalalgia* 16: 545–9. http://dx.doi.org/10.1046/j.1468-2982.1996.1608545.x

Barlow CF (1984) Symptomatic headache evalutation and investigation. In: Barlow CF, editor. *Headaches and Migraine in Childhood.* Oxford: Blackwell Scientific Publications, pp. 204–19.

Bener A, Uduman SA, Quassimi EM et al (2000) Genetic and environmental factors associated with migrtaine in schoolchildren. *Headache* 40: 152–7. http://dx.doi.org/10.1046/j.1526-4610.2000.00021.x

Beyer JE, Wells N (1989) The assessment of pain in children. *Pediatr Clin N Am* 36: 837–54.

Bhatt-Mehta V (1996) Current guidelines for the treatment of acute pain in children. *Drugs* 51: 760–76. http://dx.doi.org/10.2165/00003495-199651050-00005

Bille B (1962) Migraine in school children. A study of the incidence and short-term prognosis, and a clinical, psychological and encephalographic comparison between children with migraine and matched controls. *Acta Paediatri* 51(Suppl): 1–151.

Bille B (1995) A 40-year follow-up of school children with migraine. *Cephalalgia* 17: 488–91. http://dx.doi.org/10.1046/j.1468-2982.1997.1704488.x

Chen TC, Leviton A (1990) Asthma and eczema in children born to mothers with migraine. *Arch Neurol* 47: 1227–30. http://dx.doi.org/10.1001/archneur.1990.00530110087022

Classification Committee of the International Headache Society (1988) Classification and diagnostic criteria for headache disorders, cranial neuralgias and facial pain. *Cephalalgia* 8(Suppl7):1–96.

Devanarayana NM, Mettananda S, Liyanarachchi C et al (2011) Abdominal pain predominant functional gastrointestinal diseases in children and adolescents: prevalence, symptomatology and association with emotional stress. *J Pediatr Gastroenterol Nutr* 53: 659–65.

Elser JM, Woody RC (1990) Migraine headache in the infant and young child. *Headache* 30: 366–8. http://dx.doi.org/10.1111/j.1526-4610.1990.hed3006366.x

Ertekin V, Selimoglu MA, Altınkaynak S (2006) Prevalence of cyclic vomiting syndrome in a sample of turkish school children in an urban area. *J Clin Gastroenterol* 40: 896–8. http://dx.doi.org/10.1097/01.mcg.0000212627.83746.0b

Fichtel Å, Larsson B (2002) Psychosocial impact of headache and comorbidity with other pains among Swedish school adolescents. *Headache* 42: 766–75. http://dx.doi.org/10.1046/j.1526-4610.2002.02178.x

Friedman AP, Harter DH, Merritt HH (1962) Ophthalmoplegic migraine. *Arch Neurol* 7: 320–7. http://dx.doi.org/10.1001/archneur.1962.04210040072007

Golden GS, French JH (1975) Basilar artery migraine in young children. *Pediatrics* 56: 722–6.

Headache Classification Subcommittee of the International Headache Society (2004) The International Classification of Headache Disorders, 2nd edn. *Cephalalgia* 24(Suppl 1): 1–52.

Holguin J, Fenichel G (1967) Migraine. *J Pediatr* 70: 290–7. http://dx.doi.org/10.1016/S0022-3476(67)80429-3

Jay GW, Tomasi LG (1981) Pediatric headaches: a one year retrospective analysis. *Headache* 21: 5–9. http://dx.doi.org/10.1111/j.1526-4610.1981.hed2101005.x

Laurell K, Larsson B, Eeg-Olofsson O (2004) Prevalence of headache in Swedish schoolchildren, with a focus on tension-type headache. *Cephalalgia* 24: 380–8. http://dx.doi.org/10.1111/j.1468-2982.2004.00681.x

Le H, Tfelt-Hansen P, Russell MB, Skytthe A, Kyvik KO, Olesen J (2011) Co-morbidity of migraine with somatic disease in a large population-based study. *Cephalalgia* 31: 43. http://dx.doi.org/10.1177/0333102410373159

Lu SR, Fuh JL, Wang SJ (2000) Migraine prevalence in adolescents aged 13–15: a student population-based study in Taiwan. *Cephalalgia* 20: 479–85. http://dx.doi.org/10.1046/j.1468-2982.2000.00076.x

Mortimer MJ, Kay J, Jaron A (1993) Clinical epidemiology of childhood abdominal migraine in an urban general practice. *Dev Med Child Neurol* 35: 243–8. http://dx.doi.org/10.1111/j.1469-8749.1993.tb11629.x

Özge A, Bugdayci R, Sasmaz T et al (2003) The sensitivity and specificity of the case definition criteria in diagnosis of headache: A school-based epidemiological study of 5562 children in Mersin. *Cephalalgia* 23: 138–45. http://dx.doi.org/10.1046/j.1468-2982.2003.00474.x

Özge A, Özge C, Öztürk C et al (2006) The relationship between migraine and atopic disorders – the contribution of pulmonary function tests and immunological screening. *Cephalalgia* 26: 172–9. http://dx.doi.org/10.1111/j.1468-2982.2005.01021.x

Pothmann R, Frankenberg SV, Mueller B, Sartory G, Hellmeier W (1994) Epidemiology of headache in children and adolescents: evidence of high prevalence of migraine among girls under 10. *Int J Behav Med* 1: 76–89. http://dx.doi.org/10.1207/s15327558ijbm0101_5

Pradalier A, Weinman S, Launay JM, Baron JF, Dry J (1983) Total IgE, specific IgE and prick-tests against foods in common migraine – a prospective study. *Cephalalgia* 3: 231. http://dx.doi.org/10.1046/j.1468-2982.1983.0304231.x

Prensky AL, Sommer D (1979) Diagnosis and treatment of migraine in children. *Neurology* 29: 506–10. http://dx.doi.org/10.1212/WNL.29.4.506

Raieli V, Raimondo D, Cammalleri R, Camarda R (1995) Migraine headache in adolescents: a student population-based study in Monreale. *Cephalalgia* 15: 5–12. http://dx.doi.org/10.1046/j.1468-2982.1995.1501005.x

Rozen TD, Swanson JW, Stang PE, McDonnell SK, Rocca WA (1999) Increasing incidence of medically recognised migraine headache in a United States population. *Neurology* 53: 1468–73. http://dx.doi.org/10.1212/WNL.53.7.1468

Russell JW (1903) Case of migraine with ophthalmoplegia. *BMJ* 1: 1020. http://dx.doi.org/10.1136/bmj.1.2209.1020

Sillanpää M (1976) Prevalence of migraine and other headache in Finnish children starting school. *Headache* 15: 288–90. http://dx.doi.org/10.1111/j.1526-4610.1976.hed1504288.x

Sillanpää M (1983a) Prevalence of headache in prepuberty. *Headache* 23: 10–14. http://dx.doi.org/10.1111/j.1526-4610.1983.hed2301010.x

Sillanpää M (1983b) Changes in the prevalence of migraine and other headaches during the first seven school years. *Headache* 23: 15–19. http://dx.doi.org/10.1111/j.1526-4610.1983.hed2301015.x

Sillanpää M, Anttila P (1996) Increasing prevalence of headache in 7-year-old schoolchildren. *Headache* 36: 466–70. http://dx.doi.org/10.1046/j.1526-4610.1996.3608466.x

Sillanpää M, Aro H (2000) Headache in teenagers: comorbidity and prognosis. *Funct Neurol* 15(Suppl 3): 116–21.

Sillanpää M, Piekkala P, Kero P (1991) Prevalence of headache at preschool age in an unselected child population. *Cephalalgia* 11: 239–42. http://dx.doi.org/10.1046/j.1468-2982.1991.1105239.x

Unlap A, Dirik E, Kurul S (2007) Prevalence and clinical findings of migraine and tension-type headache in adolescents. *Pediatr Int* 49: 943–9. http://dx.doi.org/10.1111/j.1442-200X.2007.02484.x

van der Wouden JC, van der Pas P, Bruijnzeels MA, Brienen JA, van Suijlekom-Smit LW (1999) Headache in children in Dutch general practice. *Cephalalgia* 19: 147–50. http://dx.doi.org/10.1046/j.1468-2982.1999.1903147.x

Vahlquist B, Hackzell G (1949) Migraine of early onset. A study of thirty-one cases in which the disease first appeared between one and four years of age. *Acta Paediatr* 38: 622–36. http://dx.doi.org/10.1111/j.1651-2227.1949.tb17914.x

Woody RC, Blaw ME (1986) Ophthalmoplegic migraine in infancy. *Clin Pediatr (Phila)* 25: 82–4. http://dx.doi.org/10.1177/000992288602500204

Van Gessel H, Gaßmann J, Kröner-Herwig B (2011) Children in pain: recurrent back pain. Abdominal pain, and headache in children and adolescents in a four-year-period. *J Pediatr* 158: 977–83. http://dx.doi.org/10.1016/j.jpeds.2010.11.051

Watson P, Steele JC (1974) Paroxysmal dysequilibrium in the migraine syndrome of childhood. *Arch Otolaryngol* 99: 177–9. http://dx.doi.org/10.1001/archotol.1974.00780030185005

Zwart JA, Dyb G, Holmen TL, Stovner LJ, Sand T (2004) The prevalence of migraine and tension-type headaches among adolescents in Norway; the Nord-Trondelag health study (head-HUNT-youth), a large population-based epidemiological study. *Cephalalgia* 24: 373–9. http://dx.doi.org/10.1111/j.1468-2982.2004.00680.x

7
IMPACT OF HEADACHE ON QUALITY OF LIFE

Andrew D Hershey and Scott W Powers

Any disease can impact on a patient and his or her family's life through the direct effects of the disease on a patient's ability to function (disease-specific disability) and through the overall effect on the patient and family (both disease-specific and disease-non-specific quality of life).

Treatment of disease is often focused on the biological and clinical characteristics, but often the disability due to the disease and the changes in the quality of life can have an equal or greater impact on the patient. Appropriately addressing these issues is integral to the evaluation and management of any disease.

For migraine and headache, several tools have been developed to address these concerns for adults, but there is a limited number of tools for children and adolescents. These instruments include the Pediatric Migraine Disability Assessment (PedMIDAS) (Hershey et al 2001, 2004), Pediatric Quality of Life 4 (PedsQL 4.0) (Varni et al 2001, Powers et al 2004), Quality of Life Headache in Youth (Langeveld et al 1996), Functional Disability Inventory (Walker and Greene 1991) and MSQ (Migraine Specific Quality of life) (Martin et al 2000). These five instruments are all specific for children (for review see Kernick and Campbell 2009); however, additional instruments validated in adults have also been used in children including MIDAS (Stewart et al 1999, 2000) and HIT-6 (Kosinski et al 2003). From a review of the studies to date, it is clear that the lives of children with headaches and their families are impacted on to a degree that is clinically significant.

Disease characteristics

The clinical characteristics of headache, and especially migraine, have a direct impact on the quality of life of the patient. Pain by itself will limit the child's involvement in activities. The pain of migraine is directly aggravated by physical activity, and thus a child will naturally limit his or her physical activity during an attack. The associated symptoms of migraine, both those included in the International Classification of Headache Disorders, 2nd edition (Headache Classification Subcommittee of the International Headache Society 2004) and additional associated features noted to occur in children with migraine (Hershey et al 2005), may also affect a child's ability to participate in life activities. Notably, nausea and vomiting will inevitably lead to the child being removed from the activity, whether it is school, social or home related. In addition, photophobia and phonophobia may lead to a child withdrawing from his or her normal activities. As most of these associated symptoms are event specific (i.e. occur during an acute migraine), effective acute treatment (Chapter 11) and preventative treatment (Chapter 12) should assist with lessening this impact of headaches.

Disability
When the features of headache result in the child not participating in activities or participating at less than their optimal level, the result is disease-specific disability. Oftentimes this is reported as school absences. Absenteeism from school has direct educational and social implications that have a direct impact on the child's success in life. This, however, captures only a portion of the child's life.

One tool that has been developed to capture a broader reflection of the child's daily activities is PedMIDAS (Hershey et al 2001, 2004). PedMIDAS is based on MIDAS (MIgraine Disability Assessment) (Stewart et al 1999, 2000, 2001). MIDAS addresses the disability due to migraine in adults by assessing the impact on work, home and social activities.

For children and adolescents, this required modification to better incorporate a balanced assessment of a child's life. PedMIDAS includes three questions related to school (full days missed, partial days missed and days in school functioning at 50% of the optimal level), one question related to home function (inability to do homework or chores) and two questions related to social function – peer, family and sports (complete absence and partial functioning at 50% of abilities). PedMIDAS has been validated for children and adolescents with migraine and has been widely used for both clinical and research assessments (Hershey et al 2001). A grading system has been established that divides the grades into Grade I (little to none), Grade II (mild), Grade III (moderate) and Grade IV (severe) (Hershey et al 2004). It is available for download at http://www.cincinnatichildrens.org/service/h/headache-center/pedmidas/.

Clinically, PedMIDAS can be used as a useful tool for assisting in determining the need for preventative medication. We have found that a PedMIDAS score above 20 (i.e. Grade II and above), even in children with relatively few headaches per month, is a flag for the potential need of a preventative agent. Additionally, a PedMIDAS score above 140 is indicative of additional comorbidity and a lack of coping ability and would require further investigation and more comprehensive management by behavioural medicine specialists.

PedMIDAS is also very sensitive to treatment effects, can be an earlier indicator of response and can be used clinically to determine the effectiveness of the suggested medication as well as assist with adherence promotion and continuation in the treatment plan.

Quality of life
Both the pain of the individual migraine attacks and the fear of an attack occurrence can have an impact on quality of life. The direct attack impact is often captured by the disability assessment. The fear of having a headache and the impact of migraine on the child's day-to-day life – even when headache free – is best captured in a disease non-specific assessment of quality of life. PedsQL 4.0 (Varni et al 2001) is one tool that has been widely used for a large variety of paediatric illnesses. It is developmentally appropriate with four different age ranges and both parental/caregiver and child report.

PedsQL 4.0 has been used to assess the impact of migraine on the quality of life of children who seek treatment. This has identified an overall negative impact on quality of life of children with headache that is similar to that of children and adolescents with arthritis and cancer, with most profound impairments in school and emotional functioning (Powers et al 2003). While the majority of children with headache do not experience clinically diagnosable changes in psychosocial functioning, a subset of these children has more broad psychosocial/ psychiatric effects, increasing the risk for academic difficulties and emotional problems such as depression and anxiety (Powers et al 2006).

A separate, disease non-specific tool that has also been used to assess the quality of life in children with migraine is the Child Health Questionnaire (CHQ-PF50) (Raat et al 2002, 2005, 2007). This is a 50-item questionnaire covering 11 domains. From a study of 70 consecutive children with primary headache seen in a tertiary headache centre and 353 control children, 83 children with attention-deficit–hyperactivity disorder (ADHD) and 148 children with asthma, it was found that children with primary headaches were negatively affected in 10 of the 11 domains when compared with healthy individuals. In addition, although both children with asthma and children with ADHD were negatively affected when compared with healthy individuals, the impact on quality of life of primary headache was significantly worse than the impacts of these two diseases. These observations confirmed those found using PedsQL 4.0: that children with primary headaches are significantly affected similarly and oftentimes more affected when compared with other chronic illnesses of childhood.

In addition, a notable subset of children with headache continues to experience significant headaches into adulthood (Brna et al 2005, Andrasik and Schwartz 2006). When a child or adolescent presents with headache, it is imperative to consider how this pain is affecting the individual and his or her family and to assume, based upon current data, that the impact is clinically significant.

Summary

In clinical practice, management of children and adolescents with headache should incorporate the addition of headache disability and quality of life assessments to the traditional outcomes of headache intensity, duration and frequency. PedMIDAS and PedsQL 4.0 are complementary, showing a correlation of +0.34, with both adding unique information to the determination of the outcome of intervention. Assessments should occur at initial evaluation and regularly throughout treatment. Results are communicated with the children and their families, as well as described in correspondence with other healthcare providers such as the child's paediatrician.

The experience of headache by children and adolescents impacts on their lives. This impact can be measured and the data that are obtained should be used in the clinical care of these patients. It is important to assess disability and quality of life as components of an evidence-based approach to the clinical care of these children and their families.

REFERENCES

Andrasik F, Schwartz MS (2006) Behavioral assessment and treatment of pediatric headache. *Behav Modif* 30: 93–113. http://dx.doi.org/10.1177/0145445505282164

Brna P, Dooley J, Gordon K, Dewan T (2005) The prognosis of childhood headache: a 20-year follow-up. *Arch Pediatr Adolesc Med* 159: 1157–60. http://dx.doi.org/10.1001/archpedi.159.12.1157

Headache Classification Subcommittee of the International Headache Society (2004) The International Classification of Headache Disorders. *Cephalagia* 24: 1–160.

Hershey AD, Powers SW, Vockell AL, Lecates S, Kabbouche MA, Maynard MK (2001) PedMIDAS: development of a questionnaire to assess disability of migraines in children. *Neurology* 57: 2034–9. http://dx.doi.org/10.1212/WNL.57.11.2034

Hershey AD, Powers SW, Vockell AL, Lecates SL, Segers A, Kabbouche MA (2004) Development of a patient-based grading scale for PedMIDAS. *Cephalalgia* 24: 844–9. http://dx.doi.org/10.1111/j.1468-2982.2004.00757.x

Hershey AD, Winner P, Kabbouche MA et al (2005) Use of the ICHD-II criteria in the diagnosis of pediatric migraine. *Headache* 45: 1288–97. http://dx.doi.org/10.1111/j.1526-4610.2005.00260.x

Kernick D, Campbell J (2009) Measuring the impact of headache in children: a critical review of the literature. *Cephalalgia* 29: 3–16. http://dx.doi.org/10.1111/j.1468-2982.2008.01693.x

Kosinski M, Bayliss MS, Bjorner JB et al (2003) A six-item short-form survey for measuring headache impact: the HIT-6. *Qual Life Res* 12: 963–74. http://dx.doi.org/10.1023/A:1026119331193

Langeveld JH, Koot HM, Loonen MC, Hazebroek-Kampschreur AA, Passchier J (1996) A quality of life instrument for adolescents with chronic headache. *Cephalalgia* 16: 183–96. http://dx.doi.org/10.1046/j.1468-2982.1996.1603183.x

Martin BC, Pathak DS, Sharfman MI et al (2000) Validity and reliability of the migraine-specific quality of life questionnaire (MSQ Version 2.1). *Headache* 40: 204–15. http://dx.doi.org/10.1046/j.1526-4610.2000.00030.x

Powers SW, Patton SR, Hommel KA, Hershey AD (2003) Quality of life in childhood migraines: clinical impact and comparison to other chronic illnesses. *Pediatrics* 112: e1–5. http://dx.doi.org/10.1542/peds.112.1.e1

Powers SW, Patton SR, Hommel KA, Hershey AD (2004) Quality of life in paediatric migraine: characterization of age-related effects using PedsQL 4.0. *Cephalalgia* 24: 120–7. http://dx.doi.org/10.1111/j.1468-2982.2004.00652.x

Powers SW, Gilman DK, Hershey AD (2006) Headache and psychological functioning in children and adolescents. *Headache* 46: 1404–15. http://dx.doi.org/10.1111/j.1526-4610.2006.00583.x

Raat H, Landgraf JM, Bonsel GJ, Gemke RJ, Essink-Bot ML (2002) Reliability and validity of the child health questionnaire-child form (CHQ-CF87) in a Dutch adolescent population. *Qual Life Res* 11: 575–81. http://dx.doi.org/10.1023/A:1016393311799

Raat H, Botterweck AM, Landgraf JM, Hoogeveen WC, Essinkbot ML (2005) Reliability and validity of the short form of the child health questionnaire for parents (CHQ-PF28) in large random school based and general population samples. *J Epidemiol Community Health* 59: 75–82. http://dx.doi.org/10.1136/jech.2003.012914

Raat H, Mangunkusumo RT, Landgraf JM, Kloek G, Brug J (2007) Feasibility, reliability, and validity of adolescent health status measurement by the Child Health Questionnaire Child Form (CHQ-CF): internet administration compared with the standard paper version. *Qual Life Res* 16: 675–85. http://dx.doi.org/10.1007/s11136-006-9157-1

Stewart WF, Lipton RB, Whyte J et al (1999) An international study to assess reliability of the migraine disability assessment (MIDAS) score. *Neurology* 53: 988–94. http://dx.doi.org/10.1212/WNL.53.5.988

Stewart WF, Lipton RB, Kolodner KB, Sawyer J, Lee C, Liberman JN (2000) Validity of the migraine disability assessment (MIDAS) score in comparison to a diary-based measure in a population sample of migraine sufferers. *Pain* 88: 41–52. http://dx.doi.org/10.1016/S0304-3959(00)00305-5

Stewart WF, Lipton RB, Dowson AJ, Sawyer J (2001) Development and testing of the migraine disability assessment (MIDAS) questionnaire to assess headache related disability. *Neurology* 56: S20–8. http://dx.doi.org/10.1212/WNL.56.suppl_1.S20

Varni JW, Seid M, Kurtin PS (2001) PedsQL 4.0: reliability and validity of the Pediatric Quality of Life Inventory version 4.0 generic core scales in healthy and patient populations. *Med Care* 39: 800–12. http://dx.doi.org/10.1097/00005650-200108000-00006

Walker LS, Greene JW (1991) The functional disability inventory: measuring a neglected dimension of child health status. *J Pediatr Psychol* 16: 39–58. http://dx.doi.org/10.1093/jpepsy/16.1.39

8
ASSESSMENT OF CHILDHOOD HEADACHE

Shashi S Seshia

Introduction

Despite advances in investigations, specifically neuroradiological investigations and others, a detailed history and examination is still the cornerstone of diagnosis and an essential step to cost-beneficial utilisation of tests. The time spent in this task has significant paybacks for the child, family, physician and healthcare costs.

Electronic medical records are becoming the norm in many countries. The use of standardised data sheets (or electronic forms) ensures a consistent, standardised and efficient approach. However, the fields of information on any health problem need to be constantly updated as new knowledge emerges.

In 1977, Engel urged physicians to (re)adopt a biopsychosocial approach to 'illness', incorporating biological, psychological, lifestyle and social factors, rather than following a rigid biological- or disease-focused methodology (Engel 1977). Nowhere is this advice more appropriate than in the child (and adult) with recurrent or chronic headache and other pain syndromes, and as such this approach will be the focus of this chapter.

Acute headache will not be discussed. The causes of acute headache vary among geographic regions. For example, bacterial meningitis, an important cause of acute headache, has become uncommon in countries where immunisation programmes have been introduced. Some causes of viral encephalitis are region and season specific. Readers are advised to consult the most appropriate reference on acute headache for their practice setting.

Developmental and other perspectives in assessment

Paediatric professionals adapt assessment (history and examination) to the developmental level of the child, an art best learnt at the bedside. Assessments also have to be gender and culture sensitive. The professional must always introduce herself or himself and explain what he or she will do in a reassuring manner. Questions often have to be open ended and non-leading. Informed consent for the examination has to be obtained not only from the guardian but also from the child, especially if he or she is judged to be a mature or competent minor; this is even more important if the assessment is going to be done by a surrogate of the physician (e.g. medical student, resident or nurse). Informed consent is also crucial in prescribing treatment. Further discussion of consent in children and adolescents is beyond the scope of this chapter. Our principal focus is the child, but management has to be family centred. Readers are directed to paediatric texts and ethical and legal guidelines in their country of practice for more details on the approaches to examining children, including situations in which a guardian may not be acting in the child's best interests.

Paediatricians and family physicians are in the front line of child care, especially in rural areas, where they may not have ready access to social workers, psychologists or paediatric subspecialists. Therefore, they have to have greater expertise in assessment than their counterparts in urban practices. Age is only a rough estimate of development (Andrasik et al 2005), and neurodevelopmental delay may have to be factored in. With this proviso, Andrasik et al (2005) suggest three age groupings (1–6y, 7–11y and 12–18y) over which there is increasing ability to describe headache characteristics, understand the concept of an illness and causation, and give consent and participate in treatment decisions (Andrasik et al 2005). Thus, in most jurisdictions, age is not the sole criterion for informed consent.

Even adolescents may have difficulty in describing headache characteristics, including duration and severity, especially in retrospect (Seshia et al 1994). Children (the term will be used to include adolescents) are dependent on their guardians, who influence history, management and adherence even through the adolescent years. The concordance between caregivers and adolescents on the presence of headache is low (Nakamura et al 2011), highlighting the need to get a history independently from the child whenever possible. In young children, symptoms have to be inferred from behaviour, and history taking modified appropriately. Observation plays a pivotal role in the assessment of young children, and paediatric neurologists become skilled in doing a complete examination without upsetting the child.

Stressors make an important contribution to primary headache disorders, including chronic daily headache (see Chapter 20). Maltreatment, including bullying and cyber-bullying, is an important contributor to chronic pain syndromes. Hence, it is ideal and sometimes essential to interview (with informed consent) mature minors, including adolescents, separately from guardians regarding social history, school, social interactions (peers, family, teachers, etc.) and stressors (Appendix 8.1); they should be reassured that the information they provide is confidential. In the author's experience in Canada, children are generally honest communicators and often volunteer vital social history and share stressors that their guardians have not. Additionally, what is a significant stressor to a child may not be perceived as one by the guardian. Local guidelines for detailed interview and management should be followed if there is a suggestion of maltreatment or concerns about the child's welfare. The history also has to be adapted to the geographic region of practice, as stressors, lifestyles, triggers, social factors, comorbid conditions and secondary causes of headache often differ from country to country (Ravishankar 2010a). What follows is not evidence based, but a personal approach, as most clinical approaches are, and one that is similar to that described and followed by others, including our mentors.

History and examination (the first assessment)
Whenever possible, it is ideal to advise families before the first visit to (1) keep a description of representative headache types and of symptoms that concern the child and parents (Tassorelli et al 2008), and (2) bring school attendance and performance reports. Thereby, the initial

assessment becomes time effective. The history should factor in the biopsychosocial nature of primary headache, help to identify comorbid conditions (especially psychiatric) and unveil red flags. The key points in the history and examination are listed in Appendix 8.1 and summarised in Table 8.1. The temporal pattern of the headache – acute, acute recurrent, chronic progressive, chronic non-progressive or mixed – as judged from the history, can be extremely useful in determining the cause (Rothner 1995, Lewis 2002).

Other features in the history that are helpful include the past medical history, characteristics of the headache, symptoms associated with the headache, the presence of red flags (see Chapter 9) and the family history. In the context of headache, red flags usually refer to features that suggest a secondary cause. However, suggestions of anxiety and mood disorders, significant stressors, substance abuse and evidence or suspicion of maltreatment are red flags too. A general paediatric history and examination is as important as a specific headache history and neurological examination.

Discussion after the first assessment
Children and guardians come to the assessment with the expectation of finding out the cause of the headache and reassurance that a serious illness is not responsible (Raieli et al 2010). Hence, the possible diagnosis or diagnostic possibilities must be discussed or uncertainty acknowledged. Any red flags would warrant prompt, appropriate action.

If a primary headache disorder is considered definite or probable, then the multifaceted nature of the disorder, including genetic and environmental contributors, is discussed. Principles of management, particularly non-pharmacological ones (especially dealing with triggers, lifestyle issues, etc.), are outlined. The importance of keeping a prospective headache diary (Richardson et al 1983), describing each headache type and the judicious use of analgesics, is emphasised.

It is ideal not to prescribe specific treatment (pharmacological, psychological or other) until reassessment and review of the headache chart after an agreed-upon period of follow-up.

Headaches, in many children, including those with chronic daily headache, remit with basic measures including informed discussion, perhaps through a placebo effect, which is now known to have a neurobiological basis. Associated medical conditions such as obesity must be addressed, and, if there is suspicion of a psychiatric disorder (such as anxiety or mood) or if there are significant psychosocial stressors, then, with the consent of the guardians and child, referral to a child and adolescent psychiatrist/psychologist is made.

If maltreatment or a potentially serious medical cause is suspected, or if symptoms are disabling, it may be necessary to admit the child to hospital to involve qualified professionals and investigate further in a timely manner.

The child and guardians must be involved in management decisions. A succinct handout that summarises pertinent information about the particular headache type, especially triggers and precipitating/contributory factors, helps to reinforce the discussion, and facilitate compliance.

Families are advised to contact their physician before the next scheduled appointment if they feel there is urgent need to do so.

Assessment of pain and disability

Primary headache has to be assessed multidimensionally, because the symptoms (not only pain but nausea, vomiting, photophobia, mood or anxiety disorders, etc.) can affect many spheres of daily life (Sieberg et al 2011). These include school, family interactions, extracurricular activities and relationships with friends.

Pain can be assessed on a visual analogue or faces scale in young children, and on a numerical rating scale (0–10) in older children, with good intrarater reliability (Sieberg et al 2012). It is impractical to suggest that a detailed record be kept of each headache episode: compliance is likely to be poor. Rather, the child and family should be instructed to document one detailed description representative of each headache type (including possible triggers), then code them as type A, B, C, etc., and record the intensity and additional features for each (e.g. A5/10+nausea+stop activity).

The Pediatric Migraine Disability Assessment (PedMidas) and the Pediatric Quality of Life Inventory have been field tested in migraine and can be used by professionals to assess the impact of migraine on a child's life (Hershey et al 2001, Powers et al 2004, Powers and Andrasik 2005). These may need to be modified for other primary headaches. The subject is discussed further in Chapter 7.

The second assessment

The reassessment can be done by either the referring professional (family physician, nurse practitioner) or the consultant (paediatrician, paediatric neurologist or headache specialist) by mutual agreement, ensuring that individuals do not fall 'between the cracks'. Tele-health or telephone follow-up discussions can be time and cost effective for those who live far from healthcare facilities; headache records can be faxed or emailed. It has been the author's practice to always phone the family to seek an update if they fail to keep an appointment. The diagnosis of the cause of headache is a clinical one, and very dependent on the history provided. A reassessment is essential and serves to establish the diagnosis with greater certainty, identify red flags that may have been missed at the first interview and determine if more specific treatment and reassessment are necessary. Adolescents with headache (as with any other disorder) should not fall between the cracks when they are transferred from paediatric to adult care; family physicians play a pivotal role in continuity of care.

Management of specific headache types is discussed in Chapters 11–13 and 26–28.

Challenges

Even in developed countries, many parents and children fail to provide an adequate history or keep diaries. The problem is worse in developing economies, where a substantial segment of the population is still illiterate (Ravishankar 2010a,b). There also may be barriers of language. Detailed history taking is impractical in busy clinics. However, wherever possible parents and children can be encouraged to fill out data sheets ahead of the clinic appointment (perhaps in the clinic itself; we did not find good compliance with postal forms).

Therefore, each clinician has to develop his or her own system of time-effective yet adequate assessment and a checklist of red flags, specific for the population in his or her

TABLE 8.1
Assessment of child with headache – summary

Initial

Introduce self, obtain informed consent from child (mature minor) and guardian, and explain the process and goals of the assessment

Interview mature minors, especially older children, separately from guardians (respect confidential information)

Child-friendly and culturally and gender-sensitive assessment

Adapt assessment to region and nature of practice

Biopsychosocial family-centred approach

Attention to red flags

Consistent yet time-effective evaluation (standardised data sheets help)

Post assessment

If there are red flags, explain and act accordingly

If confident about absence of serious disease, reassure and discuss plan of care and goals and seek input/ acceptance; it often helps to explain the genetic, environmental and multifaceted nature of primary headache

Explain the importance of keeping a headache diary and identifying each headache type

Discuss triggers (especially stressors) and lifestyles as major contributors to primary headache and the need to recognise and address them to minimise or eliminate headache

Children and families to be their own detectives to identify their triggers

Caution against medication overuse (including herbal!)

A handout of information is extremely useful to reinforce discussion

Reassessment is essential to confirm initial impression and determine further course of care

care. Even if parents are illiterate, many children have access to education and can often read information sheets, and act as interpreters between parents and healthcare professionals.

Conclusions

The pioneers of modern medicine, including paediatrics, paediatric neurology and childhood headache, relied on astute comprehensive clinical assessment to make management decisions. Investigations, especially neuroradiological ones, have now become increasingly accessible but have to be used cost-beneficially. Collective clinical experience with childhood headache suggests that the initial basic steps of comprehensive clinical assessment (Appendix 8.1) should never be bypassed.

Addendum

Readers may be interested in the approach discussed by Claar et al to 'the difficult paediatric headache patient'. Claar RL, McDonald-Nolan L, LeBel A (2012) The pediatrician's guide to managing the difficult pediatric headache patient. *Clin Pediatr (Phila)* 51: 175–80.

REFERENCES

Andrasik F, Powers SW, McGrath PJ. (2005) Methodological considerations in research with special populations: children and adolescents. *Headache* 45: 520–5. http://dx.doi.org/10.1111/j.1526-4610.2005.05104.x

Engel GL (1977) The need for a new medical model: a challenge for biomedicine. *Science* 196: 129–36. http://dx.doi.org/10.1126/science.847460

Hershey AD, Powers SW, Vockell AL, Lecates S, Kabbouche MA, Maynard MK (2001) PedMIDAS: development of a questionnaire to assess disability of migraines in children. *Neurology* 57: 2034–9. http://dx.doi.org/10.1212/WNL.57.11.2034

Lewis DW (2002) Headaches in children and adolescents. *Am Fam Physician* 65: 625–32.

Nakamura EF, Cui L, Lateef T, Nelson KB, Merikangas KR (2011) Parent-Child Agreement in the Reporting of Headaches in a National Sample of Adolescents. *J Child Neurol* 27: 61–7. http://dx.doi.org/10.1177/0883073811413580

Powers SW, Andrasik F (2005) Biobehavioral treatment, disability, and psychological effects of pediatric headache. *Pediatr Ann* 34: 461–5.

Powers SW, Patton SR, Hommel KA, Hershey AD (2004) Quality of life in paediatric migraine: characterization of age-related effects using PedsQL 4.0. *Cephalalgia* 24: 120–7. http://dx.doi.org/10.1111/j.1468-2982.2004.00652.x

Raieli V, Compagno A, Pandolfi E et al (2010) Headache: what do children and mothers expect from pediatricians? *Headache* 50: 290–300. http://dx.doi.org/10.1111/j.1526-4610.2009.01583.x

Ravishankar K (2010a) Headache medicine in India: Past, present and future. In: Chowdhury D, Gupta M, Balta A, editors. *Headache and Related Disorders*. New Delhi: GB Pant Hospital, pp. 148–52.

Ravishankar K (2010b) The "IHS" Classification (1988, 2004) – contributions, limitations and suggestions. *J Assoc Physicians India* 58(Suppl): 7–9.

Richardson GM, McGrath PJ, Cunningham SJ, Humphreys P (1983) Validity of the headache diary for children. *Headache* 23: 184–7. http://dx.doi.org/10.1111/j.1526-4610.1983.hed2304184.x

Rothner AD (1995) The evaluation of headaches in children and adolescents. *Sem Pediatr Neurol* 2: 109–18. http://dx.doi.org/10.1016/S1071-9091(05)80021-X

Seshia SS, Wolfstein JR, Adams C, Booth FA, Reggin JD (1994) International headache society criteria and childhood headache. *Dev Med Child Neurol* 36: 419–28. http://dx.doi.org/10.1111/j.1469-8749.1994.tb11868.x

Sieberg CB, Huguet A, von Baeyer CL, Seshia SS (2012) Psychological interventions for headache in children and adolescents. *Can J Neurol Sci* 39: 26–34.

Tassorelli C, Sances G, Allena M et al (2008) The usefulness and applicability of a basic headache diary before first consultation: results of a pilot study conducted in two centres. *Cephalalgia* 28: 1023–30. http://dx.doi.org/10.1111/j.1468-2982.2008.01639.x

Appendix 8.1 Assessment of headache

Specifics of headache (each type separately)

Age at onset	Frequency (range)	Severity (range)
Duration (range)	Usual time of occurrence	Location
Quality	Nausea	Vomiting
Photophobia	Phonophobia	Osmophobia
Hyperalgesia	Allodynia	Influence of physical activity
Influence of posture	Visual/other neurological dysfunction (before, during)	
Abdominal pain (associated)	Lacrimation	Red conjunctiva
Nasal stuffiness	Ptosis/pupillary change	
Missing school because of headache (how often)		
Missing extracurricular activities (how often)		
Headache progression (same, less, worsening; which symptom)		
If chronic daily headache (≥ 15d/mo for ≥ 3mo), preceded by intermittent headache?		
Any inciting event around the time of transformation or onset (if chronic daily headache)?		
Medicines used for treatment (including overuse)		

Triggers or aggravating factors

Stressors: home-related	School-related	Friends-related, etc. (see Note at end of table)
Noise	Weather	Irregular meals/going hungry
Dietary smells	Bus or car rides	Physical activity
Menstrual periods (females)	Combing hair	
Irregular sleep/sleep deprivation	Video games/bright lights/computer	
Other (may be identified by child/family)		
Concussion (especially recreation or sports related)		

Past and other medical history

Pregnancy/birth milestones, illnesses	Travel sickness, colic
Episodes of head tilt/vomiting/vertigo	Dental issues
Smoke/alcohol/other substances	On contraceptive pill?
History to suggest anxiety/mood/other psychiatric disorder	History to suggest disorder of sleep

School and related history

School performance (grade) and stressors (bullying, teachers, school- and homework)
Worsening of school performance
Attendance (If missing school is this because of headache? How often?)
Extracurricular and recreational activities (and impact of headache on them)

Family history (especially first and second degree)

Stressors in family unit
Other relevant medical, social histories
Other family members with headache (specify type of headache if possible)
Parental history of headache (Which parent? Can headache type be determined from description?)
Anxiety, mood or other psychiatric disorders in family members

EXAMINATION

General examination

Head circumference (serial ideal)		Head circumference of parents	
Height (serial ideal)	Weight	Body mass index	
Blood pressure	Peripheral pulse and rate		
Visual acuity (must)	Tenderness over sinuses	Cough headache	
Bruit (skull, eyeballs, carotids)		Evidence of neurocutaneous disorder?	
Evidence of inherited disorder of connective tissue?		Temporomandibular joint tenderness/ discomfort	
Tender points 'in' muscles (neck, shoulder)			
Examination of abdomen and chest (lungs and heart)			
Examination of spine neck movements head tilt			

Neurological examination

Higher functions		
Cranial nerves (especially fundi, fields, squint; blind spot and colour perception may need to be tested if there is a suspicion of papilloedema)		
Motor system (tone, power, coordination, stance/gait)		Reflexes
Sensations	Hyperalgesia	Allodynia

Level of disability and quality of life assessment (see text and Chapter 7)
Note: List of some stressors (adverse psychosocial factors) one should ask about, especially in those with frequent headache (chronic daily headache) and intractable headache; in many jurisdictions such history is often part of the social history that is integral in paediatric practice.

Parental separation/discord	Relationships with siblings, parent's significant other, etc.
Financial	Illness in immediate family members
Relocation/move from familiar place	Bereavement (including loss of pet)
School related (bullying very important)	Cyber-bullying
Learning dysfunction/overachiever	Relationship with teachers/friends/boyfriend/girlfriend
Control issues at home (that are often a source of conflict during the adolescent years)	Maltreatment (emotional, physical, sexual)

9
INVESTIGATION OF THE CHILD WITH CHRONIC HEADACHE: THE RED FLAGS

Mas Ahmed

Introduction

Chronic headache is not a single disorder but a term that encompasses many conditions. A headache is considered chronic when it persists over a period of 3 months. It is reported in up to 25% of schoolchildren and it accounts for the majority of patients seen in specialist clinics (Abu-Arafeh and Russell 1994).

Red flags are clinical predictors that may distinguish patients with sinister causes of chronic headaches. A sinister cause is a pathological state that will adversely affect the patient's morbidity and/or mortality. The possibility that chronic headache might be secondary to a life-threatening disease remains a major concern to clinicians. It is important to establish assessment criteria before neuroimaging is performed for patients with chronic headaches. Such criteria include clinical red flags based on history and physical examination and the headache diagnosis.

This chapter aims to create pathways for the diagnoses of chronic headaches without overlooking uncommon serious conditions. It also aims to address the following questions: (1) what are the red flags in the history and examination of a child with chronic headaches? and (2) what are the assessment strategies in a child in whom chronic headache is probably the only symptom of a serious neurological disorder?

Red flags

A diagnostic approach to childhood headache, based on the presence of 'red flags', has been suggested (Gierris 1976, Barlow 1982, Flores et al 1986, Haas 1991, Chu and Shinnar 1992, Edgeworth et al 1996, Medina et al 1997, 2001, Battistella et al 1998, Abu-Arafeh and Macleod 2005, Wilne et al 2007). Chronic headache in childhood is rarely due to a serious intracranial pathology (Abu-Arafeh and MacLeod 2005) and headache has been found to be a common presentation of childhood brain tumours (Vazquez-Barquero et al 1994, Miltenburg et al 1996, Wilne et al 2007). Use of red flags as predictive variables of serious causes of childhood headache is not easy. First, many studies have examined red flags among patients with headaches, but none of these studies has analysed their statistical significance. Second, it might be hard to prove that some red flags are actually worrying features of an underlying serious aetiology. Finally, the complex relationship between headache and red flags might not be possible to establish with certainty. However, red flags might be especially useful when headache diagnosis remains non-specific and/or the need for brain imaging is not clear. Including red flags in the assessment of patients with headache provides a positive approach for 'what should be done' rather than 'what not to do'. Complete history and physical examination should be focused on headache by a detailed description and correct interpretation of clinical features in order to identify red flags.

General red flags

AGE OF THE CHILD AT PRESENTATION

Diagnosis of headache in children under 4 years of age can be challenging as it can be extremely difficult to obtain a detailed history, bearing in mind that the median age at diagnosis of brain tumour is 5.8 years, with almost half of patients under the age of 4 (Hayashi et al 2009). In young children, information on the child's physical activities (weakness, coordination, handedness, etc.) is valuable in the absence of a validated assessment tool. Therefore, one may argue the need to examine young children on several occasions, with a lower threshold for brain imaging (Chu and Shinnar 1992, Stilberstein 2000).

CLINICAL COURSE

The clinical course of headache is usually distinct from its onset and is categorised as acute (recurrent or not) and chronic (progressive or non-progressive). Chronic progressive headaches are not always secondary headaches, whereas acute headaches are not always primary headaches. The current literature is sparse, although overall data suggest that chronicity lowers the probability of an underlying sinister cause, provided the headaches are non-progressive and there are no associated abnormal physical findings. In patients under the age of 10 years, cranial sutures may separate to relieve symptoms of increased intracranial pressure temporarily for weeks or even months. Thus, intermittent headache does not exclude intracranial causes that might require prompt intervention. Therefore, the clinical course of childhood headache may help in some, but not all, cases to distinguish between primary and secondary chronic headaches.

COUGH HEADACHE

Headache triggered by cough may be an indication of increased intracranial pressure, which is usually due to cerebral oedema or ventricular obstruction. Arnold–Chiari malformation, cerebral aneurysm, brain tumour and carotid artery stenosis may also trigger cough headache (Haas 1991, Battistella et al 1998, Wilne et al 2007). Benign primary 'cough headache' is rare in children and the diagnosis is made on exclusion of other causes (Gierris 1976). In both primary and secondary cough headaches, the pain is bilateral, brief (few minutes), precipitated by cough and may be relieved by avoiding cough (Headache Classification Subcommittee of the International Headache Society 2004). Therefore, a detailed assessment of patients with cough headache is essential for early detection of serious causes.

SLEEP DISTURBANCE

Sleep disturbance among patients with headaches is common. Primary and secondary headaches can cause a variety of sleep disturbances such as difficulty falling asleep, interrupted sleep, poor sleep quality, daytime tiredness and parasomnia (Blau 1982).

Although evidence for the relationship between brain tumours and sleep disturbance is limited, tumours in specific areas of the brain might be associated with specific sleep problems such as snoring and obstructive sleep apnoea (Blau 1982, Sahota and Dexter 1990, Bruni et al 2008). A child with migraine may wake up at night because of headache, but, if sleep disturbances are persistent, investigations including brain imaging need to be considered.

LOCATION OF PAIN

The significance of the location of headache in children and adolescents has not been studied fully. Patients with primary headache, such as migraine, tension-type headache, new daily persistent headache and cervicogenic headache, may experience side-locked headaches. Occasionally, unilateral-locked headache is caused by brain tumours, hydrocephalus, abscess, subdural haematoma and arteriovenous malformation (Leone et al 1993, 2008). However, a multicentre study reported no significant relationship between headache location and abnormalities on brain imaging (Rho et al 2011), but a wide range of differential diagnoses should be considered on individual cases.

PARENTAL ANXIETY

Parents' anxiety may influence clinical management decisions (Gladstein and Holden 1996), and brain imaging in response to parental anxiety often returns normal results (Rho et al 2011). In a study on the value of neuroimaging in children with headache, 14% of all neuroimaging was carried out purely to allay parental concerns without abnormal findings to explain the headache (Maytal et al 1995). Following head trauma, headache is not an indicator of brain injury (Jacobs and Maconochie 2005); nevertheless, following an isolated brain concussion and mild injury, parents have heightened concerns about brain damage (Nacajauskaite et al 2006). As parental reassurance is paramount in managing childhood headache, there may be a place for imaging in selected cases.

Red flags from clinical history and physical examination

RED FLAGS IN EXAMINATION OF A PATIENT WITH CHRONIC HEADACHE

Table 9.1 shows red flags in children with headache and abnormal examination. Physical examination of a patient with chronic headaches should include all systems.

Neurological examination and neurodevelopment assessment of young children require expertise to avoid misinterpretation of the findings, and normal neurological examination may not exclude a brain tumour. The classical triad of headache, vomiting and papilloedema in children with brain tumour is uncommon (Edgeworth et al 1996). Optic nerve drusen can be a pitfall and difficult to distinguish from true papilloedema. Disparity in tendon reflexes is not uncommon among healthy young people. Plantar response is a reliable indicator of pyramidal function, but it might be difficult to distinguish it from withdrawal response. Migraine-like headaches are reported in patients with other conditions (Honig and Charney 1982, Kurita

TABLE 9.1

Red flags in children with chronic headaches and abnormal examination

Neurology

Focal neurological deficit

Positive pronation drift

Abnormal gait or tandem walk

Changes in handedness

Loss of fine motor function (e.g. writing, computer use)

Skull tenderness on gentle percussion (brain abscess?)

Occipital prominence (Dandy–Walker syndrome?)

Cranial bruit

Symptoms of increased ICP (vomiting, lethargy, double vision, etc.)

Ophthalmology

New-onset paralytic squint

Abnormal visual field

Reduction in visual acuity without refractive error

Optic disc oedema

Others

Hypertension with or without bradycardia

Delayed or precocious puberty

Polyuria, polydipsia or proved diabetes insipidus

Unsatisfactory growth (e.g. short stature, weight loss, obesity)

Neurocutaneous stigmata

Skin whorls (brain abnormalities)

Behavioural changes (tiredness, personality changes, mood swings or aggression)

Unsatisfactory school performance

Risk factors of brain tumour (family history of brain tumour, irradiation, NF 1 or 2 and tuberous sclerosis)

ICP, intracranial pressure; NF, neurofibromatosis.

et al 2000). Furthermore, symptoms such as weakness, cranial nerve palsy, ataxia, confusion and behavioural changes that may accompany migraine can make it difficult to distinguish migraine from other neurological diseases (Bickerstaff 1961, Golden and French 1975, Hansen et al 1990, Shaabat 1996, Lanzi et al 1997, Herraiz et al 1999, Anttila et al 2001).

Abnormal examination, particularly of the central nervous system, is probably the most reliable indicator that headache has a serious cause. Thorough physical examination would reveal subtle clinical findings suggestive of secondary headaches. For example, careful inspection of the skin might be needed to reveal important findings regarding the cause of chronic headaches. Also, patients with mild corticospinal lesions may have subtle abnormal signs, such as positive pronation drift, that require skills and a properly conducted neurological examination. Careful neurological examination might also show other red flags such as abnormal tandem walk, changes in handedness and loss of fine motor function such as writing or computer use.

Ophthalmological red flags include new-onset paralytic squint, reduction in visual acuity without refractive error and defects in visual field and/or optic disc oedema; however, clinical examination should also be directed towards other important clues including symptoms and signs of increased intracranial pressure, pubertal status, height and cranial bruit, and one should enquire about risk factors of brain tumour.

RED FLAGS IN HISTORY TAKING FROM A PATIENT WITH CHRONIC HEADACHE
Table 9.2 shows red flags that are headache related and whose use might be helpful, particularly for patients with normal general and neurological examination. Headache can be the first symptom before physical signs of the underlying cause become obvious. Diagnosis of chronic headache is not always straightforward, as the borders between different types of headache can be blurred. Headache-focused history and awareness of red flags would help the clinician to spawn and follow ample differentials of chronic headaches in order to reach the correct diagnosis. The main causes of secondary headache are trauma, infection, inflammation, tumour and toxins (e.g. metabolic disorders). Such causes should be debarred among neurologically healthy patients with progressive chronic headaches, headaches not yet specific and/or other headache-related red flags.

TABLE 9.2

Red flags in children with chronic headaches and normal examination

---

Persistent[a] headache occurring in a child younger than 5y

The worst headache the patient has ever had

New persistent[a] headaches

Headache for less than 1 month

Chronic progressive headaches

Headache persistently awakens the patient from sleep

Change of headache pattern

Unilateral locked headaches

Headache persistently occurring on awakening

Confusion or disorientation occurring with headache

Headache associated with cough, straining, sneezing or bending

Headache not yet specified

Atypical aura (stereotype, prolonged or shows a 'march')

Headache with persisting vomiting on awakening

No response to conventional treatment

Parental worries

---

[a]Lasting more than 4 weeks.

Rapid assessment of patients with chronic headache

The algorithms shown in Figures 9.1 and 9.2 show a rapid assessment tool for chronic headache. In some children with non-specific chronic headache, the physical examination is normal but the overall clinical evaluation raises some red flags. Although primary headaches are still possible in these cases, the differential diagnosis should include secondary headaches (see the four clinical cases).

Case 1

An 11-year-old male presents with severe recurrent alternating unilateral headache that lasts for several hours and has occurred over the past 2 years. The headache tends to occur at the end of the school day and is often associated with nausea, vomiting and photophobia. Systemic and neurological examination showed no abnormality.

Case 2

A 7-year-old female presents with an 8-month history of recurrent moderate bifrontal headache that lasts for at least a day and occurs on more than 15 days per month. The headache is associated with vomiting, phonophobia, photophobia and visual aura. On further questioning headache is reported on awakening and causes sleep disruption. Her parents have noticed personality changes. Systemic and neurological examination showed no abnormality.

Case 3

A 14-year-old female has an 8-month history of recurrent mild bitemporal headache that lasts from a few hours to a day with an average frequency of four times a week. The headache is not associated with nausea, vomiting, phonophobia, photophobia or an aura. There are no specific triggers or other concerns. Systemic and neurological examination showed no abnormality.

Case 4

A 6-year-old female presents with an 18-month history of recurrent severe headache. Headache always occurs on the left parietal site and lasts for a few hours. The headache previously occurred once a month but recently increased in frequency to four times per week. The headache is not associated with nausea, vomiting, phonophobia, photophobia or an aura. There are no specific triggers or other issues. Systemic and neurological examinations were normal.

Headaches in two of the patients from the four case studies (1 and 2) are consistent with migraine, whereas the headaches are difficult to classify in cases 3 and 4. Clinical evaluation of case 2 revealed headaches on awakening, sleep interruption and personality changes. Concerns about increased headache frequency and fixed head pain to the left parietal side were raised for the patient in case 4. All patients had a normal physical examination. Evaluation of these patients highlighted issues related to headaches that remain unclassified and also to the

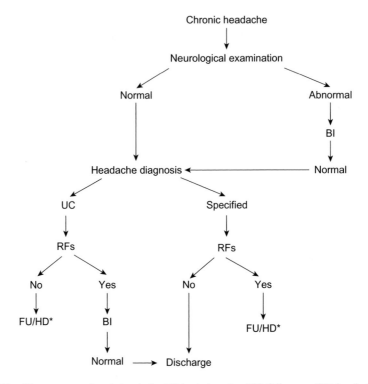

Fig. 9.1 Algorithm to assess chronic headache. BI, brain imaging; FU, follow-up; HD, headache diaries; UC, unclassified; RF, red flags; *, consider secondary causes such as brain tumour, idiopathic intracranial hypertension, chronic sinusitis, chronic meningitis, carbon monoxide poisoning, temporomandibular dysfunction, consider referral for ear, nose and throat assessment or lumbar puncture.

presence of red flags, leading to some difficulties in management decisions. The red flags in cases 2 and 4 may imply intracranial pathology.

In case 1, headache diagnosis is specific (migraine) and the patient has no red flags, so brain imaging is unnecessary. Case 4 has two red flags and lacks a headache diagnosis; therefore, brain imaging is indicated. Standard follow-up and headache diaries are necessary for cases 2 and 3 and further investigations may become indicated.

Role of investigations in the child with normal examination
Despite various recommendations, missing a life-threatening disease such as a brain tumour remains an ongoing concern. This issue incontestably emphasises an unmet clinical stipulation, and undeniably enhances the case for parents' requests for brain imaging.

BRAIN IMAGING
The role of brain imaging of patients with headache has been examined (Dooley et al 1990, Abu-Arafeh and Russell 1994, Frishberg 1994, Demaerel et al 1996, Gladstein and Holden 1996, Wober-Bingol et al 1996, Medina et al 1997, 2001, Lewis and Dorbad 2000, Alehan

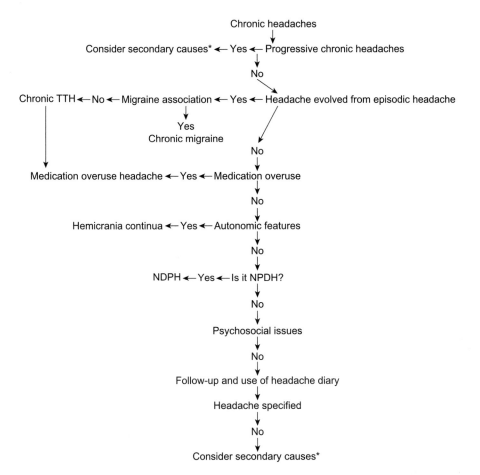

Fig. 9.2 Algorithm to diagnose chronic headache. NDPH, newly daily persistent headache; TTH, tension-type headache; *, brain tumour, idiopathic intracranial hypertension, chronic sinusitis, chronic meningitis, carbon monoxide poisoning, temporomandibular dysfunction, consider referral for ear, nose and throat assessment or lumbar puncture.

2002, Abu-Arafeh and Macleod 2005, Wilne et al 2007, Graf et al 2008, Ahmed et al 2010, Rho et al 2011).

An abnormal neurological examination in children with chronic headache constitutes an absolute indication for urgent brain imaging. Brain imaging is also indicated in children in whom the diagnosis of the headache disorder is ambiguous and in those with chronic progressive headache. Brain imaging should be carefully considered for neurologically healthy patients with non-specific headaches and red flags. Routine brain imaging is not indicated for patients with specific primary headaches and normal examination.

A decision rule on when to investigate neurologically healthy children with headaches, based on the yield of significant pathology, has recently been published (Ahmed et al 2010).

Brain computed tomography is usually used for urgent evaluation of a child with headache, and it remains the test of choice to detect acute haemorrhage and lesions containing calcium. Computed tomography has good tolerance for patient movement. Magnetic resonance imaging (MRI) has a superior resolution to computed tomography, a better grey–white matter differentiation and detects brain pathology in difficult areas, such as the posterior fossa, without repositioning the child or the machine. Additionally, there is no risk of radiation. Limitations of MRI include the child's apprehension and refusal to cooperate with the procedure, claustrophobia, the existence of metal (bracelet) and the need for sedation or a general anaesthesia.

OTHER INVESTIGATIONS

An assessment by an ear, nose and throat specialist may be necessary in the presence of nasal symptoms, allergy, use of decongestants, nasal polyps, oedema or erythema of nasal mucosa.

Carbon monoxide poisoning is not uncommon. Data from the Health Protection Agency in the UK showed that over a period of 1 year, between July 2010 and June 2011, there were 25 fatalities due to carbon monoxide poisoning. The number of non-fatal incidents and the number of patients presenting with ill health and other symptoms, of whom 90% report headache, are much higher, but are not known (Health Protection Scotland 2011). Unfortunately, specific data on the prevalence of carbon monoxide poisoning in children are not available. Carbon monoxide poisoning should be considered in patients with non-specific chronic headache associated with cherry-red skin, gastrointestinal symptoms, tiredness or family history of similar complaints, or if headaches improve when the child is away from home or worsen during winter. Diagnosis can be made with the use of a pulse carbon monoxide oximeter and venous blood sampling for carbon monoxide haemoglobin assay.

Idiopathic intracranial hypertension and raised intracranial pressure should be considered in some patients (see Chapter 23).

Clinical distinction of epilepsy and headache, particularly migraine, is often difficult, and electroencephalography can be misguiding. The value of routine paediatric electroencephalography in the diagnosis of chronic headache in children is negligible and does not merit its routine use (Kramer et al 1997).

Blood count may be necessary in some patients to exclude anaemia.

In some patients psychological and child protection issues may need to be explored as possible causes of headache chronification (Tietjen et al 2009).

Summary

The key to diagnosis is a history that should be headache focused and tailor-made to spot clinical predictors of serious neurological disorders. Thorough examination, especially of the central nervous system, is probably the strongest tool in the assessment of the child with chronic headache. When diagnostic uncertainty exists, standard follow-up and headache diaries are needed for individual cases, particularly for patients with normal physical examination and normal brain imaging.

REFERENCES

Abu-Arafeh I, Macleod S (2005) Serious neurological disorders in children with chronic headache. *Arch Dis Child* 90: 937–40. http://dx.doi.org/10.1136/adc.2004.067256

Abu-Arafeh I, Russell G (1994) Prevalence of headache and migraine in school children. *BMJ* 309: 765–9. http://dx.doi.org/10.1136/bmj.309.6957.765

Ahmed MAS, Martinez A, Cahill D, Chong K, Whitehouse WP (2010) When to image neurologically normal children with headaches: development of a decision rule. *Acta Paediatr* 99: 940–3. http://dx.doi.org/10.1111/j.1651-2227.2010.01728.x

Alehan FK (2002) Value of neuroimaging in the evaluation of neurologically normal children with recurrent headache. *J Child Neurol* 17: 807–9. http://dx.doi.org/10.1177/08830738020170110901

Anttila P, Metsahonkala L, Mikkelsson M, Helenius H, Sillanpaa MM (2001) Comorbidity of other pains in schoolchildren with migraine or nonmigrainous headaches. *J Pediatr* 138:176–80. http://dx.doi.org/10.1067/mpd.2001.112159

Barlow F (1982) Headaches and brain tumours. *Am J Dis Child* 136: 99–101.

Battistella PA, Naccarella C, Soriani S, Perilongo G (1998) Headaches and brain tumours: different features versus primary forms in juvenile patients. *Headache Q-Curr Trea* 9: 245–8.

Bickerstaff ER (1961) Basilar artery migraine. *Lancet* 1: 15–17. http://dx.doi.org/10.1016/S0140-6736(61)92184-5

Blau JN (1982) Resolution of migraine attacks: sleep and the recovery phase. *J Neurol Neurosurg Psychiatry* 45: 223–6. http://dx.doi.org/10.1136/jnnp.45.3.223

Bruni O, Rosso PM, Feri R, Novelli L, Galli F, Guidetti V (2008) Relationships between headache and sleep in a non-clinical population of children and adolescent. *Sleep Med* 9: 542–8. http://dx.doi.org/10.1016/j.sleep.2007.08.010

Chu ML, Shinnar S (1992) Headache in children younger than seven years of age. *Arch Neurol* 49: 79–82. http://dx.doi.org/10.1001/archneur.1992.00530250083020

Demaerel P, Boelaert I, Williams G, Baert AL (1996) The role of cranial camputed tomograpgy in the diagnostic work up of headache. *Headache* 36: 347–8. http://dx.doi.org/10.1046/j.1526-4610.1996.3606347.x

Dooley JM, Camfield PR, O'Neill M, Vohra A (1990) The value of CT scans for children with headaches. *Can J Neurol Sci* 17: 309–10.

Edgeworth J, Bullock P, Bailey A, Gallagher A (1996) Why are brain tumours still being missed? *Arch Dis Child* 74: 148–51. http://dx.doi.org/10.1136/adc.74.2.148

Flores L, Williams D, Bell B, O'Brien M, Rgab A (1986) Delay in the diagnosis of paediatric brain tumours. *Am J Dis Child* 140: 684–6.

Frishberg BM (1994) The utility of neuroimaging in the evaluation of headache in patients with normal neurological examinations. *Neurology* 44: 1191–7. http://dx.doi.org/10.1212/WNL.44.7.1191

Gierris F (1976) Clinical aspects and long-term prognosis of intracranial tumours in infancy and childhood. *Dev Med Child Neurol* 18: 145–9. http://dx.doi.org/10.1111/j.1469-8749.1976.tb03623.x

Gladstein J, Holden EW (1996) Chronic daily headache in children and adolescents: a 2 year prospective study. *Headache* 36: 349–51. http://dx.doi.org/10.1046/j.1526-4610.1996.3606349.x

Golden GS, French JH (1975) Basilar artery migraine in young children. *Pediatrics* 56: 722–6.

Graf WD, Kayyali HR, Alexander JJ, Simon SD, Morris MC (2008) Neuroimaging-use trends in non-acute paediatric headache before and after clinical practice parameters. *Pediatrics* 122: 1001–5. http://dx.doi.org/10.1542/peds.2008-1159

Haas DC (1991) Arteriovenous malformation and migraine: case reports and an analysis of the relationship. *Headache* 31: 509–13. http://dx.doi.org/10.1111/j.1526-4610.1991.hed3108509.x

Hansen SL, Borelli ML, Stange P, Nielsen BM, Olesen J (1990) Ophthalmologic migraine: diagnostic criteria, incidence of hospitalization and possible etiology. *Acta Neurol Scand* 81: 54–60. http://dx.doi.org/10.1111/j.1600-0404.1990.tb00931.x

Hayashi N, Kidokoro H, Miyajim Y et al (2009) How do the clinical features of brain tumours in childhood progress before diagnosis? *Brain Dev* 32: 636–41. http://dx.doi.org/10.1016/j.braindev.2009.10.001

Headache Classification Subcommittee of the International Headache Society (2004) The International Classification of Headache Disorders. Second Edition. *Cephalalgia* 24 (Suppl 1): 1–160.

Health Protection Scotland (HPS) (2011) Information on CO Poisoning. Available at: http://www.documents. hps.scot.nhs.uk/ewr/pdf2011/1142.pdf

Herraiz C, Clavin FJ, Tapia MC, de Lucas P, Arroyo R (1999) The migraine: benign paroxysmal vertigo of childhood complex. *Int Tinnitus J* 5: 50–2.

Honig P, Charney E (1982) Children with brain tumour headaches: distinguishing features. *Am J Dis Child* 136: 121–4.

Jacobs M, Maconochie I (2005) Headache in paediatric head injury. *Emerg Med J* 22: 889. http://dx.doi.org/10.1136/emj.2005.031724

Kramer U, Nevo Y, Neufeld MY, Harel S (1997) The value of EEG in children with chronic headaches. *Brain Dev* 16: 304–8. http://dx.doi.org/10.1016/0387-7604(94)90028-0

Kurita H, Ueki K, Shin M et al (2000) Headaches in patients with radiosurgically treated occipital arteriovenous malformation. *J Neurosurg* 93: 224–5. http://dx.doi.org/10.3171/jns.2000.93.2.0224

Lanzi G, Zambrino CA, Balottin U, Tagliasacchi M, Vercelli P, Termine C (1997) Periodic syndrome and migraine in children and adolescents. *Ital J Neurol Sci* 18: 283–8. http://dx.doi.org/10.1007/BF02083305

Leone M, D'Amico D, Frediani F, Torri W, Sjaastad O, Bussone G (1993) Clinical considerations of side-blocked unilaterality in long-lasting primary headaches. *Headache* 33: 381–4. http://dx.doi.org/10.1111/j.1526-4610.1993.hed3307381.x

Leone M, Cecchini AP, Mea E, Tullo V, Bussone G (2008) Epidemiology of fixed unilateral headaches. *Cephalagia* 28: 8–11. http://dx.doi.org/10.1111/j.1468-2982.2008.01607.x

Lewis DW, Dorbad D (2000) The utility of neuroimaging in the evaluation of children with migraine or chronic daily headache who have normal neurological examinations. *Headache* 40: 629–32. http://dx.doi.org/10.1046/j.1526-4610.2000.040008629.x

Maytal J, Bienkowski RS, Patel M, Eviatar L (1995) The value of brain imaging in children with headaches. *Pediatrics* 96: 413–16.

Medina LS, Pinter JD, Zurakowski D, Davis RG, Kuban K, Barnes PD (1997) Children with headache: clinical predictors of surgical space-occupying lesions and the role of neuroimaging. *Radiology* 202: 819–24.

Medina LS, Kuntz KM, Pomeroy SL (2001) Children with headache suspected of having a brain tumour: a cost effectiveness analysis of diagnostic strategies. *Pediatrics* 108: 255–63. http://dx.doi.org/10.1542/peds.108.2.255

Miltenburg D, Louw DF, Sutherland GR (1996) Epidemiology of childhood brain tumours. *Can J Neurol Sci* 23: 118–22.

Nacajauskaite O, Endziniene M, Jureniene K, Schrader H (2006) The validity of post-concussion syndrome in children: a controlled historical cohort study. *Brain Dev* 28: 507–14. http://dx.doi.org/10.1016/j.braindev.2006.02.010

Rho Y, Chung HJ, Suh ES et al (2011) The role of neuroimaging in children and adolescents with recurrent headaches – multicentre study. *Headache* 51: 403–8. http://dx.doi.org/10.1111/j.1526-4610.2011.01845.x

Sahota PK, Dexter JD (1990) Sleep and headache syndromes: a clinical review. *Headache* 30: 80–4. http://dx.doi.org/10.1111/j.1526-4610.1990.hed3002080.x

Shaabat A (1996) Confusional migraine in childhood. *Pediatr Neurol* 15: 23–5. http://dx.doi.org/10.1016/0887-8994(96)00089-6

Stilberstein SD (2000) Practice parameter: evidence-based guidelines for migraine headache (an evidence-based review): report of the Quality Standards Subcommittee of the American Academy of Neurology. *Neurology* 55: 754–62. http://dx.doi.org/10.1212/WNL.55.6.754

Tietjen GE, Brandes JL, Peterlin BL et al (2009) Allodynia in migraine: association with comorbid pain conditions. *Headache* 49: 1333–44. http://dx.doi.org/10.1111/j.1526-4610.2009.01521.x

Vazquez-Barquero A, Ibanez FJ, Herrera S, Izquierdo JM, Berciano J, Pascual J (1994) Isolated headaches as presenting clinical manifestations of intracranial tumours: a prospective study. *Cephalalgia* 14: 270–2. http://dx.doi.org/10.1046/j.1468-2982.1994.1404270.x

Wilne SH, Collier J, Kennedy C, Koller K, Grundy R, Walker D (2007) Presentation of childhood CNS tumours: a systematic review and meta-analysis. *Lancet Oncol* 8: 685–95. http://dx.doi.org/10.1016/S1470-2045(07)70207-3

Wober-Bingol C, Wober C, Prayer D et al (1996) Magnetic resonance imaging for recurrent headaches in childhood and adolescence. *Headache* 36: 83–90. http://dx.doi.org/10.1046/j.1526-4610.1996.3602083.x

10
CHILDHOOD MIGRAINE: CLINICAL FEATURES

Paul Winner

Migraine is the most common headache disorder that physicians will diagnose in their office. It also proves to be one of the most disabling medical disorders. An early accurate diagnosis is the first and most important step in controlling disability and preventing potential progression. Migraine has a significant impact not only on the patient, but also on the entire family. This chapter will address the common and the unusual presenting symptoms of migraine and its variants. The phenotypic expression of migraine from childhood, throughout adolescence, to young adulthood will be outlined. When and what diagnostic studies should be done will be reviewed.

Making the diagnosis of migraine for the first time in a child presents a unique situation that allows the physician to reassure the patient and his or her parents that the patient does not have a brain tumour or significant structural abnormality of the brain, but a chronic neurological inherited disorder. Educating patients and their parents about migraine, its potential course and available management, including a discussion on the avoidance of medication overuse, is crucial to preventing disability and possibly averting the development of comorbidities.

Epidemiology and classification of paediatric migraine

A full discussion of the epidemiology and classification can be found in the appropriate chapters of this book, but relevant points are discussed here in order to highlight specific clinical issues. The prevalence of migraine in adults is 12%; about 50% of adults report onset in childhood or adolescence. The results of the American Migraine Prevalence and Prevention Study determined the prevalence of migraine in adolescents to be 6.3% (5% in males and 7.7% and females). Overall, the incidence of migraine peaks earlier in males than in females: the mean age at onset of migraine in males is 7 years and in females 11 years. The incidence of migraine with aura peaks earlier than the incidence of migraine without aura in the paediatric population (Stewart et al 1991, 1992, Lipton et al 1994, Laurell et al 2004).

The International Classification for Headache Disorder (ICHD-II) is the currently accepted universal classification for headache disorder. Designed to primarily address headache in adults, it often lacks the sensitivity to accurately diagnose paediatric migraine. The full ICHD-II criteria for migraine and migraine variants can be found online (www.ihs-headache. org), and an abbreviated list can be found as an appendix to Chapter 5 (Headache Classification Subcommittee of the International Headache Society 2004, Lewis et al 2008).

Migraine is divided into six subtypes. The three migraine groups most often observed in paediatric patients are migraine without aura (common migraine), migraine with aura (classic migraine) and childhood periodic syndromes that are commonly precursors of migraine, which include cyclical vomiting, abdominal migraine and benign paroxysmal vertigo of childhood.

Complications of migraine include retinal migraine (uncommon in children), chronic migraine, status migraine, persistent aura without infarction and migrainous infarction. The sixth subtype of migraine is probable migraine, which was added to encompass the subset of patients whose headache patterns fail to fulfil the formal criteria for migraine, with or without aura, but most likely represent the migraine spectrum. It is common for young children to have headaches that are short (≤30 min) and which therefore cannot be classified formally as migraine. In these patients, headache falls into the category of probable migraine. Children and adolescents may not have the requisite number of associated symptoms (e.g. photophobia and phonophobia) and will be classified as having probable migraine (Lewis et al 2008).

The ICHD-II classification system does not address the migraine variants of confusional migraine or Alice in Wonderland syndrome; they will be discussed later in this chapter.

Migraine without aura

Migraine without aura is the most frequent form of migraine. The migraine attacks may include all or part of stereotyped sequential phases: premonitory phase, aura, headache and associated symptoms, and recovery (Table 10.1) (Lewis et al 2008). Not all attacks include all phases and have the same duration or severity. This is especially true in the paediatric population as the phenotypic expression of these phases varies with age. This contributes to making the diagnosis of paediatric migraine so challenging.

Premonitory features, lasting from minutes to hours to days, preceding the migraine pain include yawning, mood changes, irritability, euphoria, food cravings, increased urination or

TABLE 10.1
Migraine attack: stereotyped sequence

Premonitory phase	Headache episode	Associated (autonomic) symptoms
Yawning, sighing	Varied onset (escalates over minutes to hours)	Photophobia/photophobia
Mood changes		Nausea, vomiting, anorexia
Irritability	Duration 1–72h	Periumbilical abdominal pain
Euphoria	Bifrontal, bitemporal, retro-orbital, unilateral	Diarrhoea
Food cravings		Pallor
Increased urination	Throbbing, pulsating, pounding	Desire to sleep
Increased thirst	Intensity increased (worsened) by activity	Cool extremities
		Periorbital discolouration
		Increased or decreased blood pressure
		Dizziness
		Syncope

Reproduced courtesy of the International Headache Society (www.i-h-s.org).

increased thirst. Often the child will withdraw from activity and go to a quiet, dark room. The associated symptoms of nausea, vomiting, pallor and periumbilical abdominal pain may be intense, and are often the most disabling features (Lewis et al 2008).

The onset of migraines tends to be during the day in younger children and adolescents. Older adolescents and younger adults may often report morning headaches. Late-afternoon headaches in adolescence may be due to missed meals, altered school schedules or just the general stress of the school day. Children and adolescents report more headaches in the early part of the school week, which may be related to altered sleep schedules and/or stress at school (Lewis et al 2008).

Children under the age of 12, and especially under the age of 7, who present with occipital headaches and/or escalation of their headache frequency and severity over a short period of time (<3–4mo) require attention to rule out structural or vascular brain lesions. Focal neurological signs support the presence of a brain lesion. Headaches that wake a child from sleep may also be another warning sign. If these children were not imaged, it is suggested that they are monitored closely over a period of several weeks for the potential development of focal neurological deficits.

The formal diagnosis of migraine in the paediatric population relies on the use of the ICHD criteria. ICHD-I criteria were initially developed for the clinical and scientific study of headache, but have been criticised for a lack of sensitivity and specificity in diagnosing paediatric migraine. Some of the suggested modifications have been adopted in the footnotes to the criteria for migraine in the second edition, ICHD-II, as in Table 10.2 (Headache Classification Subcommittee of the International Headache Society 2004). This has improved the sensitivity from the ICHD-I, but further modifications are still necessary (Hershey et al 2005).

The recognised problems include the short duration of paediatric migraines, higher likelihood of a bilateral location and difficulty in describing the headache features and associated symptoms. These features may change and evolve over time as a result of the variable expression of the migraine pathophysiology in a developing brain (Virtanen et al 2007). The ICHD-II is a diagnostic tool and does not adequately address potential variables or the reduction of features secondary to effective treatment.

In a study evaluating the sensitivity of ICHD-II criteria for paediatric migraine, headache characteristics in 260 patients aged 18 years or younger and diagnosed with migraine were summarised from standard intake questionnaires, and physician-assigned clinical diagnoses were used as the criterion standard for assessing the validity of ICHD-II criteria (Table 10.2) (Hershey et al 2005, Bigal et al 2008). Among the 260 patients clinically diagnosed with migraine, 70.4% met ICHD-I criteria and 61.9% met ICHD-II criteria, including the 4- to 72-hour headache duration. When a 1- to 72-hour duration specified in the ICHD-II footnote was used, 71.9% met the criteria. The most common reasons for patients' headaches not meeting the standard criteria were the requirements for unilateral location, headache duration and number of associated symptoms. When the ICHD-II criteria were modified to the proposed criteria for paediatric migraine to include bilateral headache, headache duration of 1 to 72 hours, and nausea and/or vomiting plus two of five other associated symptoms (photophobia, phonophobia, difficulty thinking, lightheadedness or fatigue), the sensitivity for diagnosing migraine improved to 84.4% (Table 10.3). Given the significant heterogeneity in associated

TABLE 10.2
Migraine without aura (ICHD-II)

Diagnostic criteria	Comments
(A) At least five attacks fulfilling criteria B–D[a]	
(B) Headache attacks lasting 4–72h (untreated or unsuccessfully treated)	Sleeping during headache attack is included in duration[b]
	In children, attacks lasting 1–2h are allowed, supported by diary[c,d]
(C) Headache has at least two of the following characteristics:	
(1) Unilateral location	Bilateral and frontal headache are common in children[e,f]
	Exclusive occipital location is worrisome based on meta-analysis[f]
(2) Pulsating quality[g]	
(3) Moderate or severe pain intensity	
(4) Aggravated by or causes avoidance of routine physical activity (e.g. walking or climbing stairs)	
(D) During headache at least one of the following:	
(1) Nausea and/or vomiting	Can be inferred by their behaviour by the parents[h]
(2) Photophobia and phonophobia[h]	
(E) Not attributed to another disorder[i]	

[a]Differentiating *migraine without aura* and *infrequent episodic tension-type headache* may be difficult, hence at least five attacks are required. Individuals who otherwise meet the criteria for *migraine without aura* but have had fewer than five attacks should be coded *probable migraine without aura*. [b]When the patient falls asleep during migraine and wakes up without it, duration of the attack is reckoned until the time of awakening. [c]In children, attacks may last 1 to 72 hours (although the evidence for the untreated durations of less than 2 hours in children requires corroboration by prospective diary studies). [d]When attacks occur on at least 15 days per month for more than 3 months, code as *migraine without aura* and as *chronic migraine*. [e]Migraine headache is commonly bilateral in young children; an adult pattern of unilateral pain usually emerges in late adolescent or early adult life. [f]Migraine headache is usually frontotemporal. Occipital headache in *children*, whether unilateral or bilateral, is rare and calls for diagnostic caution; many cases are attributable to structural lesions. [g]*Pulsating* means throbbing or varying with the heartbeat. [h]In young children, photophobia and phonophobia may be inferred from their behaviour. [i]History and physical and neurological examinations do not suggest any of the disorders listed in groups 5 to 12, or history and/or physical and/or neurological examinations do not suggest such disorder but it is ruled out by appropriate investigations, or such a disorder is present but attacks do not occur for the first time in close temporal relation to the disorder. ICHD-II: the International Classification of Headache Disorders, 2nd edn. Reproduced from Headache Classification Subcommittee of the International Headache Society (2004).

symptoms among children, increasing the list of associated symptoms improves sensitivity further (Hershey et al 2005, Bigal et al 2008, Lewis et al 2008).

New tools and biomarkers need to be developed and integrated into the diagnostic process. Researchers have begun to examine additional tools for children to augment these criteria and include the use of drawings for the paediatric population (Chapter 31). Presently, the ICHD-II

TABLE 10.3

Proposed modified criteria for paediatric migraine without aura

(A) At least five attacks fulfilling criteria B–D

(B) Headache attacks lasting *1–72h* (untreated or unsuccessfully treated). (Sleep is also considered part of the headache duration)

(C) Headache has at least two of the following characteristics:

  (1) *Bifrontal/bitemporal* or unilateral location

  (2) Pulsating/*throbbing* quality[a]

  (3) Moderate or severe pain intensity[a,b] (numerical scale, faces scale)

  (4) Aggravation by or causing avoidance of routine physical activity[a]

(D) During headache at least one of the following:

  (1) Nausea and/or vomiting[a]

  (2) *Two of five symptoms (photophobia, phonophobia, difficulty thinking, lightheadedness or fatigue)*[a]

(E) Not attributed to another disorder

[a]May be inferred from their behaviour. [b]0 to 10 scale or faces scale can be used. Reproduced courtesy of the International Headache Society (www.i-h-s.org).

is an improvement over the initial criteria and it remains the foundation for the diagnosis and scientific study of headache and migraine (Stafstrom et al 2002, 2005, Larsson and Sund 2005, Diamond et al 2007). The clinician needs to make the diagnosis of migraine using the ICHD-II criteria as a guideline to avoid clinically underdiagnosing migraine and potentially missing the opportunity to make an early diagnosis in a patient's life.

Paediatric migraines can have a significant impact on the lives of both the child and the parents. The impact of migraine can be measured by both the disability related to the loss of ability to participate in desired activities and the effect on the individual's quality of life (Chapter 7).

Migraine with aura

Migraine with aura has special challenges when it comes to diagnosis, especially in young children. The aura is a recurrent reversible disorder that is composed of a focal neurological symptom(s) with a gradual onset over 5 to 20 minutes and lasts for less than 60 minutes in its typical form. Auras can consist of visual and/or sensory and/or speech disturbance symptoms in their typical form (Headache Classification Subcommittee of the International Headache Society 2004, Lewis et al 2008).

Abrupt onset of aura(s) and complicated visual images should prompt consideration of benign occipital epilepsy or another paroxysmal disorder. Transient visual obscurations may also be described with idiopathic intracranial hypertension. Auras associated with fully reversible motor weakness and at least one other reversible aura symptom of visual, sensory or speech disturbance are usually associated with familial hemiplegic migraine (FHM). Migraine is classified as FHM if there is a first- or second-degree relative with the condition or sporadic hemiplegic migraine if there is no family history. Auras that last more than an

TABLE 10.4
Migraine aura (fully reversible)

Aura type	Symptoms
Visual	Negative scotoma
	Fortification scotoma
	Field deficits, hemianopic, quadrantanopic, photopsia
	Visual distortions: teichopsia, metamorphopsia, prosopagnosia
Sensory	Numbness
	Tingling
	Perioral numbness
	Hemidysaesthesia
Speech	Dysphasic speech disturbance
Motor	Hemiparesis
	Monoparesis

Reproduced courtesy of the International Headache Society (www.i-h-s.org).

hour and are associated with motor deficits require attention to rule out structural vascular, metabolic or paroxysmal disorders, especially in the paediatric age group. These patients should be considered for neuroimaging, electrophysiological profiles and metabolic workups, as clinically warranted. At the very least, these patients need to be followed more frequently until the diagnosis is confirmed.

Asking the child to draw an aura can often prove diagnostically very helpful. In the paediatric population, an aura can occur in isolation of a headache or associated symptoms. As the children advance in age, more typical phenotypic presentation of migraine with aura will usually be described (Table 10.4). Several subtypes of migraine with aura are described: typical aura with migraine headache, typical aura with non-migraine headache, typical aura without headache, FHM, sporadic hemiplegic migraine and basilar-type migraine (Headache Classification Subcommittee of the International Headache Society 2004).

Typical migraine aura
The ICHD-II criteria for migraine with aura are listed in Table 10.5. Between 15% and 30% of paediatric migraine patients report aura symptoms before or as the headache begins (Lewis et al 2008). The aura is an inconsistent feature in childhood and adolescence. The majority of paediatric patients who have experienced migraine with aura have also experienced migraine without aura. Hachinski's reported three dominant visual phenomena: binocular visual impairment with scotoma (77%); distortion or hallucinations (16%); and monocular visual impairment or scotoma (7%) (Hachinski et al 1973, Lewis et al 2008).

Familial hemiplegic migraine
FHM is an uncommon autosomal dominant form of migraine with aura, which has been associated with a missense mutation in the calcium channel gene (CACNA1A) linked to

TABLE 10.5
Migraine with aura

(A) At least two attacks fulfilling the following criteria B–E

(B) Aura consisting of at least one of the following, but no motor weakness:

    (1) Fully reversible visual symptoms including positive features and/or negative features (e.g. flickering lights, spots or lines)

    (2) Fully reversible sensory symptoms including positive features (i.e. pins and needles) and/or negative features (i.e. numbness)

    (3) Fully reversible dysphasic speech disturbances

(C) At least two of the following:

    (1) Homonymous visual symptoms and/or unilateral sensory symptoms

    (2) At least one aura symptom develops gradually ≥5min and/or different aura symptoms occur in succession ≥ 5 minutes

    (3) Each symptom lasts ≥5min and ≤60min

(D) Migraine aura fulfilling criteria B and C for one of the subforms 1.2.4–1.2.6

(E) Not attributable to another disorder

Reproduced from Headache Classification Subcommittee of the International Headache Society (2004).

chromosome 19p13 (FHM1) in some individuals. FHM1 episodes can be triggered by mild head trauma. In approximately 50% of families with FHM1, chronic progressive cerebellar ataxia occurs independent of the migraine headache attack. A series of recent discoveries about the molecular genetics of FHM have broadened our understanding of the fundamental mechanisms of migraine and demonstrated the overlap with other paroxysmal disorders such as acetazolamide-responsive episodic ataxia (Joutel et al 1993). FHM2 accounts for less than 25% of the cases and is caused by a mutation in the Na/K-ATPase gene ATP1A2. FHM3 is a rare subtype that is caused by a mutation in the sodium channel α-subunit-coding gene *SCNA1*. These three subtypes account for most, but not all, the cases of FHM, supporting the existence of at least one other form, FHM4. Separate pedigrees with linkage to chromosome 1q31 (FHM4) have been reported (Gardner et al 1997).

    FHM is a subtype of migraine with aura that includes motor weakness and occurs only in patients who have at least one first- or second-degree relative who experiences similar migraine with aura including motor weakness (Table 10.6). The symptoms can often be described as stroke-like symptoms of hemiparesis. Clinically, to receive the diagnosis of hemiplegic migraine, true weakness must be demonstrated. Patients who complain about a feeling of heaviness, but without measurable weakness documented, should not be classified as having hemiplegic migraine (Lewis et al 2008).

    The appearance of acute, focal neurological deficits in the setting of headache in an adolescent necessitates vigorous investigation for disorders such as intracranial haemorrhage, stroke, tumour and vascular malformations. Complex partial seizure or drug intoxication with a sympathomimetic must also be considered. Neuroimaging [magnetic resonance imaging (MRI) and/or magnetic resonance angiography (MRA)] and electroencephalography (EEG)

TABLE 10.6

Diagnostic criteria of familial hemiplegic migraine

(A) Fulfils criteria for migraine with aura

(B) Aura consisting of fully reversible motor weakness and at least one of the following:

    (1) Fully reversible visual symptoms including positive features (e.g. flickering lights, spots or lines) and/or negative features (e.g. loss of vision)

    (2) Fully reversible sensory symptoms including positive features (e.g. pins and needles)

    (3) Fully reversible dysphasic speech disturbance

(C) At least two of the following:

    (1) At least one aura symptom develops gradually over >5min

    (2) Each aura symptom lasts >5min and <24h

    (3) Headache that fulfils criteria for migraine without aura begins during the aura or follows the onset of aura within 60min

(D) At least one first-degree or second-degree relative has had attacks fulfilling criteria A–E

(E) At least one of the following:

    (1) History, physical and neurological examinations not suggesting any organic disorder

    (2) History, physical or neurological examinations suggesting such disorder, but is ruled out by appropriate investigations

    (3) Such disorder is present, but migraine attacks do not occur for the first time in close temporal relation to the disorder

Reproduced from Headache Classification Subcommittee of the International Headache Society (2004).

may be indicated. Investigations for embolic sources/hypercoagulable or medical disorders are appropriate (Lewis et al 2008).

Transient episodes of focal neurological deficits precede the headache phase by 30 to 60 minutes but, occasionally, extend well beyond the headache itself (hours to days). The location of headache is often, but not invariably, contralateral to the focal deficits.

Sporadic hemiplegic migraine
The diagnostic criteria are the same as for FHM except for the requirement for an affected first- or second-degree relative.

Basilar-type migraine
The formal diagnosis of basilar-type migraine requires the presence of objective signs or symptoms of brainstem or posterior fossa involvement. There is a wide range because of the rigour of this diagnosis; ICHD-II criteria are shown in Table 10.7 (Bickerstaff 1961, Golden and French 1975, Lapkin and Golden 1978). Basilar-type migraine tends to present in young children, with the mean age being 7 years, although the clinical entity may present much earlier in childhood as episodic pallor, clumsiness and vomiting, possibly in association with a condition known as benign paroxysmal vertigo.

Attacks are characterised by episodes of intense dizziness, vertigo, visual disturbances,

TABLE 10.7

Diagnostic criteria for basilar-type migraine

(A) Fulfils criteria for migraine with aura

(B) Two or more symptoms of the following types

    (1) Dysarthria

    (2) Vertigo

    (3) Tinnitus

    (4) Hypacusia

    (5) Diplopia

    (6) Visual symptoms simultaneously in both the temporal and nasal fields of both eyes

    (7) Ataxia

    (8) Decreased level of consciousness

    (9) Simultaneous bilateral paraesthesias

(C) At least one of the following:

    (1) At least one aura symptom develops gradually over 5min

    (2) Different aura symptoms occur in succession over 5 min

    (3) Each aura symptom lasts ≥ 5 and ≤ 60 min

(D) Headache fulfilling criteria B–D for migraine without aura begins during the aura or follows aura within 60min

Reproduced from Headache Classification Subcommittee of the International Headache Society (2004).

ataxia and diplopia. The initial symptoms may last for minutes or up to 1 hour and are then followed by the headache phase. The head pain may include the occipital region. Some patients may describe dizziness and ataxia in association with aura after the headache symptoms have started.

There should be a low threshold for investigating a patient who presents with posterior fossa symptoms accompanied by headache, including MRI and MRA of the brain and MRI of the upper cervical cord, EEG and metabolic studies such as ammonia, lactic acid and drug screens in patients who present with the above symptom complex (Lewis et al 2008).

Confusional migraine

Confusional migraine is often termed a migraine variant that is reported in children and adolescents, but has been omitted from the ICHD criteria. It is reported, usually in males, with an abrupt onset of agitation, restlessness, disorientation, behaviour changes and, occasionally, aggression. The confusion has been reported to last from minutes to hours and there may or may not be a recollection of the events and associated headache symptoms. It has been reported to be associated with minor head trauma (Lewis et al 2008).

A patient with a sudden unexplained loss or alteration of consciousness following head injury should be evaluated for an intracranial lesion, drug intoxication, metabolic derangement or paroxysmal disorder. A diagnosis of confusional migraine is a diagnosis of exclusion and may actually be a subset presentation of basilar-type migraine.

Alice in Wonderland syndrome

Alice in Wonderland syndrome has been described as a specific form of migraine with aura, but the visual aura is quite atypical and may include bizarre visual illusions and spatial distortions preceding an otherwise non-descript headache. Affected patients will describe distorted visual perceptions similar to those experienced by Alice in the book *Through the Looking-Glass, and What Alice Found There*, such as micropsia, macropsia, metamorphopsia, teleopsia, macro/microsomatognosia (Lewis et al 2008).

Thus, Alice in Wonderland syndrome is an unusual migraine variant seen in children with visual auras. In children presenting with these symptoms, it is important to address the complex visual–perceptual abnormalities that may occur with infectious mononucleosis or complex partial seizures (particularly benign occipital epilepsy), and in drug ingestions. When a child presents with an unusual complex visual aura history, there should be a low threshold for neuroimaging of the brain with MRI and/or MRA to rule out structural or vascular lesions, electrophysiological profile to address paroxysmal disorders and appropriate metabolic evaluations, as clinically warranted by the situation.

Retinal migraine

Retinal migraine is described as repeated attacks of monocular visual disturbance including scintillations, scotomata or blindness associated with migraine headache. The migraine pain is often described as retro-orbital with ipsilateral visual disturbance (Lewis et al 2008).

Examination of the optic fundi during an attack may disclose constriction of retinal veins and arteries as well as retinal pallor. Vasoconstriction with retinal infarction is thought to be the mechanism for some patients who suffer permanent or prolonged visual dysfunction, such as scotoma, altitudinal defects or monocular blindness, in retinal migraine (Wolter and Burchfield 1971, Hupp et al 1989). Patients with retinal migraine are generally younger than those who experience amaurosis fugax from atheromatous carotid disease. Evaluation for hypercoagulable states, embolic sources and vascular disruption (carotid dissection) needs to be addressed with the appropriate medical and neurological workup (Lewis et al 2008).

Chronic migraine

Chronic migraine primarily evolves from an episodic migraine pattern in children, as it does in adults. The actual time of transformation tends to be shorter in the paediatric population. In adults, the transition time can be 10 to 11 years. In the paediatric population, the time course can be shorter than 2 years. This headache pattern has been previously referred to as transformed migraine, but the term chronic migraine has become the more accepted term over the past few years (Guitera et al 1999, Silberstein and Lipton 2001). Debate still continues regarding the formal classification of chronic migraine; the revised (ICHD-IIR) criteria in Table 10.8 are presently in use, but still spike continuing controversy (Bigal et al 2004, 2005). The observation in adults that as migraines become more frequent their severity and associated symptoms are somewhat diminished is clinically noted in the paediatric population, but this not always the case (Hershey et al 2001a, Bigal et al 2005). The ICHD-IIR criteria require only 8 days per month of headaches to qualify as migraine with a total frequency of greater

TABLE 10.8

Chronic migraine: evolution of classification and diagnosis

(A) Headache on ≥15d/mo for ≥3mo

(B) Five or more prior migraine attacks

(C) On 8 or more days per month, headache fulfils criteria for migraine

    (1) Two or more of the following: (a) unilateral; (b) throbbing; (c) moderate or severe pain; (d) aggravated by physical activity

    (2) One or more of the following: (a) nausea and/ or vomiting; (b) photophobia and phonophobia

    (3) Relieved with triptans or ergotamines

(D) Not attributed to another causative disorder

(E) Subclassified as *without* medication overuse headache as defined in section 8.2 ICHD-II

ICD-II, International Classification of Headache Disorders, 2nd edn. Reproduced courtesy of the International Headache Society (www.i-h-s.org).

than 15 days per month (Olesen et al 2006). The influence of medication overuse also remains controversial, and the application of the criteria for chronic migraine and medication overuse headache is felt to be in conflict. The clinical recommendation presently is not to require medication cessation before being able to make a diagnosis of chronic migraine (Olesen et al 2006).

CASE PRESENTATION

A 14-year-old female presents with a history of headaches since age 11. Her headaches initially were episodic, once every 2 to 3 months. They were bifrontal, throbbing and lasted 1 to 2 hours. The episodes tended to escalate quickly, with photophobia and phonophobia. She lost her appetite but denied vomiting. These headaches did not respond to acetaminophen. She would often seek out a dark, quiet room and was unable to read or exercise.

Over the last 2 years her headaches have increased in frequency, and now occur on 4 or 5 days per week. The headaches remain bifrontal with fluctuating levels of pain, primarily moderate, but occasionally severe. The headaches presently last 4 to 6 hours, and occasionally all day. Her past medical history is unremarkable. Her mother and brother have been diagnosed with migraine, which reportedly occurs once or twice a month. She is a good student and active in extracurricular activity when she is not disabled by the headaches. She denies the use of drugs, alcohol or cigarettes. She denies sexual activity. Medical and neurological examinations are normal.

This patient's history is most consistent with chronic migraine.

Now that she has a diagnosis, this patient will need appropriate treatment algorithms for both acute and preventive therapy. The first step in managing this, or any, patient is to make an accurate diagnosis, and then to educate the patient and his or her parents as to the mechanism of migraine/chronic migraine.

CLINICAL CHARACTERISTICS

Patients with chronic migraine often complain of severe migraine episodes superimposed on milder headaches (Wang et al 2006). These milder headaches are often misdiagnosed as tension-type or even sinus headaches by the patient or parent(s). The severe episodes can occur multiple times a week.

Many adolescents with chronic migraine will complain of continuous headaches that are present daily. Some of these patients will experience a headache for only a few hours each day, whereas others describe continuous headache that waxes and wanes in severity, often being worse in the morning or at the end of the school day. The clinical characteristics of the continuous headache pain are similar to the episodes of severe headaches, only much less intense (Wang et al 2006).

Other features of chronic migraine include allodynia and ice-pick pain. Chronic migraine patients may experience allodynia over all or part of their head. Allodynia is hypersensitivity to touch on part of the scalp or face that occurs with severe migraines. Some patients may experience ice-pick head pain symptoms, intermittently, oftentimes multifocal, occurring for seconds at a time and happening many times during the day (Hershey et al 2008).

Patients with chronic migraine can also experience symptoms that include dizziness, sleep disturbance, neck pain, abdominal pain, fatigue, difficulty in concentration and altered mood (Hershey et al 2008).

Those patients who do experience dizziness often deny vertigo. The dizziness is often positional, and patients will complain of near-syncope symptoms. The dizziness is particularly prominent in the morning, and if patients are dehydrated. It is important to consider postural orthostatic tachycardia syndrome in the differential diagnosis if they experience tachycardia on standing. If they experience a decrease in systolic blood pressure with standing, consider neurocardiogenic syncope. A tilt-table test will help confirm these diagnoses. Orthostatic symptoms can be treated by increasing the patient's fluid and salt intake and, when medically indicated, by the use of beta-blockers (Hershey et al 2008).

The physician is responsible for addressing and ruling out secondary causes of headache and for providing appropriate reassurance to the patients and their families whenever the diagnosis of chronic migraine is made. The most important step in making an accurate diagnosis of chronic daily headache in a young person is a comprehensive and thorough history and physical examination. When medically indicated, neuroimaging, laboratory studies, electrophysiology evaluations and occasionally a lumbar puncture may need to be obtained. Some patients may require other medical evaluations such as a tilt-table test or sleep studies depending on the clinical situation (Hershey et al 2008).

The majority of patients who present with chronic daily headache will have a history consistent with ICHD-IIR chronic migraine. But for those who do not fit the criteria, it is important to address the appropriate medical workup for the differential diagnoses (Hershey et al 2008).

The majority of patients presenting with chronic migraine will have a normal medical and neurological physical examination, which should include measurement of blood pressure for hypertension and head circumference for macrocephaly, a clue of unrecognised chronic hydrocephalus or subdural collections. Examination should also include the skin, to look for hints of neurofibromatosis, tuberous sclerosis or other neurocutaneous disorder (Hershey et al 2008), and fundoscopic examination to rule out the presence of papilloedema and increased intracranial pressure. Examination of the spine with attention to the cervical region may reveal trigger points. In the presence of focal neurological signs or a history of seizures, there will often be abnormal neuroimaging (Meskunas et al 2006). Fortunately, in the majority of patients with chronic migraine, neuroimaging is normal. Occasional abnormalities such as vascular anomalies, white matter abnormalities, arachnoid cysts or pineal cysts are generally of little or no clinical significance (Mathew et al 1990).

Clinical assessment for idiopathic intracranial hypertension is discussed in Chapter 23 and post-traumatic headache in Chapter 25. Other investigations will be considered as clinically appropriate, such as thyroid function tests, inflammatory markers (erythrocyte sedimentation rate), serology for viral diseases and Lyme disease, lumbar puncture and cerebrospinal fluid pressure and antibodies for systemic lupus erythematosus (Hershey et al 2008).

The first step in managing chronic migraine is an accurate diagnosis and reassurance to both the patient and his or her parents that this is not a life-threatening illness. It is important to discuss current understanding of the mechanism of chronic migraine and how it influences the potential development of comorbidities. It is often difficult for both patients and parents to comprehend that headaches can persist for such a long time and be so disabling, even though diagnostic studies are negative. In order to limit the patient and family's frustration it is important to spend adequate time reviewing the comprehensive management of chronic migraine, including the avoidance of excessive usage of over-the-counter medication and the proper use of pharmacological and non-pharmacological treatments (Hershey et al 2008).

Migraine disability
Migraine results in significant disability in children and adolescents, causing absence from school, absence from social opportunities and disruption of family activities. Several tools have been developed to evaluate the disability of migraine (Chapter 7). In adults this can be addressed by using the MIDAS (Migraine Disability Assessment) tool (Stewart et al 1999, 2000, 2001, Lipton et al 2001). The Pediatric Migraine Disability Assessment Score (PedMIDAS) can be used to identify the impact of migraine on children as well as the children's responses to treatment (Hershey et al 2001b, 2004).

The impact of migraine can also be assessed by measuring the child's quality of life. The Pediatric Quality of Life 4 (PedsQL 4.0) (Osterhaus et al 1994) is a 23-question tool, with separate sex-appropriate versions for those aged between 5 and 17 years, that uses responses from both the child and the parents (Varni et al 2001, Powers et al 2004).

Conclusion
Migraine and chronic migraine are common in the paediatric population. The high incidence and prevalence of migraine in children and adolescents has a significant impact on both patients and their families. Early accurate diagnosis coupled with a comprehensive management plan is essential to help minimise the disability associated with migraine, to potentially prevent its progression and for the development of comorbid disorders.

Migraine with aura and its many subtypes represent a fascinating and challenging group of disorders characterised by the onset of focal neurological signs and symptoms such as hemiparesis, altered consciousness or ophthalmoparesis followed by headache. Often, these ominous neurological signs initially lead the clinician in the direction of epileptic, cerebro-vascular, traumatic or metabolic disorders, and only after a thorough history and physical examination, and appropriate neurodiagnostic studies, does the diagnosis become apparent. Some of these entities occur in infants and young children, in whom the history is limited, thus making accurate diagnosis even more challenging.

REFERENCES

Bickerstaff ER (1961) Basilar artery migraine. *Lancet* 1:15–17. http://dx.doi.org/10.1016/S0140-6736(61)92184-5

Bigal ME, Tepper SJ, Sheftell FD, Rapoport AM, Lipton RB (2004) Chronic daily headache: correlation between the 2004 and the 1988 International Headache Society diagnostic criteria. *Headache* 44: 684–91. http://dx.doi.org/10.1111/j.1526-4610.2004.04128.x

Bigal ME, Rapoport AM, Tepper SJ, Sheftell FD, Lipton RB (2005) The classification of chronic daily headache in adolescents – a comparison between the second edition of the international classification of headache disorders and alternative diagnostic criteria. *Headache* 45: 582–9.

Bigal ME, Lipton RB, Winner P (2008) Epidemiology and classification of headache. In: Winner P, Lewis DW, Rothner AD, editors. *Headache in Children and Adolescents,* 2nd edn. Hamilton: BC Decker, pp. 1–18.

Diamond S, Bigal ME, Silberstein S, Loder E, Reed M, Lipton RB (2007) Patterns of diagnosis and acute and preventive treatment for migraine in the United States: results from the American Migraine Prevalence and Prevention study. *Headache* 47: 355–63.

Gardner K, Barmada MM, Ptacek LJ, Hoffman EP (1997) A new locus for hemiplegic migraine maps to chromosome 1q31. *Neurology* 49: 1231–8. http://dx.doi.org/10.1212/WNL.49.5.1231

Golden GS, French JH (1975) Basilar artery migraine in young children. *Pediatrics* 56: 722–6.

Guitera V, Muñoz P, Castillo J, Pascual J (1999) Transformed migraine: a proposal for the modification of its diagnostic criteria based on recent epidemiological data. *Cephalalgia* 19: 847–50. http://dx.doi.org/10.1046/j.1468-2982.1999.1910847.x

Hachinski VC, Porchawka J, Steele JC (1973) Visual symptoms in the migraine syndrome. *Neurology* 23: 570–9. http://dx.doi.org/10.1212/WNL.23.6.570

Headache Classification Subcommittee of the International Headache Society (2004) The International Classification of Headache Disorders. *Cephalalgia* 24 (Suppl 1): 16–36.

Hershey AD, Powers SW, Bentti AL, LeCates S, deGrauw TJ (2001a) Characterization of chronic daily headaches in children in a multidisciplinary headache center. *Neurology* 56: 1032–7. http://dx.doi.org/10.1212/WNL.56.8.1032

Hershey AD, Powers SW, Vockell AL, LeCates S, Kabbouche MA, Maynard MK (2001b) PedMIDAS: development of a questionnaire to assess disability of migraines in children. *Neurology* 57: 2034–9. http://dx.doi.org/10.1212/WNL.57.11.2034

Hershey AD, Powers SW, Vockell AL, LeCates SL, Segers A, Kabbouche MA (2004) Development of a patient-based grading scale for PedMIDAS. *Cephalalgia* 24: 844–9. http://dx.doi.org/10.1111/j.1468-2982.2004.00757.x

Hershey AD, Winner P, Kabbouche MA et al (2005) Use of the ICHD-II criteria in the diagnosis of pediatric migraine. *Headache* 45: 1288–97. http://dx.doi.org/10.1111/j.1526-4610.2005.00260.x

Hershey A, Gladstein J, Mack K, Winner P, Lewis D (2008) Chronic daily headaches in children and adolescents. In: Winner P, Lewis D, Rothner AD, editors. *Headache in Children and Adolescents*. Hamilton: McGraw-Hill Medical, pp. 127–43.

Hupp SL, Kline LB, Corbett JJ (1989) Visual disturbances of migraine. *Surv Ophthalmol* 33: 221–36. http://dx.doi.org/10.1016/0039-6257(82)90149-7

Joutel A, Bousser M-G, Biousse V et al (1993) A gene for familial hemiplegic migraine maps to chromosome 19. *Nat Genet* 5: 40–5. http://dx.doi.org/10.1038/ng0993-40

Lapkin ML, Golden GS (1978) Basilar artery migraine, a review of 30 cases. *Am J Dis Child* 132: 278–81.

Larsson B, Sund AM (2005) One-year incidence, course, and outcome predictors of frequent headaches among early adolescents. *Headache* 45: 684–91. http://dx.doi.org/10.1111/j.1526-4610.2005.05137a.x

Laurell K, Larsson B, Eeg-Olofsson O (2004) Prevalence of headache in Swedish schoolchildren, with a focus on tension-type headache. *Cephalalgia* 24: 380–8. http://dx.doi.org/10.1111/j.1468-2982.2004.00681.x

Lewis D, Bigal M, Winner P (2008) Migraine and the childhood periodic syndromes. In: Winner P, Lewis D, Rothner AD, editors. *Headache in Children and Adolescents*. Hamilton: McGraw-Hill Medical, pp. 37–55.

Lipton RB, Silberstein SD, Stewart WF (1994) An update on the epidemiology of migraine. *Headache* 34: 319–28. http://dx.doi.org/10.1111/j.1526-4610.1994.hed3406319.x

Lipton RB, Stewart WF, Sawyer J, Edmeads JG (2001) Clinical utility of an instrument assessing migraine disability: the Migraine Disability Assessment (MIDAS) questionnaire. *Headache* 41: 854–61.

Mathew NT, Kurman R, Perez F (1990) Drug induced refractory headache – clinical features and management. *Headache* 30: 633–7. http://dx.doi.org/10.1111/j.1526-4610.1990.hed3010634.x

Meskunas CA, Tepper SJ, Rapoport AM, Sheftell FD, Bigal ME (2006) Medications associated with probable medication overuse headache reported in a tertiary care headache center over a 15-year period. *Headache* 46: 766–72. http://dx.doi.org/10.1111/j.1526-4610.2006.00442.x

Olesen J, Bousser MG, Diener HC, et al (2006) New appendix criteria open for a broader concept of chronic migraine. *Cephalalgia* 26: 742–6. http://dx.doi.org/10.1111/j.1468-2982.2006.01172.x

Osterhaus JT, Townsend RJ, Gandek B, Ware JE Jr (1994) Measuring the functional status and well-being of patients with migraine headache. *Headache* 34: 337–43. http://dx.doi.org/10.1111/j.1526-4610.1994.hed3406337.x

Powers SW, Patton SR, Hommel KA, Hershey AD (2004) Quality of life in paediatric migraine: characterization of age-related effects using PedsQL 4.0. *Cephalalgia* 24: 120–7. http://dx.doi.org/10.1111/j.1468-2982.2004.00652.x

Silberstein S, Lipton R (2001) Chronic daily headache including transformed migraine, chronic tension-type headache, and medication over-use. In: Silberstein SD, Lipton RB, Dalessio DJ, editors. *Wolff's headache and other head pain.* New York: Oxford University Press, pp. 247–82.

Stafstrom CE, Rostasy K, Minster A (2002) The usefulness of children's drawings in the diagnosis of headache. *Pediatrics* 109: 460–72. http://dx.doi.org/10.1542/peds.109.3.460

Stafstrom CE, Goldenholz SR, Dulli DA (2005) Serial headache drawings by children with migraine: correlation with clinical headache status. *J Child Neurol* 20: 809–13. http://dx.doi.org/10.1177/08830738050200100501

Stewart WF, Linet MS, Celentano DD, Van Natta M, Siegler D (1991) Age and sex-specific incidence rates of migraine with and without visual aura. *Am J Epidemiol* 34: 1111–20.

Stewart WF, Lipton RB, Celentano DD, Reed ML (1992) Prevalence of migraine headache in the United States. *JAMA* 267: 64–9. http://dx.doi.org/10.1001/jama.1992.03480010072027

Stewart WF, Lipton RB, Whyte J et al (1999) An international study to assess reliability of the Migraine Disability Assessment (MIDAS) score. *Neurology* 53: 988–94. http://dx.doi.org/10.1212/WNL.53.5.988

Stewart WF, Lipton RB, Kolodner KB, Sawyer J, Lee C, Liberman JN (2000) Validity of the Migraine Disability Assessment (MIDAS) score in comparison to a diary-based measure in a population sample of migraine sufferers. *Pain* 88: 41–52. http://dx.doi.org/10.1016/S0304-3959(00)00305-5

Stewart WF, Lipton RB, Dowson AJ, Sawyer J (2001) Development and testing of the Migraine Disability Assessment (MIDAS) questionnaire to assess headache-related disability. *Neurology* 56 (Suppl 1): S20–8. http://dx.doi.org/10.1212/WNL.56.suppl_1.S20

Varni JW, Seid M, Kurtin PS (2001) PedsQL 4.0: reliability and validity of the Pediatric Quality of Life Inventory version 4.0 generic core scales in healthy and patient populations. *Med Care* 39: 800–12. http://dx.doi.org/10.1097/00005650-200108000-00006

Virtanen R, Aromaa M, Rautava P et al (2007) Changing headache from preschool age to puberty. A controlled study. *Cephalalgia* 27: 294–303. http://dx.doi.org/10.1111/j.1468-2982.2007.01277.x

Wang SJ, Fuh JL, Lu SR, Juang KD (2006) Chronic daily headache in adolescents: prevalence, impact, and medication overuse. *Neurology* 66: 193–7. http://dx.doi.org/10.1212/01.wnl.0000183555.54305.fd

Wolter JR, Burchfield WJ (1971) Ocular migraine in a young man resulting in unilateral transient blindness and retinal edema. *J Pediatr Ophthalmol* 8: 173–6.

11
MANAGEMENT OF ACUTE ATTACKS OF MIGRAINE

Mirja Hämäläinen

Non-pharmacological management
To guarantee a sound basis for the treatment of migraine attacks in children, one must ensure that the child adopts a lifestyle that reduces the trigger factors of migraine attacks. The child should be encouraged to maintain a good state of hydration, drink adequate amounts of fluids, eat regular meals with high fibre intake, especially for breakfast, adopt a good sleeping pattern and participate in suitable physical activity and outdoor life (Millichap and Yee 2003).

Sunglasses and a brim hat to protect against bright light and sunlight, especially on the water and in a snowy environment, have been suggested to reduce the effects of light as a strong trigger factor, although the evidence to support this advice is weak. The head should also be protected against heavy concussions in contact sports. One trigger for migraine attacks may be computer use (Rossi et al 2001, Oksanen et al 2005).

General principles
Patients and parents may have already found that some non-pharmacological factors can alleviate pain and suffering during attacks of migraine. Patients tend to seek rest in a darkened and quiet room. Some children find sleep to be a very good relieving factor and tend to go to bed hoping to have recovered upon awakening. Other children report that vomiting relieves or alleviates the pain of migraine.

The symptoms of migraine, including visual aura and vomiting in addition to the severe pain, can be very disabling and may last for several hours (Mortimer et al 1992, Hämäläinen et al 1996). Therefore, if the attack is not relieved simply by sleeping, drug treatment is necessary. An adequate dose of the drug should be given as early as possible after the onset of the symptoms for maximum benefit. Several studies have shown that the earlier the treatment is given, the better the response will be, especially if nausea and vomiting are early features in the course of the attacks. The early administration of paracetamol or ibuprofen seems to diminish the nausea occurring during the migraine attack.

A second dose can be given after 2 hours. The recommended daily doses and adult doses should not be exceeded.

SIMPLE ANALGESICS

Paracetamol (acetaminophen) and ibuprofen are the only two analgesic medications that were shown to be effective and safe in the treatment of migraine attacks in children in double-blind, placebo-controlled trials (Hämäläinen et al 1997b, Lewis et al 2002, Evers et al 2006). There is no evidence to support the use of other analgesics.

Paracetamol (acetaminophen) and ibuprofen

Paracetamol (15mg/kg, maximum 60mg/kg/d) and ibuprofen (10mg/kg, maximum 40mg/kg/d) given orally are safe and effective in the treatment of migraine attack in children. The effect of paracetamol begins sooner than that of ibuprofen, but ibuprofen is twice as likely as paracetamol to induce complete resolution of symptoms, as shown in several double-blind, placebo-controlled trials. Paracetamol is suitable for children of all ages and ibuprofen is recommended for children over the age of 1 year. Their simultaneous use is not encouraged.

It is important to use the formulation most acceptable for the child, such as solutions and effervescent tablets if the child has difficulties in swallowing solid tablets or capsules. Suppositories or rectal solutions may be used in young children who have a problem in accepting oral medications or when nausea and vomiting interfere with the absorption of oral preparation.

Although simple analgesics are safe and effective, they are not suitable for the treatment of frequent migraine attacks or chronic migraine. The frequent use of simple analgesics and especially the use of combination products containing caffeine or codeine increases the risk of medication overuse headache.

Non-steroidal anti-inflammatory drugs

Except for ibuprofen, there is no evidence for the safety and effectiveness of non-steroidal anti-inflammatory drugs; however, in clinical practice, diclofenac may have good analgesic effects in migraine. Naproxen is shown to be effective in adults, but there is no evidence for its efficacy or safety in children. Aspirin is not recommended in children under the age of 15 years because of the risk of Reye syndrome.

Codeine and other narcotics

The use of codeine and other narcotics is not recommended for routine use in childhood migraine because of the risk of side effects and dependence. Preparations with a combination of analgesics containing codeine are also not recommended.

SPECIFIC ANTIMIGRAINE MEDICATIONS (TRIPTANS)

Triptans are serotonin (5-hydroxytryptamine) 1B and D receptor agonists and their actions are specific for migraine. Their exact mechanism of action is not known but involves both vaso-constriction of cerebral blood vessels and neuronal inhibition on the trigeminovascular system.

Triptans are effective in the treatment of acute migraine attacks from the onset of head-ache phase, but they seem to be less effective when given during the aura phase (when the brain vessels may be constricted). Owing to their vasoconstrictive properties on the cerebral

TABLE 11.1

Drugs used in the treatment of acute migraine attack in children and adolescents

Drug	Licensed for	Single dose	Maximum dose, must not exceed adult dose	Minimum dose interval (h)	Dosing form
Ibuprofen[a]	All ages	10–20mg/kg	40mg/kg/d	2	Oral suspension Effervescent tablet
Paracetamol[a]	All ages	10–15mg/kg	60mg/kg/d	2	Rapid tablet Oral suspension tablet
Sumatriptan[a]	>12y	10mg (20–39kg)[a] 2mg (>39kg)	20mg/d 40mg/d	2	Nasal spray
Rizatriptan	>18y	5mg (20–39kg) 10mg (>39kg)	10mg/d 20mg/d	2	Tablet
Zolmitriptan	>18y	5mg 2.5mg	10mg/d 5mg/d	2	Nasal spray Tablet
Prochlorperazine	Weight >10kg	0.10–0.30mg/kg 0.1–0.15mg/kg	0.4–0.5mg/kg/d Max. single dose 10mg	4	Tablet Injection solution

[a]Drugs and dosages licensed for children and adolescents in the UK.

circulation, triptans are particularly not recommended in the treatment of hemiplegic and basilar artery-type migraine.

Data on the use of oral triptans in children are very limited. The small number of trials of oral triptans have shown a poor response to active medications compared with the high placebo response rate (Winner et al 2007).

Sumatriptan

Several double-blind, placebo-controlled trials have shown sumatriptan nasal spray to be effective in the treatment of acute migraine attacks in children and adolescents (Ueberall and Wenzel 1999, Winner et al 2000, 2006, Ahonen et al 2004). Sumatriptan nasal spray has been shown to be superior to placebo in relieving pain within 2 hours and has an excellent safety profile. Bitter or bad taste is the most common side effect reported by children. Sumatriptan nasal spray is licensed for the treatment of migraine in children and adolescents of 12 years of age in the European Union but not in the USA. In order to avoid the sensitisation of the central pain pathways, which decreases the efficacy of sumatriptan (Burstein et al 2005), a dose of 10mg or 20mg (maximum twice daily) should be given within 30 minutes of the onset of the headache.

Sumatriptan oral preparations are available in 25mg, 50mg and 100mg tablets for therapy-resistant migraine attacks, but they are not as effective in children and adolescents as they are in adults. In comparative trials, no difference has been shown between oral sumatriptan and the placebo (Hämäläinen et al 1997a).

Sumatriptan subcutaneous injections are ineffective in children and not recommended, as it is available only in one preloaded auto-injector adult dose of 6mg (Linder 1996). However, some benefit of its use was reported from an open study.

Rizatriptan

Rizatriptan tablets may be effective in the treatment of migraine attacks in children, but further evidence is needed before it can be recommended. Rizatriptan is not yet licensed for children and adolescents (Winner et al 2002, Ahonen et al 2006).

Zolmitriptan

Zolmitriptan nasal spray may relieve migraine attacks in adolescents aged 12 to 17 years – based on limited evidence – but it is not licensed for this age group (Lewis et al 2007).

Zolmitriptan tablets may have a role to play in the treatment of migraine attacks in children aged 6 to 18 years, even if the evidence is contradictory (Evers et al 2006, Rothner et al 2006).

Eletriptan

There is no evidence for eletriptan's effectiveness in children, and studies have found children's responses to eletriptan and placebo to be similar.

ANTIEMETICS

Antiemetic drugs may be useful in the treatment of acute migraine attacks in some children if nausea and vomiting are early symptoms and impair the absorption of oral medications. The selection of antiemetic medications available varies in different countries, but may include metoclopramide, domperidone and prochlorperazine.

Prochlorperazine has been studied in an emergency setting (Kabbouche et al 2001, Brousseau et al 2004). In the treatment of prolonged severe migraine attacks, intravenous prochlorperazine (0.1–0.3mg/kg, maximum single dose 10mg) may be beneficial, at least temporarily.

The extrapyramidal and dystonic adverse events are distressing when they occur. Although such side effects are temporary and disappear upon clearance of drug from the body, their occurrence discourages the use of antiemetic medications.

Summary

Medications and their doses for the treatment of acute migraine attacks are listed in Table 11.1. In the treatment of migraine attacks, oral paracetamol (acetaminophen) and ibuprofen are effective first-line treatments. Their simultaneous use is not recommended.

Nasal sumatriptan is effective against migraine attacks in children and adolescents. It is licensed for children 12 years of age and over (in Europe). The highest effect is attained if the spray is insufflated within the first 30 minutes of the onset of headache.

Oral rizatriptan may be effective but further studies are needed. Nasal zolmitriptan has shown efficacy in adolescents, but further studies are needed. Oral zolmitriptan may be effective in 6- to 18-year-olds, even if evidence is contradictory. The response to oral eletriptan was similar to that to placebo in adolescents.

Prochlorperazine has been studied in the treatment of therapy-resistant migraine attacks in an emergency clinic.

REFERENCES

Ahonen K, Hämäläinen ML, Rantala H, Hoppu K (2004) Nasal sumatriptan is effective in treatment of migraine attacks in children: a randomized trial. *Neurology* 62: 883–7. http://dx.doi.org/10.1212/01. WNL.0000115105.05966.A7

Ahonen K, Hämäläinen ML, Eerola M, Hoppu K (2006) A randomized trial of rizatriptan in migraine attacks in children. *Neurology* 67: 1135–40. http://dx.doi.org/10.1212/01.wnl.0000238179.79888.44

Brousseau DC, Duffy SJ, Anderson AC, Linakis JG (2004) Treatment of pediatric migraine headaches: a randomized, double-blind trial of prochlorperazine versus ketorolac. *Ann Emerg Med* 43: 256–62. http://dx.doi.org/10.1016/S0196-0644(03)00716-9

Burstein R, Levy D, Jakubowski M (2005) Effects of sensitization of trigeminovascular neurons to triptan therapy during migraine. *Rev Neurol (Paris)* 161: 658–60. http://dx.doi.org/10.1016/S0035-3787(05)85109-4

Evers S, Rahmann A, Kraemer C et al (2006) Treatment of childhood migraine attacks with oral zolmitriptan and ibuprofen. *Neurology* 67: 497–9. http://dx.doi.org/10.1212/01.wnl.0000231138.18629.d5

Hämäläinen ML, Hoppu K, Santavuori P (1996) Pain and disability in migraine or other recurrent headaches as reported by children. *Eur J Neur* 3: 528–32. http://dx.doi.org/10.1111/j.1468-1331.1996.tb00268.x

Hämäläinen ML, Hoppu K, Santavuori P (1997a) Sumatriptan for migraine attacks in children: a randomized placebo-controlled study. Do children with migraine respond to oral sumatriptan differently from adults? *Neurology* 48: 1100–3. http://dx.doi.org/10.1212/WNL.48.4.1100

Hämäläinen ML, Hoppu K, Valkeila E, Santavuori P (1997b) Ibuprofen or acetaminophen for the acute treatment of migraine in children – a double-blind, randomized, placebo-controlled, crossover study. *Neurology* 48: 103–7. http://dx.doi.org/10.1212/WNL.48.1.103

Kabbouche MA, Vockell AL, LeCates S, Powers SW, Hershey AD (2001) Tolerability and effectiveness of prochlorperazine for intractable migraine in children. *Pediatrics* 107: E62. http://dx.doi.org/10.1542/peds.107.4.e62

Lewis DW, Kellstein D, Dahl G et al (2002) Children's ibuprofen suspension for the acute treatment of pediatric migraine. *Headache* 42: 780–6. http://dx.doi.org/10.1046/j.1526-4610.2002.02180.x

Lewis DW, Winner P, Hershey AD, Wasiewski WW, Adolescent Migraine Steering Committee (2007) Efficacy of zolmitriptan nasal spray in adolescent migraine. *Pediatrics* 120: 390–6. http://dx.doi.org/10.1542/peds.2007-0085

Linder SL (1996) Subcutaneous sumatriptan in the clinical setting–the first 50 consecutive patients with acute migraine in a pediatric neurology office practice. *Headache* 36: 419–22. http://dx.doi.org/10.1046/j.1526-4610.1996.3607419.x

Millichap JG, Yee MM (2003) The diet factor in pediatric and adolescent migraine. *Pediatr Neurol* 28: 9–15. http://dx.doi.org/10.1016/S0887-8994(02)00466-6

Mortimer MJ, Kay J, Jaron A (1992) Childhood migraine in general practice: clinical features and characteristics. *Cephalalgia* 12: 238–43. http://dx.doi.org/10.1046/j.1468-2982.1992.1204238.x

Oksanen A, Metsahonkala L, Anttila P et al (2005) Leisure activities in adolescents with headache. *Acta Paediatr* 94: 609–15. http://dx.doi.org/10.1080/08035250410023331

Rossi LN, Cortinovis I, Menegazzo L, Brunelli G, Bossi A, Macchi M (2001) Classification criteria and distinction between migraine and tension-type headache in children. *Dev Med Child Neurol* 43: 45–51. http://dx.doi.org/10.1017/S001216220100007X

Rothner AD, Wasiewski W, Winner P, Lewis D, Stankowski J (2006) Zolmitriptan oral tablet in migraine treatment: high placebo responses in adolescents. *Headache* 46: 101–9. http://dx.doi.org/10.1111/j.1526-4610.2006.00313.x

Ueberall MA, Wenzel D (1999) Intranasal sumatriptan for the acute treatment of migraine in children. *Neurology* 52: 1507–10. http://dx.doi.org/10.1212/WNL.52.7.1507

Winner P, Rothner AD, Saper J et al (2000) A randomized, double-blind, placebo-controlled study of sumatriptan nasal spray in the treatment of acute migraine in adolescents. *Pediatrics* 106: 989–97. http://dx.doi.org/10.1542/peds.106.5.989

Winner P, Lewis D, Visser WH, Jiang K, Ahrens S, Evans JK (2002) Rizatriptan 5 mg for the acute treatment of migraine in adolescents: a randomized, double-blind, placebo-controlled study. *Headache* 42: 49–55. http://dx.doi.org/10.1046/j.1526-4610.2002.02013.x

Winner P, Rothner AD, Wooten JD, Webster C, Ames M (2006) Sumatriptan nasal spray in adolescent migraineurs: a randomized, double-blind, placebo-controlled, acute study. *Headache* 46: 212–22. http://dx.doi.org/10.1111/j.1526-4610.2006.00339.x

Winner P, Linder SL, Lipton RB, Almas M, Parsons B, Pitman V (2007) Eletriptan for the acute treatment of migraine in adolescents: results of a double-blind, placebo-controlled trial. *Headache* 47: 511–18. http://dx.doi.org/10.1111/j.1526-4610.2007.00755.x

12
PREVENTATIVE TREATMENT FOR MIGRAINE AND OTHER HEADACHE DISORDERS

Ishaq Abu-Arafeh

Patients and parents want a treatment that can achieve complete cessation of all migraine attacks for all patients. However, doctors know that it is not possible to achieve this goal and, therefore, it makes sense to aim to reduce the number and duration of attacks as much as possible and to reduce the severity and misery of migraine to the minimum.

In order to achieve the best results from the treatment and an adequate compliance with the advice, it is important to ensure that the following general objectives are achieved before attempting to start treatment:

- An accurate diagnosis of the primary headache disorder is made on the basis of reliable, widely acceptable clinical criteria such as those of the International Classification for Headache Disorder, 2nd edn (ICHD-II).
- Patients and parents have fully understood the diagnosis and been reassured of its benign nature by taking a full clinical history and complete physical examination and have carried out any necessary investigations.
- The doctor understands the patient and his or her family's concerns and addresses them before starting treatment. It is not uncommon for patients and families to express fear of a sinister cause of the headache, such as a brain tumour, and, unless this fear has been adequately assuaged, it will continue to cause anxiety and make the treatment of migraine ineffective. If brain imaging is needed, it should be done early in the management process to avoid prolonged hidden anxieties.
- Patients and parents are given appropriate education about the headache disorder including the natural course of migraine, which is characterised by spells of remissions and relapses.
- Patients, parents and doctors agree on realistic goals and expectations from treatment.
- Patients and parents are aware of the treatment options, the choice of drugs and their efficacy and side effects.
- The roles of patients and relatives in helping the child during headache attacks and in the implementation of prevention strategies is clearly set out.
- A formal, individualised management plan is developed.
- The family doctor, practice nurse and a psychologist, as necessary, are involved in creating the management plan.
- Specific issues such as pregnancy, smoking and trigger factors are discussed.

Non-pharmacological strategies in the prevention of migraine
Non-pharmacological measures should be offered to all children with recurrent headache and particularly those with migraine. Pharmacological prevention of migraine should be reserved for patients with severe, frequent and long attacks of migraine.

HEALTHY LIFESTYLE
Poor lifestyle can be associated with a higher frequency and greater severity of headache in children and adults. A limited number of high-quality randomised studies have shown the importance of a healthy lifestyle in modifying disease course in migraine, but there are many open, uncontrolled studies that can illustrate the relationship between the severity of headache and the poor adherence to a healthy lifestyle in children and in adults.

A study of 344 schoolchildren between 13 and 16 years of age found 22% to have frequent headache of at least one episode per week, and females with frequent headache were more likely to smoke [odds ratio (OR) 6.6; 95% confidence interval (CI) 1.2–35.5], to go to bed later than 11 p.m. (OR 4.4; 95% CI 1.1–18.0) and to take part in few sports activities (OR 3.0; 95% CI 1.2–7.5). In males, frequent headache was highly associated with smoking (OR 12.0; 95% CI 1.5–101). The same study found that headaches improved in pupils participating in a healthy lifestyle programme (Leonardsson-Hellgren 2001). Similar findings were reported for adult patients, with emphasis on the impact of headache on work productivity, and showing reduction in the frequency and severity of headache attacks upon implementation of a healthy lifestyle in the workplace (Parker and Waltman 2012). In addition, the initiation of a migraine education programme on avoiding trigger factors and adopting a healthy lifestyle is shown to improve quality of life in migraine patients (Smith et al 2010).

Children should be encouraged to adopt a healthy lifestyle for its wide range of benefits and not least the reduction of migraine attacks. The following elements are particularly useful for children with migraine:

1 *Regular meals.* Missing a meal is a common trigger factor for migraine attacks in children (Abu-Arafeh and Russell 1994), in particular the morning and midday meals. Children give many reasons for missing meals, but it is important to emphasise the importance of regular meals in order to reduce the number of headache attacks in general and migraine in particular. Children should be encouraged to have a predictable eating pattern by having breakfast before going to school and making reliable arrangements for a lunch, either by taking a packed meal to school or by subscribing to school lunch. If children have their family dinner early in the evening, it may be helpful to take a small supper before going to bed to avoid long periods of fasting during sleep and in order to reduce the occurrence of headache in the morning.

2 *Regular sleep.* Missing out on sleep has also been reported as one of the common triggers of migraine attacks in children (Abu-Arafeh and Russell 1994). Encouraging children to adopt a good bedtime routine, including going to bed at an appropriate time and adhering to it, will help to reduce the frequency of migraine attacks. Feeling fresh in the morning is an indication that the children have had good sleep the previous night. Some children will need the help of a specialist nurse, psychologist or a counsellor to achieve a change

in sleeping routine. Occasionally medical treatment may be necessary to help children initiate sleep and maintain it over a period of time.

3   *Regular exercise and appropriate rest.* It is common for adults and children with sedentary lifestyles to experience an increased frequency of headache, especially if most leisure time is spent watching television, playing video games or working on computers. Children and adults with frequent headache and migraine can reduce the headache attacks by adopting an active lifestyle and participating in sports, social interactions and physical exercise. Strenuous exercise should be avoided and the child should have adequate rest afterwards. Children should also avoid dehydration and ensure a sufficient intake of water on a daily basis.

AVOIDING FOOD TRIGGERS

Although the proportion of children who can identify food triggers is relatively small as compared with adult patients, it is always worth exploring the possible triggers and avoiding them. This is fully discussed in Chapter 28.

ADDRESSING EMOTIONAL AND PSYCHOLOGICAL ISSUES

Episodes of migraine cause misery and disruption to the child and family's life. Frequent migraine attacks impact on the child's education, school attendance and social life. An unpleasant and stressful environment caused by migraine may lead to the worsening of migraine attacks, leading to a vicious circle. Also, migraine can be associated with psychological comorbidities that will further impact on the child and family.

Chapters 26 and 27 look in details at these aspects and their roles in the prevention of migraine.

Pharmacological strategies in the prevention of migraine

Before deciding on the use of medications to prevent migraine attacks, it is important to explore the child and his or her parents' expectations from treatment and explain the less than perfect nature of all antimigraine drugs. Emphasis should be given to education of the child and the family on the roles of medications in reducing the number, duration and severity of migraine attacks, but not to expect cessation of the headache completely, though it would be desirable. Some medications are more suitable for certain children than others, and the aim is to use the drug that is most likely to help the child with the fewest side effects. It is possible that a child may not respond to the first-choice drug and a trial of a second or third drug with different doses may be necessary (Table 12.1).

An important part of the education for the child and family is the nature of preventative treatment, which should be taken regularly over a period of not less than 8 weeks in an optimum dose, before it can be judged effective or ineffective. If proven to be effective, the preventative medication may be taken for at least 6 months before withdrawal is attempted. It is important to avoid any misunderstanding and avoid the use of preventative medications as rescue treatment or for brief courses in small doses.

TABLE 12.1
Drugs for the prevention of migraine in children (see also Chapters 19 and 29)

Drug	Total daily dose	Dose frequency	Evidence
Flunarizine	5–10mg	Once per day	DB, PC, RTs
Topiramate	1–2mg/kg	Once per day	DB, PC trials
Pizotifen	0.5–1.5mg	Once per day	DB, open trials
Propranolol	1–3mg/kg	Twice per day	DB, open trials
Amitriptyline	0.25–1mg/kg	Once per day	Open trials
Sodium valproate	500–1000mg	Twice per day	DB, open trials
Cyproheptadine	2–8mg	One or two doses per day	Open trials

DB, double-blind; PC, placebo controlled; RTs, randomised trials.

EVIDENCE OF EFFICACY OF MIGRAINE-PREVENTATIVE MEDICATIONS

Randomised, double-blind, placebo-controlled trials remain the cornerstone in evaluating the efficacy of medications in migraine prophylaxis. A review of the available evidence of medications for the prevention of migraine in children (Lewis et al 2004a) showed that flunarizine is the only drug that has been properly evaluated and shown to be superior to placebo. Recently, topiramate was also shown to be effective (Lewis et al 2009). Unfortunately, there has been little research into the efficacy of new drugs in childhood migraine; a lack of commercial interest in old orphan drugs and the high cost of randomised studies have made the availability of evidence-based medications for the prevention of migraine in children extremely limited (Abu-Arafeh 2012). Also, the high placebo effects in childhood migraine trials make it necessary for any study to recruit a large number of patients, adding more difficulties and incurring a high cost. For all the above reasons, many drugs used in the prevention of migraine in children have been used on the basis of open studies or evidence of efficacy derived from studies in adult patients.

INDICATIONS FOR DRUG TREATMENT

There are no agreed criteria on when to start preventative medication for children with migraine. The European Federation of Neurological Societies Task Force (Evers et al 2006) suggested that prophylaxis should be considered if
- quality of life, business duties or school attendance are severely impaired – although there is an element of subjectivity in this criterion that should be acknowledged;
- the frequency of attacks is at least two per month;
- migraine attacks do not respond to acute drug treatment;
- migraine attacks are frequent, very long or associated with uncomfortable auras.

FLUNARIZINE

Flunarizine has been shown to be superior to placebo in several controlled trials in adults (Evers et al 2006), in one controlled trial in children for the prevention of migraine (Sorge et al 1988) and particularly in hemiplegic migraine in an open study (Peer Mohammed et al 2012). Flunarizine is a calcium channel blocker with selective effects on the cerebrovascular circulation. It has also been tried in peripheral vascular disease and vertigo of central or peripheral origin. Its mechanism of action in the prevention of migraine may involve both vascular (smooth muscle inhibition) and neuronal effects (5-hydroxytryptamine antagonism). Flunarizine is widely prescribed for the prevention of migraine in continental Europe, but it is not licensed in the UK or the USA. However, clinicians in the UK can prescribe the drug on a named-patient basis with the patient's and family's knowledge of its off-licence use.

Concerns about the associated side effects (despite its effectiveness) was the main limiting factor for its use in the UK, though a recent study has shown a favourable side effect profile and the drug is rarely associated with major side effects, although depression, extrapyramidal symptoms, drowsiness (may be avoided by taking the dose at night) and excessive weight gain have been reported.

Flunarizine has a long half-life, and thus it can be taken once a day in the evening, so the effect of drowsiness is reduced and adherence to treatment is improved.

The usual dose of flunarizine is between 5 and 10mg per day and it should be taken for 2 to 3 months before its efficacy is judged. Once proven effective, the course of treatment may continue for 6 to 12 months, but longer if necessary. Regular clinical reviews are necessary while the child is on treatment for early detection of side effects, mainly low mood and depression. No blood tests are needed.

TOPIRAMATE

Topiramate is an antiepileptic drug with an uncertain mechanism of action on pain. It exerts its anticonvulsant properties by modulating GABA (gamma-aminobutyric acid) receptors, increasing the availability of GABA, blocking sodium and calcium channels and by inhibiting carbonic anhydrase. It has been shown to have pain-modulating properties, particularly in migraine.

Topiramate was found to be superior to placebo in the prevention of migraine in double-blind, placebo-controlled trials in children aged 6 to 15 years (Winner et al 2005, Lakshmi et al 2007) and in adolescents 12 to 17 years old (Lewis et al 2009). It has also been shown to reduce the number and severity of basilar migraine attacks in children (Lewis and Paradiso 2007).

The usual starting dose of topiramate is 25mg per day and the dose is increased every 2 weeks, as necessary, to a maximum dose of 2mg/kg/day. Topiramate is generally safe and well tolerated by patients. The most commonly reported side effects are loss of appetite, weight loss, gastrointestinal upset and sleepiness. The treatment can be given as a single dose at night to increase adherence and reduce the effect of sleepiness. The treatment course is usually between 6 and 12 months and can be repeated if symptoms relapse.

PIZOTIFEN

Pizotifen was one of the early drugs to be used in the prevention of migraine. Its antimigraine properties are due to its antagonist function on 5-hydroxytryptamine 2-receptor (5-HT2) and, to a lesser degree, its function as an antihistamine. Pizotifen was shown in clinical trials to be more effective than placebo in the prevention of migraine in adult patients; however, the number of randomised, placebo-controlled trials in children is very low (Gillies et al 1986). It is widely used in Europe but not in the USA. The usual dose varies between 0.5mg and 1.5mg per day, but higher doses of up to 3.5mg per day, especially in abdominal migraine, have been used (Symon and Russell 1995). Pizotifen has a relatively good safety profile and the main side effects are weight gain and sedation, making it unsuitable for children with weight problems. Giving it in a single daily dose at night would reduce the effect of sedation on the child.

PROPRANOLOL

Propranolol and other non-selective beta-blockers have been evaluated in adult patients for the prevention of migraine. Several placebo-controlled trials have shown propranolol to be superior to placebo in adults, but the evidence in children is lacking. A double-blind, placebo-controlled, crossover study of children (7–16y) with migraine showed a significant reduction in migraine attacks in 28 children receiving propranolol in a dose of 60 to 120mg per day, compared with 28 children taking placebo (Ludvigsson 1974). Two other studies failed to show efficacy of propranolol over placebo (Lewis et al 2004a, Damen et al 2005).

Despite the conflicting evidence for its efficacy, propranolol may still have a role in the treatment of children with migraine and there are some children who will benefit. The optimum dose in paediatrics is between 1 and 3mg/kg/day and the course of treatment should be at least 3 months. The need to continue with treatment should be evaluated every 6 months.

Propranolol is contraindicated in children with asthma because of its potential to induce an asthma attack. Propranolol can also cause weight gain, mood disturbances and nightmares. Children should be monitored while on treatment and have their blood pressure measured.

AMITRIPTYLINE

Amitriptyline is a tricyclic antidepressant and has pain-modulating properties that are not specific to migraine. There are no controlled trials to assess amitriptyline as a prophylactic drug in childhood migraine. A large open study of the efficacy of amitriptyline in the prevention of migraine in children showed that amitriptyline caused a significant reduction in headache attacks at a dose of up to 1mg/kg/day (Hershey et al 2000). Amitriptyline is well tolerated and occasional side effects may include drowsiness, weight gain and dry mouth. No serious side effects were observed at this low dose.

Amitriptyline is a useful preventative drug in children with migraine and in those with mixed headache disorders presenting with chronic daily headache.

SODIUM VALPROATE

Sodium valproate is an antiepileptic drug that was shown to have a role in the prevention of migraine in adult patients. A recent large double-blind, placebo-controlled study of extended-release valproate in the prophylaxis of migraine, in adolescents 12 to 17 years of age, found that the drug had no benefit over placebo, but an equal safety profile (Apostol et al 2008).

Traditionally, the evidence for valproate in the prevention of migraine in children was based on open clinical observational studies (Caruso et al 2000, Serdaroglu et al 2002), in comparison with propranolol (Bidabadi and Mashouf 2010) or with topiramate (Unalp et al 2008). Valproate was also shown to be helpful in the prevention of cyclical vomiting syndrome in an open observational study (Hikita et al 2009). A suggested effective dose is between 500 and 1000mg per day with a reasonable safety profile. Side effects include sleepiness and weight gain.

CYPROHEPTADINE

Cyproheptadine is mainly used in North America for the prevention of migraine in children and is rarely used in the UK or Europe. The efficacy of cyproheptadine is not well established and the only evidence of efficacy is derived from an open observational study. There is no recommended dose, but doses at 2 to 8 mg per day were used (Lewis et al 2004b). Cyproheptadine has a similar profile of side effects to pizotifen and may cause sleepiness and weight gain.

Other medications

MAGNESIUM OXIDE (SEE CHAPTER 28)

The use of magnesium in the prevention of migraine is based on the hypothesis that migraine patients may have lower blood and brain magnesium levels and correction of such a deficiency may help reduce headache attacks (Sun-Edelstein and Mauskop 2009). Therefore, magnesium oxide may provide an option for prophylaxis of migraine in some patients, as shown in early studies in adult patients (Peikert et al 1996). A randomised study of magnesium oxide in children, 3 to 17 years of age, using a dose of 9mg/kg/day versus placebo showed a statistically significant improvement in headache frequency and headache severity (Wang et al 2003). However, the study population was too small for a firm conclusion to be drawn. However, magnesium oxide (300mg/d) used in combination with feverfew (100mg) and riboflavin (400mg) was not superior to riboflavin (25mg) alone in reducing headache frequency in adult patients (Maizels et al 2004).

RIBOFLAVIN

Riboflavin (vitamin B2) is a precursor of two coenzymes necessary for the electron transfer in oxidation–reduction reactions. Such a role was found in an open study to be of benefit in some patients with mitochondrial myopathies or encephalomyopathies and may benefit patients with migraine (Schoenen et al 1994). A further open-label study using high-dose riboflavin (400mg/d) in adult patients with migraine, showed a reduction in headache frequency and in the use of rescue medications after 3 to 6 months of treatment (Boehnke et al 2004).

FEVERFEW

Daily intake of dried leaves of feverfew was found to be effective in reducing the frequency and severity of migraine attacks in a double-blind, placebo-controlled, crossover study in adult patients (Murphy et al 1988, Pfaffenrath et al 2002, Diener et al 2005), but a similar study failed to show any benefit (De Weerdt et al 1996). No similar studies are available in children.

CO-ENZYME Q10

See Chapter 28.

Summary

Successful preventative treatment depends on accurate diagnosis, reassurance to child and parents, adopting a healthy lifestyle, avoidance of trigger factors and appropriate use of medications. Pharmacological prophylaxis should be considered in patients with disabling headache and migraine with attacks that are severe, long and frequent enough to impact on quality of life. The choice of medications should reflect the disease profile of each patient and potential side effects. Medications should be given in appropriate dose and appropriate length of course in order to assess response.

REFERENCES

Abu-Arafeh I (2012) Flunarizine for prevention of migraine: a new look at an old drug. *Dev Med Child Neurol* 54: 204–5.

Abu-Arafeh I, Russell G (1994) Prevalence of headache and migraine in schoolchildren. *BMJ* 309: 765–9.

Apostol G, Cady RK, Laforet GA et al (2008) Divalproex extended-release in adolescent migraine prophylaxis: results of a randomized, double-blind, placebo-controlled study. *Headache* 48: 1012–25. http://dx.doi.org/10.1111/j.1526-4610.2008.01081.x

Bidabadi E, Mashouf M (2010) A randomized trial of propranolol versus sodium valproate for the prophylaxis of migraine in pediatric patients. *Pediatr Drugs* 12: 269–75. http://dx.doi.org/10.2165/11316270-000000000-00000

Boehnke C, Reuter U, Flach U, Schuh-Hofer S, Einhäupl KM, Arnold G (2004) High-dose riboflavin treatment is efficacious in migraine prophylaxis: an open study in a tertiary care centre. *Eur J Neurol* 11: 475–7. http://dx.doi.org/10.1111/j.1468-1331.2004.00813.x

Caruso JM, Brown WD, Exil G, Gascon GG (2000) The efficacy of divalproex sodium in the prophylactic treatment of children with migraine. *Headache* 40: 672–6. http://dx.doi.org/10.1046/j.1526-4610.2000.040008672.x

Damen L, Bruijn J, Verhagen AP, Berger MY, Passchier J, Koes BW (2005) Prophylactic treatment of migraine in children, Part 2. A systematic review of pharmacological trials. *Cephalalgia* 26: 497–505. http://dx.doi.org/10.1111/j.1468-2982.2005.01047.x

De Weerdt CJ, Bootsma HPR, Hendriks H (1996) Herbal medicines in migraine prevention: randomized double-blind placebo-controlled crossover trial of a feverfew preparation. *Phytomedicine* 3: 225–30. http://dx.doi.org/10.1016/S0944-7113(96)80057-2

Diener HC, Pfaffenrath V, Schnitker J, Friede M, Henneicke-von Zepelin HH (2005) Efficacy and safety of 6.25 mg t.i.d. feverfew CO$_2$-extract (MIG-99) in migraine prevention – a randomized, double-blind, multicentre, placebo-controlled study. *Cephalalgia* 25: 1031–41. http://dx.doi.org/10.1111/j.1468-2982.2005.00950.x

Evers S, Afra J, Frese A et al (2006) EFNS guideline on the drug treatment of migraine – report of an EFNS task force. *Eur J Neurol* 13: 560–72. http://dx.doi.org/10.1111/j.1468-1331.2006.01411.x

Gillies D, Sills M, Forsythe I (1986) Pizotifen (Sanomigran) in childhood migraine. A double-blind controlled trial. *Eur Neurol* 25: 32–5. http://dx.doi.org/10.1159/000115983

Hershey AD, Powers SW, Bentti AL, deGrauw TJ (2000) Effectiveness of amitriptyline in the prophylactic management of childhood headaches. *Headache* 40: 539–49. http://dx.doi.org/10.1046/j.1526-4610.2000.00085.x

Hikita T, Kodama H, Nakamoto N et al (2009) Effective prophylactic therapy for cyclic vomiting syndrome in children using valproate. *Brain Dev* 31: 411–13. http://dx.doi.org/10.1016/j.braindev.2008.07.005

Lakshmi CVS, Singhi P, Malhi P, Ray M (2007) topiramate in the prophylaxis of pediatric migraine: a double-blind placebo-controlled trial. *J Child Neurol* 22: 829–35. http://dx.doi.org/10.1177/0883073807304201

Leonardsson-Hellgren M, Gustavsson UM, Lindblad U (2001) Headache and associations with lifestyle among pupils in senior level elementary school. *Scand J Prim Health Care* 19: 107–11. http://dx.doi.org/10.1080/028134301750235349

Lewis D, Paradiso E (2007) A double-blind, dose comparison study of topiramate for prophylaxis of basilar-type migraine in children: a pilot study. *Headache* 47: 1409–17.

Lewis D, Ashwal S, Hershey A, Hirtz D, Yonker M, Silberstein S (2004a) Practice parameter: pharmacological treatment of migraine headache in children and adolescents: children and adolescents report of the

American Academy of Neurology Quality Standards Subcommittee and the Practice Committee of the Child Neurology Society. *Neurology* 63: 2215–24. http://dx.doi.org/10.1212/01.WNL.0000147332.41993.90

Lewis D, Diamond S, Scott D, Jones V (2004b) Prophylactic treatment of pediatric migraine. *Headache* 44: 230–7. http://dx.doi.org/10.1111/j.1526-4610.2004.04052.x

Lewis D, Winner P, Saper J et al (2009) Randomized, double-blind, placebo-controlled study to evaluate the efficacy and safety of topiramate for migraine prevention in pediatric subjects 12 to 17 years of age. *Pediatrics* 123: 924–34. http://dx.doi.org/10.1542/peds.2008-0642

Ludvigsson J (1974) Propranolol used in prophylaxis of migraine in children. *Acta Neurol* 50: 109–15. http://dx.doi.org/10.1111/j.1600-0404.1974.tb01350.x

Maizels M, Blumenfeld A, Burchette R (2004) A combination of Riboflavin, Magnesium, and Feverfew for migraine prophylaxis: a randomized trial. *Headache* 44: 885–90. http://dx.doi.org/10.1111/j.1526-4610.2004.04170.x

Murphy JJ, Heptinstall S, Mitchell JRA (1988) Randomised double-blind placebo-controlled trial of feverfew in migraine prevention. *Lancet* 332: 189–92. http://dx.doi.org/10.1016/S0140-6736(88)92289-1

Parker C, Waltman N (2012) Reducing the frequency and severity of migraine headaches in the workplace, implementing evidence-based interventions. *Workplace Health Saf* 60: 12–18. http://dx.doi.org/10.3928/21650799-20111227-02

Peer Mohamed B, Goadsby PJ, Prabhakar P (2012) Safety and efficacy of flunarizine in childhood migraine: 11 years' experience, with emphasis on its effect in hemiplegic migraine. *Dev Med Child Neurol* 54: 274–7. http://dx.doi.org/10.1111/j.1469-8749.2011.04154.x

Peikert A, Wilimzig C, Kohne-Volland R (1996) Prophylaxis of migraine with oral magnesium: results from a prospective, multi-center, placebo-controlled and double-blind randomized study. *Cephalalgia* 16: 257–63. http://dx.doi.org/10.1046/j.1468-2982.1996.1604257.x

Pfaffenrath V, Diener HC, Fischer M, Friede M, Henneicke-von Zepelin HH (2002) The efficacy and safety of Tanacetum parthenium (feverfew) in migraine prophylaxis – a double-blind, multicentre, randomized placebo-controlled dose–response study. *Cephalalgia* 22: 523–32. http://dx.doi.org/10.1046/j.1468-2982.2002.00396.x

Schoenen J, Lenaerts M, Bastings E (1994) High-dose riboflavin as a prophylactic treatment of migraine: results of an open pilot study. *Cephalalgia* 14: 328–9. http://dx.doi.org/10.1046/j.1468-2982.1994.1405328.x

Serdaroglu G, Erhan E, Tekgul et al (2002) Sodium valproate prophylaxis in childhood migraine. *Headache* 42: 819–22. http://dx.doi.org/10.1046/j.1526-4610.2002.02186.x

Smith TR, Nicholson RA, Banks JW (2010) Migraine education improves quality of life in a primary care setting. *Headache* 50: 600–12. http://dx.doi.org/10.1111/j.1526-4610.2010.01618.x

Sorge F, De Simone R, Marano E, Nolano M, Orefice G, Carrieri P. (1988) Flunarizine in prophylaxis of childhood migraine. A double-blind, placebo-controlled, crossover study. *Cephalalgia* 8: 1–6. http://dx.doi.org/10.1046/j.1468-2982.1988.0801001.x

Sun-Edelstein C, Mauskop A (2009) Role of magnesium in the pathogenesis and treatment of migraine. *Expert Rev Neurother* 9: 369–79. http://dx.doi.org/10.1586/14737175.9.3.369

Symon DN, Russell G (1995) Double blind placebo controlled trial of pizotifen syrup in the treatment of abdominal migraine. *Arch Dis Child* 72: 48–50.

Unalp A, Uran N, Oztürk A (2008) Comparison of the effectiveness of topiramate and sodium valproate in pediatric migraine. *J Child Neurol* 23: 1377–81. http://dx.doi.org/10.1177/0883073808318547

Wang F, Van Den Eeden SK, Ackerson LM, Salk SE, Reince RH, Elin RJ (2003) Oral magnesium oxide prophylaxis of frequent migrainous headache in children: a randomized, double-blind, placebo-controlled trial. *Headache* 43: 601–10. http://dx.doi.org/10.1046/j.1526-4610.2003.03102.x

Winner P, Pearlman EM, Linder SL et al (2005) Topiramate for migraine prevention in children: a randomized, double-blind, placebo-controlled trial. *Headache* 45: 1304–12. http://dx.doi.org/10.1111/j.1526-4610.2005.00262.x

13
POTENTIAL DRUGS FOR THE TREATMENT OF MIGRAINE IN CHILDREN

Part 1: Medications for the prevention of chronic headache: botulinum toxin as a treatment in childhood headache

Kamran A Ahmed and Kenneth J Mack

In adult patients, botulinum toxin has been studied as a potentially effective treatment for chronic daily headache. Recent double-blind, placebo-controlled trials of onabotulinumtoxinA have shown promise in adults with chronic migraine (Aurora et al 2010, Deiner et al 2010). In the UK, the recent guidelines of the National Institute for Health and Clinical Excellence on the diagnosis and management of headache in young people and adults have accepted onabotulinumtoxinA as a treatment option for adults with chronic migraine (NICE 2012).

In a large multicentre trial in which the primary end point was reduction in the number of headache days over a 28-day period relative to baseline, it was found that 155 (up to 195) international units of onabotulinumtoxinA was statistically significantly superior to placebo injection (onabotulinumtoxinA, −9.0d; placebo, −6.7d; $p<0.001$) (Deiner et al 2010). Another study found that, compared with placebo, 155 IU of onabotulinumtoxinA resulted in a significant reduction in the Headache Impact Test (HIT-6) score and improvement in quality of life measures (Lipton et al 2011).

In adult patients, a consistent clinical profile of likely botulinum toxin type A (BoNT-A) responders has not yet been obtained from either currently published, randomised, double-blind, placebo-controlled trials or open studies. However, subgroup analysis suggests that patients who are severely impaired may be able to benefit from BoNT-A (Binder et al 2000, 2001, Silberstein et al 2000, Evers 2006). The pooled analyses of two phase 3, 24-week, double-blind, parallel-group, placebo-controlled multicentre studies (PREEMPT 1 and 2), followed by a 32-week open-label phase, found BoNT-A to be a safe and effective long-term (>24wk) prophylactic treatment for chronic migraine in adults (Aurora et al 2010). The method of action of BoNT-A involves inhibiting synaptic vesicle release into the synaptic cleft. BoNT-A's antinociceptive effect is believed to result from inhibition of the release of nociceptive mediators, such as glutamate, substance P and calcitonin gene-related peptide, from nociceptive fibres (Aoki 2003, Cui et al 2004, Durham et al 2004).

There are currently no published prospective placebo-controlled studies analysing the potential benefit or tolerability of BoNT-A in children with chronic daily headache. However, analyses have shown BoNT-A to be effective in the treatment of chronic daily headache in a select group of the medically intractable paediatric population. In a study conducted by Kabbouche et al (2005) on the treatment of adolescents (mean age 16.0y) with chronic daily headache, about half of the patients experienced some relief with BoNT-A (Botox) at an average dose of 88 units. In an uncontrolled, prospective study on the use of BoNT-A in six adolescent females (aged 14–18y), who received standard 3-month-interval injections over 3 to 29 months, there was an average improvement of 33% to 75% in quality of life (Chan et al 2009). A study at our institution revealed that 4 of 10 (40%) patients experienced a subjective, but clinically significant, relief of headache symptoms post injection (Ahmed et al 2010). Additionally, two of these patients experienced a decrease in headache frequency. Three of five of our patients with the chronic migraine subtype of chronic daily headache experienced significant clinical improvement, suggesting that these patients may be more likely to experience pain relief.

A clear dosing regimen for the use of BoNT-A in paediatric patients has not yet been determined. The dose of BoNT-A is preparation dependent and the usual dose of Botox, for the treatment of children with spasticity, is between 3 and 6 units/kg of body weight and the maximum safe dose is up to 12 units/kg per session. The most common dosing regimen at our institution is 100 units of onabotulinumtoxinA (Botox), with dosing at 3-month intervals, using a protocol frequently used in adults with chronic migraine (Fig. 13.1; Ahmed et al 2010). The dosing regimen includes 2.5 units into each corrugator and procerus muscle (7.5 units total); 1.25 units into the right and left frontalis muscles (2.5 units total); 7.5 units into each temporalis muscle (left and right) (15 units total); 12.5 units into each splenius capitis muscle (left and right) (25 units total); and 25 units into each trapezius muscle (50 units total).

The safety of BoNT-A has not been determined in children. OnabotulinumtoxinA (Botox) is used in multiple neurological disorders; however, its safety has not been well established in those younger than 16 years of age with cervical dystonia; in those younger than 18 years of age with hyperhidrosis; and in those younger than 12 years of age with strabismus or blepharospasm (PDR-Staff 2009). Based on a recently published evidence-based review from the American Academy of Neurology, BoNT-A appears to be generally safe for localised/ segmental spasticity (Delgado et al 2010). The majority of the class I and II studies included

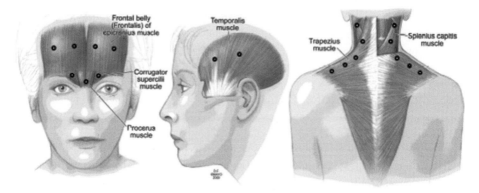

Fig. 13.1 Anatomical injection sites for botulinum toxin type A. (Reproduced from Garza and Cutrer 2010 with permission from the Mayo Foundation for Medical Education and Research. All rights reserved.)

children as young as 2 years of age; however, many received abobotulinumtoxinA (Dysport). Doses of abobotulinumtoxinA (Dysport) are not equivalent to onabotulinumtoxinA (Botox). Research is needed to further establish the potential safety and proper dosing of BoNT-A products in children.

In the USA, many insurance companies will demand that the patient be tried on and fail at least two preventative medications before consideration is given to Botox. Botox treatment is particularly useful for patients with complicated medical regimens, or those who seem to be extremely sensitive to the side effects of oral medications.

There may be a potential benefit from BoNT-A in paediatric patients with medically intractable chronic daily headache, particularly in those with chronic migraine. BoNT-A appears to be very well tolerated in this population. Controlled studies are clearly needed, however, to confirm efficacy and tolerability.

Part 2: Medications for the relief of acute migraine attacks: calcitonin gene-related peptide receptor antagonists

Ishaq Abu-Arafeh

Calcitonin gene-related peptide (CGRP) is one of several neuropeptides found in the human trigeminal sensory neurons, pericranial vascular nerves and the trigeminal ganglion. As shown in Chapter 3, CGRP plays an important part in the pathogenesis of migraine and its concentration rises in the trigeminovascular complex during attacks of migraine. CGRP release is associated with vascular dilatation in the cerebral and dural vessels. Inhibition or reversal of CGRP action may, in principle, abort the attack of migraine and relieve symptoms. The use of such compounds would overcome the problem of vasoconstriction induced by other treatments of migraine, such as the group of triptans, and make them useable in conditions such as hemiplegic migraine and basilar-type migraine for which triptans may have a potential risk (Edvinsson and Linde 2010).

Early research on BIBN 4096 BS (olcegepant), a non-peptide CGRP receptor antagonist given by the intravenous route, has shown its potential in the treatment of migraine. Several phase 1, phase 2 and phase 3 studies have shown the drug to be effective and safe in a proof of concept (Olesen et al 2004).

Large, multicentre, double-blind, placebo-controlled trials on MK-0974 (telcagepant), an oral CGRP receptor antagonist, confirmed its efficacy and safety profile. In a study of 1380 adult patients who were randomly assigned to receive telcagepant 150mg ($n=333$) or 300mg (354), zolmitriptan (345) or placebo (348), telcagepant 300mg was more effective than placebo in producing pain freedom, pain relief and absences of phonophobia, photophobia and nausea. Efficacy of telcagepant 300mg and zolmitriptan 5mg were much the same. Adverse events were recorded in 37% of patients taking telcagepant 300mg, 51% taking zolmitriptan 5mg and 32% taking placebo (Ho et al 2009).

Studies in children are not yet available and future post-marketing studies may help inform paediatric practice.

REFERENCES

Ahmed, KA, Oas KH, Mack KJ, Garza I (2010) Experience with botulinum toxin type A in medically intractable pediatric chronic daily headache. *Pediatr Neurol* 43: 316–19. http://dx.doi.org/10.1016/j. pediatrneurol.2010.06.001

Aoki KR (2003) Evidence for antinociceptive activity of botulinum toxin type A in pain management. *Headache* 43: S9–S15. http://dx.doi.org/10.1046/j.1526-4610.43.7s.3.x

Aurora SK, Dodick DW, Turkel CC et al (2010) OnabotulinumtoxinA for treatment of chronic migraine: results from the double-blind, randomized, placebocontrolled phase of the PREEMPT-1 trial. *Cephalalgia* 30: 793–803. http://dx.doi.org/10.1177/0333102410364676

Binder WJ, Brin MF, Blitzer A, Schoenrock LD, Pogoda JM (2000) Botulinum toxin type A (BOTOX) for treatment of migraine headaches: an open-label study. *Otolaryngol Head Neck Surg* 123: 669–76. http:// dx.doi.org/10.1067/mhn.2000.110960

Binder WJ, Brin MF, Blitzer A, Pogoda JM. (2001) Botulinum toxin type A (BOTOX) for treatment of migraine. *Semin Cutan Med Surg* 20: 93–100. http://dx.doi.org/10.1053/sder.2001.24423

Chan VW, McCabe EJ, MacGregor DL (2009) Botox treatment for migraine and chronic daily headache in adolescents. *J Neurosci Nurs* 41: 235–43. http://dx.doi.org/10.1097/JNN.0b013e3181aaa98f

Cui M, Khanijou S, Rubino J, Aoki KR (2004) Subcutaneous administration of botulinum toxin A reduces formalin-induced pain. *Pain* 107: 125–33. http://dx.doi.org/10.1016/j.pain.2003.10.008

Delgado MR, Hirtz D, Aisen M et al (2010) Practice parameter: pharmacologic treatment of spasticity in children and adolescents with cerebral palsy (an evidence-based review): report of the Quality Standards Subcommittee of the American Academy of Neurology and the Practice Committee of the Child Neurology Society. *Neurology* 74: 336–43. http://dx.doi.org/10.1212/WNL.0b013e3181cbcd2f

Diener HC, Dodick DW, Aurora SK et al (2010). OnabotulinumtoxinA for treatment of chronic migraine: results from the double-blind, randomized, placebocontrolled phase of the PREEMPT 2 trial. *Cephalalgia* 30: 804–14. http://dx.doi.org/10.1177/0333102410364677

Durham PL, Cady R, Cady R (2004) Regulation of calcitonin gene-related peptide secretion from trigeminal nerve cells by botulinum toxin type A: implications for migraine therapy. *Headache* 44: 35–42. http://dx.doi. org/10.1111/j.1526-4610.2004.04007.x

Edvinsson L, Linde M (2010) New drugs in migraine treatment and prophylaxis: telcagepant and topiramate. *Lancet* 376: 21–7. http://dx.doi.org/10.1016/S0140-6736(10)60323-6

Evers S (2006) Status on the use of botulinum toxin for headache disorders. *Curr Opin Neurol* 19: 310–15.

Garza I, Cutrer F (2010) Pain relief and persistence of dysautonomic features in a patient with hemicrania continua responsive to botulinum toxin type A. *Cephalalgia* 30: 500–3.

Ho TW, Ferrari MD, Dodick DW et al (2009) Efficacy and tolerability of MK-0974 (telcagepant), a new oral antagonist of calcitonin gene-related peptide receptor, compared with zolmitriptan for acute migraine: a randomised, placebo-controlled, parallel-treatment trial. *Lancet* 372: 2115–23. http://dx.doi.org/10.1016/ S0140-6736(08)61626-8

Kabbouche MA, Hershey AD, Powers SW (2005) Botulinum toxin A in the treatment of migraine headache in children. *Headache* 45: 786.

Lipton RB, Varon SF, Grosberg B et al (2011) OnabotulinumtoxinA improves quality of life and reduces impact of chronic migraine. *Neurology* 77: 1465–72. http://dx.doi.org/10.1212/WNL.0b013e318232ab65

Olesen J, Diener H-C, Husstedt IW et al (2004) Calcitonin gene–related peptide receptor antagonist BIBN 4096 BS for the acute treatment of migraine. *N Engl J Med* 350: 1104–10. http://dx.doi.org/10.1056/ NEJMoa030505

NICE (National Institute for Health and Clinical Excellence) (2012) Diagnosis and Management of Headache in Young People and Adults – CG150. Available at: www.guidance.nice.org.uk/cg150

PDR-Staff (2009). Botox. PDR: Physicians Desk Reference 2010, PDR Network, LLC: 596–601.

Silberstein S, Mathew N, Saper J, Jenkins S (2000) Botulinum toxin type A as a migraine preventive treatment. For the BOTOX Migraine Clinical Research Group. *Headache* 40: 445–50. http://dx.doi. org/10.1046/j.1526-4610.2000.00066.x

14
HEADACHE AND COMORBIDITY IN CHILDREN: STROKE, PATENT FORAMEN OVALE AND EPILEPSY

Benedetta Bellini, Alessandra Cescut, Franco Lucchese, Francesca Craba and Vincenzo Guidetti

The clinical nature of recurrent headaches in childhood and their association with comorbidities and biological correlates highlight paediatric headache as a significant and important disease.

Comorbidity may be defined either as the presence of one or more disorders in addition to the primary condition or as the effect of such an additional disorder (Feinstein 1970). The presence of a comorbidity may complicate diagnosis because of overlapping symptoms. As stated by Lipton and Silberstein (1994), comorbidity may arise by coincidence or selection bias, one condition may cause the other, both conditions may be related and share environmental and genetic risk factors, and the same environmental or genetic risk factors may determine the state that gives rise to both conditions.

Comorbidity of migraine has been extensively studied and comprehensive reviews have been published for both adults and children. An association has been reported with allergies, mitral valve prolapse, hypotension, hypertension, stroke, depression and anxiety (Merikangas and Rasmussen 2000). Based on all the current data, Breslau and Rasmussen (2001) emphasised the co-occurrence of migraine with psychiatric conditions, epilepsy and stroke.

For example, in a study of the families of Finnish migraine patients (Artto et al 2006), the patients with migraine reported significantly more hypotension, allergies and psychiatric disorders than their family members without migraine; in particular, women, and those fulfilling the criteria for both migraine with and without aura were likely to have additional disorders besides their migraine. Male migraineurs with aura reported a significant association with stroke and epilepsy. In children and adolescents too, headache and migraine are commonly associated with different diseases, such as psychiatric comorbidities, atopic diseases, attention-deficit–hyperactivity disorder, epilepsy, stroke and patent foramen ovale (PFO) (Chen and Leviton 1990, Breslau et al 1991, Mortimer et al 1993, Guidetti 1998).

Migraine and stroke
The association between migraine and cerebrovascular disease is less recognised in children, although migraine is a recognised cause of cerebral infarction in adults. The average annual incidence of stroke in children is about 2.5 per 100 000, excluding strokes associated with birth, intracranial infection or trauma (Ebinger et al 1999).

The causes of cerebral infarction in childhood are heart diseases, vascular diseases, hae-matological disorders, primary hypercoagulable states or inborn metabolic disorders, but 50% of strokes are regarded as idiopathic (Dusser et al 1986). In the adult population, it is gener-ally accepted that cerebral infarction can occur during a migraine attack (Biller et al 1994); between 10% and 27% of ischaemic strokes in young adults could be the result of migraine (Olesen et al 1993). In contrast, in childhood the diagnosis of migrainous stroke is still called into question, and only a few patients less than 16 years of age with migraine-related ischaemic stroke have been reported (Garg and De Myer 1995, Nezu et al 1997). In most patients the ischaemic stroke occurred in a territory of the middle cerebral artery (Nezu et al 1997), but brain regions supplied by the posterior cerebral and basilar arteries can be afflicted as well.

In particular, a complex bidirectional relationship exists between migraine and stroke, including migraine as a risk factor for cerebral ischaemia, migraine caused by cerebral isch-aemia, migraine as a cause of stroke, migraine mimicking cerebral ischaemia, migraine and cerebral ischaemia sharing a common cause and migraine associated with subclinical vascular brain lesions.

Confirming that migraine may be associated with cerebrovascular disease, there are some studies that consider migraine as a cause of stroke in young patients (Wober-Bingol et al 1995). A history of migraine with aura seems to be more common among victims of ischaemic stroke than among comparison individuals, and an acute migraine attack or migraine-like headache may precede, accompany or follow a thromboembolic transient ischaemic attack or stroke, and this headache seems to occur more often among migraineurs than among migraine-free patients (Welch and Levine 1990, Ebinger et al 1999, Rasul et al 2009). Olesen et al (1993) discussed the relationship between migraine and stroke carefully; it seems reason-able to assume a causal relationship between migraine and stroke, either ischaemia-triggered symptomatic migraine or a migraine-induced ischaemic insult.

Owing to a lack of objective and measurable diagnostic criteria, the diagnosis of migrain-ous infarction is impossible to prove, and therefore it can be made partly by the exclusion of other causes and partly on positive evidence. It is also difficult to distinguish short-lasting symptoms of cerebral thromboembolism from migrainous manifestations. Therefore, it is necessary to apply strict criteria in order to study the relationship between migraine and stroke. In 1988 the Headache Classification Committee of the International Headache Society (IHS) defined the criteria for migrainous infarction; however, these criteria were considered too restrictive to account for the majority of migrainous strokes, especially those of child-hood (Welch and Levine 1990, Wober-Bingol et al 1995, Ebinger et al 1999). In fact, the IHS criteria require not only that a patient has migraine with aura, but that the episode, end-ing in stroke, must be typical of the patient's attacks. However, some degree of variability in symptoms from one episode to another in the same patient is well known, even in patients with aura (Barlow 1984). A single migraine patient can manifest migraine with or without aura (Garcia and Pantoni 1995) and the aura might occur in silent areas of the brain as well (Welch and Levine 1990). Finally, as already mentioned, several well-documented reports exist of migraine-related stroke during the first episode of migraine (Caplan 1991, Wober-Bingol et al 1995). Thus, from the literature, we can say that a history of migraine with or without aura is acceptable for the diagnosis of migrainous stroke. However, when the stroke is the first manifestation of migraine, the diagnosis of migrainous stroke can be made only retrospectively.

Although the pathophysiology of migraine is still under discussion (Post and Silberstein 1994, D'Andrea 2010), the IHS demands that a history of migraine with aura in migrainous stroke is based upon the supposition of pathophysiological differences between those episodes with aura and those without. A unifying concept of migraine is that of the cortical spreading depression of Leao (Leao 1944). According to this theory, the spread of the cortical depression produces the 'creeping' development of neurological symptoms, and the accompanying spreading oligaemia could contribute to the neurological disabilities. It could generate headache via trigeminovascular mechanisms. One mechanism of propagation of the spreading depression is the action of glutamate on N-methyl-D-aspartate (NMDA) receptors (Lauritzen 1994). NMDA receptors, of course, occupy a crucial position in the cascade of cell death due to cerebral ischaemia (Rothman and Olney 1987). Thus, during cortical spreading depression, two mechanisms might contribute to the generation of a migrainous stroke (Lauritzen 1994): the calibre changes in arterioles and capillaries associated with a reduction in profusion (Rothrock et al 1993) and the changes in cellular metabolism, which could be directly provoked or enhanced by the activation of NMDA receptors.

Moreover, known risk factors for cardiovascular and cerebrovascular disease include dyslipidaemia, obesity (Wilson et al 2008), and elevated blood levels of C-reactive protein (CRP) (Makita et al 2009) and homocysteine (Towfighi et al 2008). Adults with migraine or other headache disorders have elevated levels of these factors (Moschiano et al 2008). Adult migraineurs with aura are at increased risk of cardiovascular disease and stroke (Bigal et al 2009). But we must keep in mind that in adults the analysis of the association of these factors with headache disorders and other outcomes is complicated by the frequent presence of such additional risk factors as smoking, hypertension and diabetes mellitus. In children, these and other potential confounders are much less common. There are reports from small clinical samples that paediatric migraine is associated with dyslipidaemia (Glueck et al 1986) and hyperhomocysteinaemia, and genetic variants relating to homocysteine are risk factors for stroke in children (Bottini et al 2006). In addition, in a representative national sample of children, severe or recurrent headache was associated with higher levels of adiposity as measured by body mass index (BMI) (Lateef et al 2009). There seems to be no report on CRP levels in children with migraine.

In this regard, Nelson et al (2010) examined the association between headaches and vascular or inflammatory biomarkers including CRP, homocysteine, folate, lipid and uric acid levels and platelet counts and their interrelationships in children. Other well-established correlates of headaches and/or vascular biomarkers include age, sex, ethnicity, poverty–income ratio (proxy for social class) and BMI. Asthma was also considered in the risk profile because previous work, in both adults (Kalaydjian and Merikangas 2008) and children (Lateef et al 2009), showed a strong relationship between asthma and headache disorders. Nelson et al (2010) found that many of these biomarkers clustered more closely in children with than in those without severe or recurrent headaches or migraine.

In this large and representative American sample (analytical sample was of 11 770 children and adolescents aged 4–19y), children and adolescents with severe or recurrent headache or migraine had higher mean BMIs, higher levels of CRP and homocysteine and lower levels of serum and red blood cell folate. More children with headache were in the quintile of highest risk for each of these biomarkers, and more were in the highest quintile of risk for three or more. These results suggest that there may be two subgroups of children with headaches: one characterised by elevated levels of homocysteine and lower serum folate levels and another characterised by relatively high CRP levels and asthma. These observations suggest that different mechanisms may contribute to vascular changes in these two groups, and these subgroups may have index potential endophenotypes that could be examined in future genetic research.

An elevated CRP level is a marker of inflammation; its concentration in blood correlates with levels of inflammatory cytokines, and it is a biomarker of risk for cardiovascular disease and stroke (Kampoli et al 2009). The results of the study presented herein are consistent with a previous one showing increased CRP levels in young adults with migraine (Vanmolkot and de Hoon 2007). There is a strong relationship between CRP levels and BMI in children and adolescents, such that a single standard deviation increase in BMI associates with a 52% increase in CRP concentration (Lambert et al 2004). Indeed, adiposity was the major determinant of CRP levels in children (Cook et al 2000). People with an elevated CRP level at initial measurement tend to continue to have elevated levels of CRP in subsequent years (Glynn et al 2009). Abnormalities in homocysteine levels are also associated with vascular risk. Risk of asymptomatic vascular disease can be identified early and its severity rises with an increasing number of risk factors (Berenson et al 1998). Nelson et al (2010) suggest that biomarkers of risk for vascular disease appear to cluster in children and adolescents with severe or recurrent headaches or migraine. Such young people may be an appropriate target for further studies and for screening, follow-up and efforts to prevent long-term vascular pathology and resulting cardiovascular disease and stroke.

Migraine and patent foramen ovale

It is reasonable to say that for those under the age of 55, migraine with aura is a risk factor for ischaemic stroke, but that a proportion of ischaemic stroke is due to PFO. PFO is the result of incomplete fusion of the septum primum and septum secundum, which normally occurs shortly after birth, when left atrial pressures exceed those in the right atrium.

Epidemiological studies have shown a clear comorbidity between migraine with aura and PFO. Indeed, available data suggest that PFO is more common in migraineurs with aura (approximately 50%) and that migraine with aura is more common in patients with PFO (Schwerzmann et al 2004, Dalla Volta et al 2005, Anzola et al 2006a,b).

The underlying mechanism of the possible relationship between PFO and migraine remains speculative: is it causally related to migraine attacks, or is it a fortuitous association due to common genetic factors? The pathophysiological mechanism is speculated to be passage of microemboli and vasoactive chemicals through the PFO, thereby evading pulmonary filtration and triggering migraine symptoms. Cortical spreading depression, which is the underlying mechanism of the migrainous aura, could be favoured by a PFO. In particular, it has been postulated that PFO may allow venous-circulating, migraine-triggering, vasoactive chemicals to bypass the pulmonary filter and reach the cerebral circulation to induce a migraine attack (Wilmshurst et al 2000).

Paradoxical emboli themselves appear to have a propensity for the posterior circulation, the area in which hypoperfusion occurs during a migraine aura (Venketasubramanian et al 1993). Perhaps the most compelling suggestion is that a particular genetic composition might govern co-development of atrial septal abnormalities and migraine (Pierangeli et al 2004).

Still, possible explanations of a PFO leading to stroke are insufficient. If the aura was due to malfunction of cerebral perfusion, symptoms would occur with a sudden onset and not gradually. It is likely that the association of migraine and PFO is coincidental, because both disorders are frequent. It is also discussed whether the disposition of PFO and migraine with aura could be inherited and transmitted simultaneously (Willis 1965).

Several retrospective and uncontrolled studies have suggested that percutaneous closure of a PFO for stroke or decompression illness in divers reduces the frequency of migraine attacks with, but also without, aura, but there is no rationale for proposing PFO closure for migraine, despite several studies showing a better course of migraine in migraine headache patients undergoing patent PFO transcatheter closure (Wilmshurst et al 2005, Chessa et al 2009, Fuller and Jesurum 2009).

Migraine and epilepsy

This association has been demonstrated in several studies, mainly based on adults affected by epilepsy (Haut et al 2006). In children, an association between migraine and some epilepsy syndromes has been reported, but data are conflicting and studies have been limited by the small numbers of patients and the lack of clearly stated diagnostic criteria of childhood migraine (Wirrell and Hamiwka 2006).

The growing knowledge of the genetic basis of familial hemiplegic migraine (FHM) (Thomsen et al 2007), and the findings of epileptic seizures occurring independent of the migraine attacks in FHM families (Ducros 2008), have stimulated interest in migraine and epilepsy comorbidity.

In previous studies, the prevalence of migraine in epileptic populations was estimated to be 8% to 24% and the risk of migraine was 2.4 times higher among adults with epilepsy than in those without (Haut et al 2006). The prevalence of migraine among children with partial epilepsy was 21% in those with benign rolandic epilepsy and 17% in those with cryptogenic/symptomatic epilepsy (Wirrell and Hamiwka 2006).

Toldo et al (2010), in a recent study, analysed the headache and epilepsy comorbidity in a large series of patients under 18 years of age with headache (1795), using the recent International Classification for Headache Disorder, 2nd edition (ICHD-II) criteria. Fifty-six patients (3.1%) suffered from idiopathic headache and idiopathic or cryptogenic epilepsy or unprovoked seizures.

There was a strong association between migraine and epilepsy: in migraineurs (46/56) the risk of epilepsy was 3.2 times higher than the risk of tension-type headache, without significant difference between migraine with and without aura; among children with epilepsy the risk of developing migraine was 4.5 times higher than the risk of tension-type headache. Among those with comorbidity, focal epilepsies prevailed (43/56; 76.8%). Among migraineurs affected by focal epilepsies (36/56), the risk of cryptogenic epilepsy (27/36; 75%) was three times higher risk than the risk of idiopathic epilepsy (9/36; 25%) (*p*=0.003). Migraine with aura was preceded by epilepsy in 71% of cases. Photosensitivity (7/56; 12.5%) and a positive family history of epilepsy (22/56; 39%) were frequent in patients with comorbidity.

As above, in Toldo's cases, migraine with aura did not increase the risk of epilepsy compared with migraine without aura and the prevalence of epilepsy was similar across the two groups of migraineurs (migraine without aura: 5.4%; migraine with aura: 5.8%), whereas in Ludvigsson et al's (2006) case–control study in children, the risk of unprovoked seizures was increased in migraine with aura (3.7-fold) but not in cases of migraine without aura. Moreover, in the majority of Toldo's cases (71%) epilepsy preceded migraine with aura and this finding is not consistent with a causative role for migraine with aura in epilepsy, as previously suggested in other studies, such as in Ludvigsson's. Therefore, Toldo supposes that it is more likely that migraine with aura and epilepsy share a common antecedent factor. More generally, in the past years, three alternative models have been proposed to explain the comorbidity between migraine and epilepsy: (1) a simple unidirectional causal explanation; (2) shared environmental risk factors; or (3) shared genetic risk factors (Ottman and Lipton 1996).

Similar to previous studies (De Romanis et al 1991, De Simone et al 2007), Toldo's results are consistent with rejecting these three possibilities because epilepsy preceded migraine in the majority of cases, and he did not find any statistically significant correlation between a positive family history of migraine and type of headache or epilepsy in the probands.

At present, many authors believe that increased brain excitability might increase the risk of both migraine and epilepsy and could explain the comorbidity (Leniger et al 2003, Rogawski 2008). There is considerable interest in the possibility that genetic polymorphisms in ion channels, or in genes encoding other molecules involved in the generation and the maintenance of membrane, contribute to epilepsy and migraine susceptibility (Rogawski 2008).

Therefore, the association between epilepsy and headache/migraine has been long recognised, but the common molecular mechanisms so far remain elusive. Indeed, recent data suggest shared genetic substrates and phenotypical–genotypical correlations with mutations in some ion transporter genes, including *CACNA1A*, *ATP1A2* and *SCN1A* (Bianchin et al 2010, Toldo et al 2011, Verrotti et al 2011), and neuronal hyperexcitability and increased susceptibility to cortical spreading depression remain important molecular mechanisms in the pathophysiology of this association.

Conclusions

The identification of comorbid disorders in migraineurs is important as it may impose therapeutic challenges and limit treatment options. Moreover, the study of comorbidity might lead to an improvement in our knowledge of the causes and consequences of migraine.

Antiepileptic medications may be good choices for migraine prophylaxis, especially if there is a family history of comorbid epilepsy or if there is a tendency towards low blood pressure in a family, for whom beta-blockers would not be appropriate.

From a pathophysiological point of view, studies involving ion channels (epilepsy), mechanisms related to the autonomic nervous system (hypotension), immunology (allergy) and serotonergic transmission (psychiatric conditions) are indicated (Artto et al 2006).

REFERENCES

Anzola GP, Frisoni GB, Morandi E, Casilli F, Onorato E (2006a) Shunt-associated migraine responds favorably to atrial septal repair: a case–control study. *Stroke* 37: 430–4. http://dx.doi.org/10.1161/01. STR.0000199082.07317.43

Anzola GP, Morandi E, Casilli F, Onorato E (2006b) Different degrees of right-to-left shunting predict migraine and stroke: data from 420 patients. *Neurology* 66: 765–7. http://dx.doi.org/10.1212/01. wnl.0000201271.75157.5a

Artto V, Wessman M, Nissila M et al (2006) Comorbidity in Finnish migraine families. *J Headache Pain* 7: 324–30. http://dx.doi.org/10.1007/s10194-006-0319-x

Barlow CF (1984) *Headaches and Migraine in Childhood.* Oxford: Spastics International Medical Publications.

Berenson GS, Srinivasan SR, Bao W, Newman WP III, Tracy RE, Wattigney WA (1998) Association between multiple cardiovascular risk factors and atherosclerosis in children and young adults: the Bogalusa Heart Study. *N Engl J Med* 338: 1650–6. http://dx.doi.org/10.1056/NEJM199806043382302

Bianchin MM, Londero RG, Lima JE, Bigal ME (2010) Migraine and epilepsy: a focus on overlapping clinical, pathophysiological, molecular, and therapeutic aspects. *Curr Pain Headache Rep* 14: 276–83. http://dx.doi.org/10.1007/s11916-010-0121-y

Bigal ME, Kurth T, Hu H, Santanello N, Lipton RB (2009) Migraine and cardiovascular disease: possible mechanisms of interaction. *Neurology* 72: 1864–71. http://dx.doi.org/10.1212/WNL.0b013e3181a71220

Biller J, Mathews KD, Love BB (eds) (1994) *Stroke in Children and Young Adults.* Boston: Butterworth-Heinemann.

Breslau N, Rasmussen BK (2001) The impact of migraine: epidemiology, risk factors, and co-morbidities. *Neurology* 56: S4–12. http://dx.doi.org/10.1212/WNL.56.suppl_1.S4

Breslau N, Davis GC, Andreski P (1991) Migraine, psychiatric disorders, and suicide attempts: an epidemiological study of young adults. *Psychiatry Res* 37: 11–23. http://dx.doi.org/10.1016/0165-1781(91)90102-U

Bottini F, Celle ME, Calevo MG et al (2006) Metabolic and genetic risk factors for migraine in children. *Cephalalgia* 26: 731–7. http://dx.doi.org/10.1111/j.1468-2982.2006.01107.x

Caplan LR (1991) Migraine and vertebrobasilar ischemia. *Neurology* 41: 55–61. http://dx.doi.org/10.1212/ WNL.41.1.55

Chen TC, Leviton A (1990) Asthma and eczema in children born to women with migraine. *Arch Neurol* 47: 1227–30. http://dx.doi.org/10.1001/archneur.1990.00530110087022

Chessa M, Colombo C, Butera G et al (2009) Is it too early to recommend patent foramen ovale closure for all patients who suffer from migraine? A single-centre study. *J Cardiovasc Med* 10: 401–5. http://dx.doi. org/10.2459/JCM.0b013e328329caf5

Cook DG, Mendall MA, Whincup PH et al (2000) C-reactive protein concentration in children: relationship to adiposity and other cardiovascular risk factors. *Atherosclerosis* 149: 139–50. http://dx.doi.org/10.1016/ S0021-9150(99)00312-3

Dalla Volta G, Guindani M, Zavarise P, Griffini S, Pezzini A, Padovani A (2005) Prevalence of patent foramen ovale in a large series of patients with migraine with aura, migraine without aura and cluster headache, and relationship with clinical phenotype. *J Headache Pain* 6: 328–30. http://dx.doi.org/10.1007/ s10194-005-0223-9

D'Andrea G, Leon A (2010) Pathogenesis of migraine: from neurotransmitters to neuromodulators and beyond. *Neurol Sci* 31 (Suppl 1): S1–7. http://dx.doi.org/10.1007/s10072-010-0267-8

De Romanis F, Buzzi MG, Cerbo R, Feliciani M, Assenza S, Agnoli A (1991) Migraine and epilepsy with infantile onset and electroencephalographic findings of occipital spike-wave complexes. *Headache* 31: 378–83. http://dx.doi.org/10.1111/j.1526-4610.1991.hed3106378.x

De Simone R, Ranieri A, Marano E et al (2007) Migraine and epilepsy: clinical and pathophysiological relations. *Neurol Sci* 28 (Suppl 2): 150–5. http://dx.doi.org/10.1007/s10072-007-0769-1

Ducros A (2008) Familial and sporadic hemiplegic migraine. *Rev Neurol* 164: 216–24. http://dx.doi. org/10.1016/j.neurol.2007.10.003

Dusser A, Goutieres F, Aicardi J (1986) Ischemic strokes in children. *J Child Neurol* 1: 131–6. http://dx.doi. org/10.1177/088307388600100207

Ebinger F, Boor R, Gawehn J, Reitter B (1999) Ischemic stroke and migraine in childhood: coincidence or causal relation? *J Child Neurol* 14: 451–5. http://dx.doi.org/10.1177/088307389901400708

Feinstein AR (1970) The pre-therapeutic classification of comorbidity in chronic disease. *J Chronic Dis* 23: 455–68. http://dx.doi.org/10.1016/0021-9681(70)90054-8

Fuller CJ, Jesurum JT (2009) Migraine and patent foramen ovale: state of the science. *Crit Care Nurs Clin North Am* 21: 471–91. http://dx.doi.org/10.1016/j.ccell.2009.07.011

Garcia JH, Pantoni L (1995) Strokes in childhood. *Sem Pediatr Neurol* 2: 180–91. http://dx.doi.org/10.1016/S1071-9091(05)80029-4

Garg BP, De Myer WE (1995) Ischemic thalamic infarction in children: clinical presentation, etiology, and outcome. *Pediatr Neurol* 13: 46–9. http://dx.doi.org/10.1016/0887-8994(95)00108-R

Glueck CJ, Bates SR (1986) Migraine in children: association with primary and familial dyslipoproteinemias. *Pediatrics* 77: 316–21.

Guidetti V, Galli F (1998) Psychiatric comorbidity and childhood migraine. *Cephalalgia* 18: 455–62. http://dx.doi.org/10.1046/j.1468-2982.1998.1807455.x

Glynn RJ, MacFadyen JG, Ridker PM (2009) Tracking of high sensitivity C-reactive protein after an initially elevated concentration: the JUPITER Study. *Clin Chem* 55: 305–12. http://dx.doi.org/10.1373/clinchem.2008.120642

Haut SR, Bigal ME, Lipton RB (2006) Chronic disorders with episodic manifestations: focus on epilepsy and migraine. *Lancet Neurol* 5: 148–57. http://dx.doi.org/10.1016/S1474-4422(06)70348-9

Headache Classification Committee of the International Headache Society (1988) Classification and diagnostic criteria for headache disorders, cranial neuralgias and facial pain. *Cephaialgia* 8 (Suppl 7): 1–93.

Kalaydjian A, Merikangas K (2008) Physical and mental comorbidity of headache in a nationally representative sample of US adults. *Psychosom Med* 70: 773–80. http://dx.doi.org/10.1097/PSY.0b013e31817f9e80

Kampoli AM, Tousoulis D, Antoniades C, Siasos G, Stefanadis C (2009) Biomarkers of premature atherosclerosis. *Trends Mol Med* 15: 323–32. http://dx.doi.org/10.1016/j.molmed.2009.06.001

Lambert M, Delvin EE, Paradis G, O'Loughlin J, Hanley JA, Levy E (2004) C-reactive protein and features of the metabolic syndrome in a population-based sample of children and adolescents. *Clin Chem* 50: 1762–8. http://dx.doi.org/10.1373/clinchem.2004.036418

Lateef TM, Merikangas KR, He J et al (2009) Headache in a national sample of American children: prevalence and comorbidity. *J Child Neurol* 24: 536–43. http://dx.doi.org/10.1177/0883073808327831

Lauritzen M (1994) Pathophysiology of the migraine aura. *Brain* 117: 199–210. http://dx.doi.org/10.1093/brain/117.1.199

Leao AAP (1944) Spreading depression of activity in the cerebral cortex. *J Neurophysiol* 7: 359–90.

Leniger T, von den Driesch S, Isbruch K, Diener HC, Hufnagel A (2003) Clinical characteristics of patients with comorbidity of migraine and epilepsy. *Headache* 43: 672–7. http://dx.doi.org/10.1046/j.1526-4610.2003.03111.x

Lipton RB, Silberstein SD (1994) Why study the comorbidity of migraine? *Neurology* 44 (Suppl 7): S4–5.

Ludvigsson P, Hesdorffer D, Olafsson E, Kjartansson O, Hauser WA (2006) Migraine with aura is a risk factor for unprovoked seizures in children. *Ann Neurol* 59: 210–13. http://dx.doi.org/10.1002/ana.20745

Makita S, Nakamura M, Satoh K et al (2009) Serum C-reactive protein levels can be used to predict future ischemic stroke and mortality in Japanese men from the general population. *Atherosclerosis* 204: 234–8. http://dx.doi.org/10.1016/j.atherosclerosis.2008.07.040

Merikangas KR, Rasmussen BK (2000) Migraine comorbidity. In: Olesen J, Tfelt-Hansen P, Welch KMA, editors. *The Headaches*, 2nd edn. Philadelphia: Lippincott Williams & Wilkins, pp. 235–40.

Mortimer MJ, Kay J, Grawkrodger DJ, Jaron A, Barker DC (1993) The prevalence of headache and migraine in atopic children: an epidemiological study in general practice. *Headache* 33: 427–31. http://dx.doi.org/10.1111/j.1526-4610.1993.hed3308427.x

Moschiano F, D'Amico D, Usai S et al (2008) Homocysteine plasma levels in patients with migraine with aura. *Neurol Sci* 29 (Suppl 1): S173–5. http://dx.doi.org/10.1007/s10072-008-0917-2

Nelson KB, Richardson AK, He J, Lateef TM, Khoromi S, Merikangas KR (2010) Headache and biomarkers predictive of vascular disease in a representative sample of us children. *Arch Pediatr Adolesc Med* 164: 358–62. http://dx.doi.org/10.1001/archpediatrics.2010.17

Nezu A, Kimura S, Ohtsuhi N, Tanaka M, Takebayashi S (1997) Acute confusional migraine and migrainous infarction in childhood. *Brain Dev* 19: 148–51. http://dx.doi.org/10.1016/S0387-7604(96)00551-7

Olesen J, Friberg L, Olsen TS et al (1993) Ischaemia-induced (symptomatic) migraine attacks may be more frequent than migraineinduced ischaemic insults. *Brain* 116: 187–202. http://dx.doi.org/10.1093/brain/116.1.187

Ottman R, Lipton RB (1996) Is the comorbidity of epilepsy and migraine due to a shared genetic susceptibility? *Neurology* 47: 918–24. http://dx.doi.org/10.1212/WNL.47.4.918

Pierangeli G, Cevoli S, Zanigni S et al (2004) The role of cardiac diseases in the comorbidity between migraine and stroke. *Neurol Sci* 25 (Suppl 3): S129–31. http://dx.doi.org/10.1007/s10072-004-0270-z

Post RM, Silberstein SD (1994) Shared mechanisms in affective illness, epilepsy and migraine. *Neurology* 44 (Suppl 7): S37–47.

Rasul CH, Mahboob AA, Hossain SM, Ahmed KU (2009) Predisposing factors and outcome of stroke in childhood. *Indian pediatr* 46: 419–21.

Rogawski MA (2008) Common pathophysiologic mechanisms in migraine and epilepsy. *Arch Neurol* 65: 709–14. http://dx.doi.org/10.1001/archneur.65.6.709

Rothman SM, Olney JW (1987) Excitotoxicity and the NMDA receptor. *Trends Neurosci* 10: 299–302. http://dx.doi.org/10.1016/0166-2236(87)90177-9

Rothrock J, North J, Madden K, Lyden P, Fleck P, Dittrich H (1993) Migraine and migrainous stroke. *Neurology* 43: 2473–6. http://dx.doi.org/10.1212/WNL.43.12.2473

Schwerzmann M, Wiher S, Nedeltchev K et al (2004) Percutaneous closure of patent foramen ovale reduces the frequency of migraine attacks. *Neurology* 62: 1399–401. http://dx.doi.org/10.1212/01.WNL.0000120677.64217.A9

Thomsen LL, Kirchmann M, Bjornsson A et al (2007) The genetic spectrum of a population-based sample of familial hemiplegic migraine. *Brain* 130: 346–56. http://dx.doi.org/10.1093/brain/awl334

Toldo I, Perissinotto E, Menegazzo F et al (2010). Comorbidity between headache and epilepsy in a pediatric headache center. *J Headache Pain* 11: 235–40. http://dx.doi.org/10.1007/s10194-010-0191-6

Toldo I, Bruson A, Casarin A et al (2011) Polymorphisms of the SCN1A gene in children and adolescents with primary headache and idiopathic or cryptogenic epilepsy: is there a linkage? *J Headache Pain* 12: 435–41. http://dx.doi.org/10.1007/s10194-011-0359-8

Towfighi A, Saver JL, Engelhardt R, Ovbiagele B (2008) Factors associated with the steep increase in latemidlife stroke occurrence among US men. *J Stroke Cerebrovasc Dis* 17: 165–8. http://dx.doi.org/10.1016/j.jstrokecerebrovasdis.2007.12.007

Vanmolkot FH, de Hoon JN (2007) Increased C-reactive protein in young adult patients with migraine. *Cephalalgia* 27: 843–6. http://dx.doi.org/10.1111/j.1468-2982.2007.01324.x

Venketasubramanian N, Sacco RL, Di Tullio M, Sherman D, Homma S, Mohr JP (1993) Vascular distribution of paradoxical emboli by transcranial Doppler. *Neurology* 43: 1533–5. http://dx.doi.org/10.1212/WNL.43.8.1533

Verrotti A, Coppola G, Di Fonzo A et al (2011) Should "migralepsy" be considered an obsolete concept? A multicenter retrospective clinical/EEG study and review of the literature. *Epilepsy Behav* 21: 52–9. http://dx.doi.org/10.1016/j.yebeh.2011.03.004

Welch KMA, Levine SR (1990) Migraine-related stroke in the context of the International Headache Society classification of head pain. *Arch Neurol* 47: 458–62. http://dx.doi.org/10.1001/archneur.1990.00530040114027

Willis T (1965) Cerebre anatome: cui accesit nervorum descripto et usus (1664) Reproduced in facsimile. In: Feindel W (ed) Thomas Willis: the anatomy of the brain and nerves. McGill University Press, Montreal.

Wilmshurst PT, Nightingale S, Walsh KP, Morrison WL (2000) Effect on migraine of closure of cardiac right-toleft shunts to prevent recurrence of decompression illness or stroke or for haemodynamic reasons. *Lancet* 356: 1648–51. http://dx.doi.org/10.1016/S0140-6736(00)03160-3

Wilmshurst P, Pearson M, Nightingale S (2005) Re-evaluation of the relationship between migraine and persistent foramen ovale and other right-to-left shunts. *Clin Sci (Lond)* 108: 365–7. http://dx.doi.org/10.1042/CS20040338

Wilson PW, Bozeman SR, Burton TM, Hoaglin DC, Ben-Joseph R, Pashos CL (2008) Prediction of first events of coronary heart disease and stroke with consideration of adiposity. *Circulation* 118: 124–30. http://dx.doi.org/10.1161/CIRCULATIONAHA.108.772962

Wirrell EC, Hamiwka LD (2006) Do children with benign rolandic epilepsy have a higher prevalence of migraine than those with other partial epilepsies or nonepilepsy controls? *Epilepsia* 47: 1674–81. http://dx.doi.org/10.1111/j.1528-1167.2006.00639.x

Wober-Bingol C, Wober C, Karwautz A, Feucht M, Brandtner S, Scheidinger H (1995) Migraine and stroke in childhood and adolescence. *Cephalalgia* 15: 26–30. http://dx.doi.org/10.1046/j.1468-2982.1995.1501026.x

15
CYCLICAL VOMITING SYNDROME

Jean-Christophe Cuvellier

Introduction

First described by Heberden in the French literature in 1806 and by Samuel Gee in the English literature in 1882 (Heberden 1806, Gee 1882), cyclical vomiting syndrome (CVS) is a disorder characterised by recurrent, discrete, self-limited episodes of severe nausea and vomiting interspersed with symptom-free periods. CVS may be the second most common cause of recurrent vomiting after gastro-oesophageal reflux in children, affecting approximately 2% of the paediatric population (Scotland 1.9%, Western Australia 2.3%) (Abu-Arafeh and Russell 1995, Fitzpatrick et al 2007).

Affected children are more often females than males (60:40). CVS has been described in all races and ethnicities, but seems to disproportionately affect white persons. A family history of migraine is present in 39% to 82% of cases (Li and Misiewicz 2003, Abell et al 2008). CVS typically begins between the ages of 2 and 9 years, and the mean delay to diagnosis is 2.7 years (20 episodes) (Li 2000, Prakash et al 2001, Li and Misiewicz 2003).

Clinical features and evaluation

Affected children usually experience a stereotypical pattern of vomiting typified by a consistent time of onset, duration and symptoms, which can be divided into four phases: (1) interepisodic phase; (2) prodromal phase; (3) emetic phase; and (4) recovery phase (Fig. 15.1). In most patients, the episodes are similar in time of onset, duration and symptomatology over months or years, but about 15% of patients have attacks of variable length and type (Li and Misiewicz 2003). The duration of the total episode ranges between 2 hours and 10 days (mean 2.0d). During the interepisodic phase, which lasts a mean of 4 weeks, the patient has relatively few symptoms (Li 2000, Prakash et al 2001, Li and Misiewicz 2003).

Episodes often commence in the early morning (usually 2–4 a.m.) or upon awakening (6–8 a.m.) and are frequently triggered by psychological (e.g. birthdays, school related, emotional excitement) and physical stress (e.g. infections, lack of sleep). The prodromal phase lasts a median of 1.5 hours and is heralded by the patient sensing an impending episode that evolves to nausea accompanied by dramatic autonomic dysfunction, decreased muscle tone, pallor and lethargy and/or apathy causing total incapacitation persisting throughout the duration of the emetic phase, but with some children being still able to take and retain oral medications (Li 2000, Prakash et al 2001, Li and Misiewicz 2003).

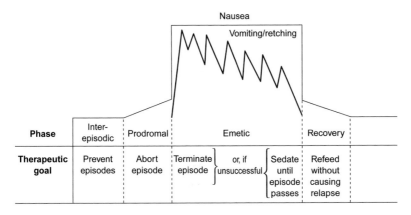

Fig. 15.1 Schematic representation of the four phases of cyclical vomiting syndrome and their therapeutic goals. Fleisher DR, Gornowicz B, Adams K, Burch R, Feldman EJ (2005) Cyclic vomiting syndrome in 41 adults: the illness, the patients, and problems of management. *BMC Med* 3: 20.

The emetic phase lasts a mean of 41 hours and a median of 24 hours. Nausea is unrelenting, completely unrelieved by vomiting, disappearing only when the episode is over, and leads to behavioural strategies designed to lessen it (e.g. fetal positioning). The vomiting is intense (median 6 times/hour at peak, but may be more than 10 times/hour), often bilious, accompanied by disabling and persistent nausea and may provoke haematemesis. Abdominal pain, which may be periumbilical or epigastric, is present in 80% of patients and may be severe enough to mimic an acute abdomen. Other accompanying symptoms include anorexia, retching, drooling, diarrhoea, headache, pallor, flushing, vertigo, photophobia and phonophobia. Patients may become irritable, verbally abusive, demanding or listless. Signs and symptoms of an intense stress response are also common (Li 2000, Prakash et al 2001, Li and Misiewicz 2003). The frequency of vomiting may gradually decrease as the attack progresses.

The recovery phase starts as soon as nausea remits and ends with resumption of normal appetite, oral intake and baseline clinical status. It is remarkably brief, 6 hours, and often typified by sleep. Some parents note such an instantaneous transition from misery to playfulness that they describe it as 'turning off a switch'. Shortly afterwards the child is likely to demand food. It is important in clinical practice to recognise this phasic pattern as it may have consequences in making the diagnosis as well as in management. Over time, a pattern emerges that can be identified as CVS. The frequency of attacks ranges from 1 to 70 per year, with a mean of 12 attacks per year.

Diagnostic approach

The diagnosis of CVS is based on a typical clinical presentation and by exclusion of other possible causes with a similar presentation (Haghighat et al 2007). Table 15.1 shows the ICHD-II criteria for the diagnosis of CVS (Headache Classification Subcommittee of the International Headache Society 2004). The North American Society for Pediatric Gastroenterology, Hepatology and Nutrition (NASPGHAN) also developed its own diagnostic criteria (Li et al

TABLE 15.1
ICHD-II criteria for cyclical vomiting

(A) At least five attacks fulfilling criteria B and C

(B) Episodic attacks, stereotypical in the individual patient, of intense nausea and vomiting lasting from 1h to 5d

(C) Vomiting during attacks occurs four or more times per hour for ≥1h

(D) Symptom free between attacks

(E) Not attributed to another disorder

ICHD-II, Second edition of the International Classification of Headache Disorders (Headache Classification Subcommittee of the International Headache Society 2004).

2008). A pattern of recurrent, episodic vomiting in children that fulfils the NASPGHAN criteria is likely (about 90%) to be ultimately diagnosed as idiopathic CVS (Li et al 2008).

The challenge to the practitioner is to differentiate individuals with specific and serious underlying causes of vomiting (about 10–12%), for whom prompt treatment may alter the outcome (Li et al 1998). A thorough history and physical examination at presentation helps identify physical findings including the following (Li et al 2008):

- Bilious vomiting, haematemesis, abdominal tenderness and/or severe abdominal pain should raise the possibility of a serious underlying disorder such as intermittent bowel obstruction from malrotation with volvulus and prompt an oesophagogastroduodeno-scopy, abdominal ultrasound or computed tomography.
- Attacks precipitated by intercurrent illness, fasting and/or a high-protein meal, or acidosis should raise the possibility of a metabolic disorder.
- Persistent headache or abnormalities on neurological examination, including severe alteration of mental status, abnormal eye movements, papilloedema, motor asymmetry and/or gait abnormality, should lead the clinician to suspect increased intracranial pressure, warranting magnetic resonance imaging.
- Progressively worsening symptoms with increased frequency and duration of episodes, weight loss or conversion to a continuous or chronic pattern.
- Caution is warranted in children younger than 2 years. Munchausen by proxy syndrome may sometimes mimic CVS.

Using decision analysis software, Olson and Li (2002) compared the cost-effectiveness of the following three approaches: (1) extensive diagnostic evaluation, (2) empirical treatment alone and (3) upper gastrointestinal radiology with small-bowel follow-through plus empirical treatment. Upper gastrointestinal radiology with small-bowel follow-through plus empirical antimigraine treatment for an initial period of 2 months was the most cost-effective strategy.

Pathophysiology

Although the pathophysiology of CVS is so far incompletely understood, it points to potential brain–gut mechanisms involving dysregulated central neural pathways and neuroendocrine mediators involved in the afferent and efferent brain–gut pathways of nausea and vomiting. CVS may be seen as the consequence of altered brain responses to visceral and emotional stimuli. Recent hypotheses have focused on the role of autonomic instability as a primary pathogenic factor. Other aetiologies that have been proposed include disturbances in the hypo-thalamic–pituitary–adrenal (HPA) axis, a mitochondrial disorder and migraine association.

Psychological or infectious stressors would initiate central arousal and the cascade of HPA axis activation. More precisely, the corticotrophin-releasing factor (CRF) signalling system would be activated by stressors and play an important role in mediating autonomic alterations that impact on gut motility, causing delayed gastric emptying and nausea (Taché 1999). CRF stimulates adrenocorticotrophic hormone production by the anterior pituitary, thus activating the HPA axis and the stress response. It also mediates anxiogenic, autonomic (sympathetic activation, vagal inhibition and sacral parasympathetic activation) and visceral responses (inhibition of gastric transit and stimulation of colonic secretory and motor func-tion) to stress. Marcus et al (2006) found elevated peripheral CRF levels in affected children during active vomiting episodes. Tricyclic antidepressants, such as amitriptyline, inhibit the promoter activity of the CRF gene, thus reducing the frequency of vomiting episodes (Stout et al 2002, Basta-Kaim et al 2005). Other potential neuroendocrine mediators, such as cortisol production and prostaglandins E_2 as well as autonomic alterations, may participate in initiating or sustaining vomiting in CVS.

Recent diagnostic investigations, such as functional magnetic resonance imaging and positron emission tomography studies, have shown evidence of an altered responsiveness of central arousal circuits involving the amygdala, cingulated cortical subregions and pontine regions, including the periaqueductal grey matter and the locus coeruleus complex in several functional gastrointestinal stress-sensitive disorders (Mayer et al 2009). Altered brainstem regulation of these autonomic signals may be the necessary abnormality that allows the dys-autonomia to feed forward and become self-sustained for days on end.

The 'autonomic nervous system' is a key factor in the responses to a range of emetic activators. Many associated symptoms, such as pallor, flushing, fever, lethargy, salivation and diarrhoea, are mediated by the autonomic nervous system (Fleisher et al 2005, Chelimsky and Chelimsky 2007). Several studies, using such tests of autonomic function as postural adjustment ratio, heart rate variability, tilt table and sudomotor testing, have shown sympa-thetic hyperresponsivity, with relative preservation of the parasympathetic nervous system, in children with CVS (Rashed et al 1999, To et al 1999, Chelimsky and Chelimsky 2007). Sympathetic autonomic imbalance may render patients more susceptible to overresponse to central emetic signals (Gordan 1994). Emetic stimulation may activate, via vagal and sym-pathetic afferent nerves, various brainstem nuclei, which would initiate the stereotypic and coordinated muscular actions involved in vomiting.

Interestingly, distinctive adrenergic autonomic abnormalities associated with CVS are similar to those in individuals with migraine headaches, adding support to the linkage between the conditions. Patients with CVS have a significantly higher prevalence of family members with migraine headaches (39–82% vs 14% of comparison individuals with a chronic vomiting pattern) (Li and Misiewicz 2003). Furthermore, 28% of patients with CVS whose vomiting resolved subsequently developed migraine headaches (Li and Misiewicz 2003). Finally, 80% of affected patients with family histories positive for migraine respond to antimigraine therapy (Li and Misiewicz 2003).

The presence of mitochondrial dysfunction, which leads to cellular energy deficits, may be an additional mechanism that could explain the link between migraine and autonomic dysfunction in paediatric CVS. Defects in mitochondrial energy production due to mutations may predispose individuals to the onset of vomiting during periods of heightened demand for energy (e.g. stress, infections) (Boles et al 2003, 2005). Boles et al have demonstrated that, among children with CVS and neuromuscular disease, 86% have a history of migraines on the maternal side (Boles et al 2003). In children with CVS, two mtDNA polymorphisms (16519T and 3010A) have been associated with CVS and these may account for the clustering of conditions (Zaki et al 2009). The mtDNA polymorphism 16519T was found to be six times more common in children with CVS than in comparison populations, whereas the mtDNA polymorphism 3010A was noted to increase the odds ratio for developing CVS in individuals with 16519T by as much as 17 times. These mtDNA polymorphisms may account for the clustering of functional conditions and symptoms in the same individuals and families.

How these pathways fit together is still unclear. Li and Misiewicz (2003) have proposed that heightened neuronal excitability, resulting from enhanced membrane ion permeability, mitochondrial energy deficits or hormonal state (e.g. menstrual periods), may be present. Stressors can initiate a known cascade that releases hypothalamic CRF, resulting in vomiting. Altered brainstem regulation of these autonomic signals may be the necessary abnormality that allows the dysautonomia to feed forward and become self-sustained for days on end.

Treatment

The management of CVS requires an individually tailored regimen that takes into consideration the clinical course, frequency and severity of attacks and resultant disability, balanced against the potential side effects of treatment. Through a trial and error process, treatment aims to customise a solution for the individual. It can be divided into supportive therapy (during episodes), prophylactic therapy (to prevent episodes) and abortive therapy (to prevent progression from prodromal symptoms to the vomiting phase). Strategies for management of CVS during the interepisodic period include avoidance of identified triggers, lifestyle changes and psychological interventions.

Rigorous therapeutic investigations have been difficult to perform, as most centres have identified only a few cases. Moreover, multicentre studies are difficult because of the acuity of the disease. Because of the absence of double-blind, controlled studies and a placebo response as high as 70%, the NASPGHAN recently issued guidelines for management of CVS in children, based mainly upon small clinical trials and expert opinion (Li et al 2008).

During the well phase, lifestyle changes such as proper management of anxiety, excessive excitement and menstrual problems, and avoidance of energy-depleted states (e.g. fasting, illness), physical overexertion, sleep deprivation, triggering foods (e.g. chocolate, cheese) and motion sickness may reduce episode frequency. Helping anxiety-prone patients to recognise anticipatory anxiety and adopting behavioural self-management techniques may prove beneficial (Forbes and Fairbrother 2008).

PROPHYLAXIS

Prophylaxis should be considered if abortive therapy or supportive measures fail consistently or if episodes are frequent, severe, debilitating and/or disabling. The ultimate goal of prophylaxis is to prevent attacks altogether, but at the very least to reduce the frequency, duration or intensity of episodes. In practice, a sequential trial of agents over periods that will cover two or three attacks is appropriate (Li 2000).

Prophylactic medications used to treat CVS include antimigraine (cyproheptadine, pizotifen, amitriptyline, propranolol), antiepileptic (phenobarbital, valproate, gabapentin and carbamazepine) and prokinetic agents (e.g. erythromycin).

Alternative prophylactic approaches include carnitine, coenzyme Q, low-dose oestrogen (catamenial CVS), acupuncture at the P6 (pericardial) point and psychotherapy (Johnston 2000, Van Calcar et al 2002). The NASPGHAN task force recommended cyproheptadine or propranolol as first choice for children 5 years old and younger (Li et al 2008). In older children, it recommended amitriptyline or propranolol.

ABORTIVE TREATMENT

Early intervention within the first several hours of onset of a CVS attack is essential. Once the vomiting starts, evaluation in an emergency department or direct admission to the hospital ward before dehydration ensues is appropriate in some patients for treatment protocols specifying intravenous fluids, medications and admission criteria. Providing the patient with a letter that specifies an individualised management protocol can facilitate prompt initiation of therapy.

Prophylactic therapy in the prodromal phase includes the control of stressful lifestyles (lying down in a dark, quiet environment or a hot bath), high carbohydrate ingestion and replacement of fluids and electrolytes. The mainstay of medications relies on both antimigraine (5-HT1B/1D agonists) and antiemetic agents (5-HT3 antagonists) (Sunku 2009). The NASPGHAN task force recommends a trial of 5-HT1B/1D agonists in children 12 years and older who have infrequent and/or mild episodes – sumatriptan (intranasal, sublingual or intravenous) or zolmitriptan (intranasal) (Li et al 2008). Success rates (around 50%) are higher in children with migraine-associated CVS when used early in the episode and in those with episodes with a duration of less than 24 hours (Li et al 1999). Ondansetron, given at a dose of 0.3 to 0.4mg/kg/dose, has an efficacy rate of around 62%, and its side effect profile is excellent (drowsiness, dry mouth and headache) (Sunku 2009). Other recommended medications during the prodromal phase include antihistamines (diphenhydramine), phenothiazines (promethazine) and benzodiazepines (lorazepam).

In the acute phase of emetic episodes, patients should be admitted to the hospital to provide supportive measures and to treat nausea, vomiting and severe abdominal pain. Supportive measures include placing children in less stimulating environments and replenishing fluids (10% dextrose or normal saline), electrolytes and energy.

Abortive agents have to be parenterally administered because the intractable emesis precludes the effective use of the oral route (ondansetron, 0.3–0.4mg/kg/dose intravenous every 4–6h, upper limit of 20mg/dose) (Fleisher 1995). When antiemetics fail to control unrelenting nausea and vomiting, expert opinion recommends adding sedatives such as the antihistamine diphenhydramine (1.0–1.25mg/kg/dose every 6h), lorazepam (0.05–0.1mg/kg/dose every 6h) or chlorpromazine. Gastric acid-suppressing agents, including proton pump inhibitors (omeprazole) and H2 receptor antagonists (ranitidine), may be helpful in preventing damage to the mucosa of the oesophagus. Relaxation techniques (e.g. deep breathing, guided imagery) have been reported anecdotally to abort episodes (Fleisher 1995, McRonald and Fleisher 2005).

SUPPORTIVE CARE

Supportive care is required when both prophylactic and abortive pharmacological therapies fail. Family support is crucial to deal with the high level of family frustration in coping with an unpredictable, disruptive, unexplained illness that not only is typically misdiagnosed, but for which there are few definitive answers. A close relationship between the family and the general practitioner is essential for optimal management (Li et al 2008). The help of a mental health professional experienced with CVS can be useful for the entire family in selected patients (Forbes and Fairbrother 2008). Families should be strongly encouraged to obtain information from one of several available online and print sources.

Evolution

The natural history of CVS in children is variable: the majority of patients will ultimately cease to have emetic episodes, at a median age of 10 years, and approximately one-third switch from having vomiting episodes to having migraine headaches. In some children, CVS progresses to abdominal migraine and then to migraine headache.

A survey by Abu-Arafeh and Russell (1995) revealed the mean ages of children with CVS, abdominal migraines and migraine headaches to be 5.3 years, 10.3 years and 11.5 years, respectively. A few patients continue to have vomiting episodes in adulthood (Dignan et al 2001). Li and Misiewicz's (2003) prediction analysis estimated that 75% would develop migraine by age 18 years. Up to 70% of adults with CVS have comorbid psychiatric diagnoses such as mood disorders, anxiety disorders and substance abuse (Fleisher 2005).

Case report

A 14-year-old female was admitted to our hospital with a diagnosis of CVS. Since the age of 24 months, she had suffered about three to five times per year from episodic attacks of frequent and severe vomiting lasting for a few days. The attacks lasted between 12 hours and 4 days. Before admission, she was evaluated by many doctors to determine the causes of her vomiting. Following extensive evaluation, at the age of 6 she was diagnosed with CVS. Attacks were greatly shortened with the antiemetic ondansetron. Numerous preventive medications were given that proved ineffective: sodium valproate, cyproheptadine, flunarizine, topiramate, propranolol, pizotifen, amitriptyline and gabapentin. Following the introduction of erythromycin, the attacks became less frequent, with a 15-month period free of attacks. A slow reduction in the dosage resulted in relapse with four attacks occurring in 6 months, which prompted a return to the previous dose. Since then, attacks have been mild and rare.

This case report illustrates that no single preventive medication is effective in all patients, warranting a successive trial of each until the adequate solution for the individual is found.

REFERENCES

Abell TL, Adams KA, Boles RG et al (2008) Cyclic vomiting syndrome in adults. *Neurogastroenterol Motil* 20: 269–84. http://dx.doi.org/10.1111/j.1365-2982.2008.01113.x

Abu-Arafeh I, Russell G (1995) Cyclical vomiting syndrome in children: a population based study. *J Pediatr Gastroenterol Nutr* 21: 454–8. http://dx.doi.org/10.1097/00005176-199511000-00014

Basta-Kaim A, Budziszewska B, Jaworska-Feil L et al (2005) Inhibitory effect of imipramine on the human corticotropin-releasinghormone gene promoter activity operates through a PI3-K/AKT mediated pathway. *Neuropharmacology* 49: 156–64. http://dx.doi.org/10.1016/j.neuropharm.2005.02.008

Boles RG, Adams K, Ito M, Li BU (2003) Maternal inheritance in cyclic vomiting syndrome with neuromuscular disease. *Am J Med Genet A* 120: 474–82. http://dx.doi.org/10.1002/ajmg.a.20126

Boles RG, Adams K, Li BUK (2005) Maternal inheritance in cyclic vomiting syndrome. *Am J Med Genet A* 133: 71–7. http://dx.doi.org/10.1002/ajmg.a.30524

Chelimsky TC, Chelimsky GG (2007) Autonomic abnormalities in cvs. *J Pediatr Gastroenterol Nutr* 44: 326–30. http://dx.doi.org/10.1097/MPG.0b013e31802bddb7

Dignan F, Symon DN, AbuArafeh I, Russell G (2001) The prognosis of cyclical vomiting syndrome. *Arch Dis Child* 84: 55–7. http://dx.doi.org/10.1136/adc.84.1.55

Fitzpatrick E, Bourke B, Drumm B, Rowland M. (2007) The incidence of cyclic vomiting syndrome in children: population based study. *Am J Gastroenterol* 103: 991–5. http://dx.doi.org/10.1111/j.1572-0241.2007.01668.x

Fleisher DR (1995) The cyclic vomiting syndrome described. *J Pediatr Gastroenterol Nutr* 21 (Suppl 1): S1–5. http://dx.doi.org/10.1097/00005176-199501001-00003

Fleisher DR, Gornowicz B, Adams K, Burch R, Feldman EJ (2005) Cyclic Vomiting Syndrome in 41 adults: the illness, the patients, and problems of management. *BMC Med* 3: 20. http://dx.doi.org/10.1186/1741-7015-3-20

Forbes D, Fairbrother S (2008) Cyclic nausea and vomiting in childhood. *Aust Fam Physician* 37: 33–6.

Gee S (1882) On fitful or recurrent vomiting. *Saint Bartholomew's Hospital Rep* 18: 1–6.

Gordon N (1994) Recurrent vomiting in childhood, especially of neurological origin. *Dev Med Child Neurol* 36: 463–7. http://dx.doi.org/10.1111/j.1469-8749.1994.tb11873.x

Haghighat M, Rafie SM, Dehghani SM, Fallahi GH, Nejabat M (2007) Cyclic vomiting syndrome in children: experience with 181 cases from southern Iran. *World J Gastroenterol* 13: 1833–6.

Heberden W (1806) *Commentaries on the History and Causes of Diseases*, 3rd Ed. London: Payne and Foss.

Headache Classification Subcommittee of the International Headache Society (2004) The International Classification of Headache Disorders, Cranial Neuralgia and Facial Pain, 2nd edn. *Cephalalgia* 24 (Suppl 1): 1–160.

Johnston W (2000) Acupuncture may treat cyclic vomiting syndrome. *Anesthesiology News* 5.

Li BUK (2000) Cyclic vomiting syndrome: the evolution of understanding of a brain-gut disorder. *Adv Pediatr* 47: 1–44.

Li BU, Misiewicz L (2003) Cyclic vomiting syndrome: a brain-gut disorder. *Gastroenterol Clin North Am* 32: 997–1019. http://dx.doi.org/10.1016/S0889-8553(03)00045-1

Li BUK, Murray R, Heitlinger L, Robbins JL, Hayes JR (1998) Heterogeneity of diagnosis presenting as cyclic vomiting. *Pediatrics* 102: 583–7. http://dx.doi.org/10.1542/peds.102.3.583

Li BUK, Murray R, Heitlinger L, Robbins J, Hayes J (1999) Is cyclic vomiting related to migraine? *J Pediatrics* 134: 567–72. http://dx.doi.org/10.1016/S0022-3476(99)70242-8

Li BU, Lefevre F, Chelimsky GG et al (2008) North American Society for Pediatric Gastroenterology, Hepatology, and Nutrition consensus statement on the diagnosis and management of cyclic vomiting syndrome. *J Pediatr Gastroenterol Nutr* 47: 379–93. http://dx.doi.org/10.1097/MPG.0b013e318173ed39

McRonald FE, Fleisher DR (2005) Anticipatory nausea in cyclical vomiting. *BMC Pediatr* 5: 3. http://dx.doi.org/10.1186/1471-2431-5-3

Marcus SB, Agiabe-Willia SM, Grigoriadis D, Tache Y, Zimmerman D, Li BU (2006) Corticotropin-releasing factor (CRF) levels are elevated during episodes of cyclic vomiting syndrome. *Gastroenterology* 130 (Suppl 2): A4.

Mayer EA, Aziz Q, Coen S et al (2009) Brain imaging approaches to the study of functional GI disorders: a Rome working team report. *Neurogastroenterol Motil* 21: 579–96. http://dx.doi.org/10.1111/j.1365-2982.2009.01304.x

Olson AD, Li BU (2002) The diagnostic evaluation of children with cyclic vomiting: a costeffectiveness assessment. *J Pediatr* 141: 724–8. http://dx.doi.org/10.1067/mpd.2002.129300

Prakash C, Staiano A, Rothbaum RJ, Clouse RE (2001) Similarities in cyclic vomiting syndrome across age groups. *Am J Gastroenterol* 96: 684–8. http://dx.doi.org/10.1111/j.1572-0241.2001.03606.x

Rashed H, Abell TL, Familoni BO, Cardoso SR (1999) Autonomic function in cyclic vomiting syndrome and classic migraine. *Dig Dis Sci* 44 (8 Suppl): 74–8S.

Stout SC, Owens MJ, Nemeroff CB (2002) Regulation of corticotropin-releasing factor neuronal systems and hypothalamic–pituitary-adrenal axis activity by stress and chronic antidepressant treatment. *J Pharmacol Exp Ther* 300: 1085–92. http://dx.doi.org/10.1124/jpet.300.3.1085

Sunku B (2009) Cyclic Vomiting Syndrome: a disorder of all ages. *Gastroenterol Hepatol* 5: 507–15.

Taché Y(1999) Cyclic vomiting syndrome: the corticotropin-releasing-factor hypothesis. *Dig Dis Sci* 44 (8 Suppl): 79–86S.

To J, Issenman RM, Kamath MV (1999) Evaluation of neurocardiac signals in pediatric patients with cyclic vomiting syndrome through power spectral analysis of heart rate variability. *J Pediatr* 135: 363–6. http://dx.doi.org/10.1016/S0022-3476(99)70135-6

Van Calcar S, Harding C, Wolff J (2002) L-carnitine administration reduces number of episodes in cyclic vomiting syndrome. *Clin Pediatr* 41: 171–4. http://dx.doi.org/10.1177/000992280204100307

Zaki EA, Freilinger T, Klopstock T et al (2009) Two common mitochondrial DNA polymorphisms are highly associated with migraine headache and cyclic vomiting syndrome. *Cephalalgia* 29: 719–28. http://dx.doi.org/10.1111/j.1468-2982.2008.01793.x

16
ABDOMINAL MIGRAINE

Donald Lewis

Introduction

Recurrent abdominal pain occurs in 9% to 15% of all children and adolescents. Affected children consume an enormous amount of healthcare resources and their episodic symptoms often lead to significant disability, including interference with family, school and social activities. Accurate diagnosis of the cause of the pain is essential in order to provide the necessary reassurance to the patient and family, to optimise therapeutic interventions and to minimise functional disability (Bentley et al 1995, Rasquin et al 2006, Russell et al 2007).

According to the American Academy of Pediatrics, 'functional abdominal pain' is the most common cause of chronic, recurring abdominal pain in children and is a practical and specific diagnosis derived following exclusion of other anatomical, infectious, inflammatory or other metabolic causes of abdominal pain (American Academy of Paediatrics Subcommittee on Chronic Abdominal Pain 2005).

Functional abdominal pain is subdivided into four categories as one, or a combination, of the following (American Academy of Paediatrics Subcommittee on Chronic Abdominal Pain 2005):

* functional dyspepsia
* irritable bowel syndrome
* functional abdominal pain syndrome
* abdominal migraine.

Clinical features

Case history

A 10-year-old female presents with recurrent bouts of moderate to severe, periumbilical abdominal pain. Her pain is vague, aching and constant and she holds her stomach with both hands, bent forward slightly at the waist. The episodes typically last several hours but are not usually associated with vomiting or diarrhoea. During the episodes, she is pale, sweaty and photophobic and occasionally complains of a frontal headache. She has undergone repeated gastrointestinal and renal evaluations without a firm diagnosis. Her frustrated mother has suffered with migraine without aura since her teenage years.

Although first described nearly a century ago, abdominal migraine has received variable and insufficient attention as one of many potential aetiologies of recurrent abdominal pain in children (Liveing 1873, Buchanan 1921, Brams 1922, Wyllie and Schlesinger 1933). Identifying abdominal migraine among the myriad of other potential causes of recurrent abdominal pain can be challenging, but the first step is to consider the diagnosis when evaluating a patient with a clinical history similar to that described above.

The key clinical feature of abdominal migraine is recurrent, stereotyped episodes of unexplained disabling periumbilical pain that last from 1 to 72 hours, separated by periods of interval wellness. The pain is typically midline or periumbilical in location, but, in younger children, it may be quite poorly localised. The pain is typically not crampy or colicky in nature, but more vague in description, with a dull or 'just sore' description. However, by definition, the pain is moderate to severe in intensity and produces some degree of functional disability. There may be a variety of associated symptoms such as anorexia, nausea, vomiting, pallor, frontal headache, phonophobia and/or photophobia (Table 16.1) (Symon and Russell 1986).

The age at onset is generally between 3 and 10 years of age, but, as with cyclical vomiting syndrome, there is typically a significant time lag between onset of symptoms and establishment of the diagnosis, which for abdominal migraine is made between 6 and 10 years of age (Table 16.2) (Symon and Russell 1986). Equal numbers of males and females are affected by this condition (Bentley et al 1995).

TABLE 16.1
Symptoms associated with abdominal migraine (*n*=40)

Symptoms	Percentage of children with the symptoms
Vasomotor	97.5
Pallor	92.5
Flushing	5
Gastrointestinal	97.5
Anorexia	85
Vomiting	50

Compiled from Symon and Russell (1986).

TABLE 16.2
Presentation of abdominal migraine

	Mean age at presentation (y)	Mean duration of symptoms (y)
Males	9.4	2.4
Females	8.4	1.4
Range	2.7–12.4	

Compiled from Symon and Russell (1986).

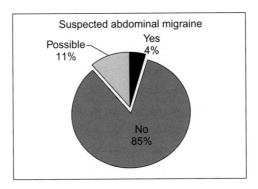

Fig. 16.1 Proportion of children with unexplained recurrent abdominal pain who have abdominal migraine or possible abdominal migraine (*n*=600) (Carson et al 2011).

The majority of epidemiological data are derived from the UK, where the prevalence of abdominal migraine was found to be 2.4% (Mortimer et al 1993). In a survey using diagnostic criteria similar to ICHD-II (Headache Classification Subcommittee of the International Headache Society 2004), Abu-Arafeh and Russell (1995) reported the prevalence of abdominal migraine to be 4.1% among 2165 children aged 5 to 15 years. There has been a transatlantic disparity in that the diagnosis of abdominal migraine is made quite commonly in Europe but quite infrequently in the USA. A recent report from one US paediatric gastroenterology practice found the prevalence rate of abdominal migraine among a population of patients with recurrent abdominal pain (*n*=600) to be 4%, with another 11% of patients deemed as having 'probable' abdominal migraine during a 2-year period during which no child was diagnosed with abdominal migraine in this clinic (Fig. 16.1) (Carson et al 2011).

The conclusion of this report was that abdominal migraine is underdiagnosed and under-recognised in the USA. The limited recognition by clinicians can be explained, in part, by the lack of awareness of abdominal migraine among primary-care physicians and among their gastrointestinal consultants, to whom children with unexplained abdominal pain are typically referred. Furthermore, expertise in the diagnosis of abdominal migraine has traditionally rested with neurologists, who are infrequently called upon in the evaluation of recurrent abdominal pain (Russell et al 2007).

Abdominal migraine is more common in those with a family history of migraine headaches. In a 10-year prospective study of nearly 150 children referred for recurrent abdominal pain, Bentley et al (1995) identified 70 children whose symptoms were consistent with abdominal migraine and 90% had a positive family history of migraines in a first-degree relative (Mortimer et al 1992).

Criteria for diagnosis
We have known for decades that abdominal pain is part of the paediatric migraine phenomenon. In fact, one of the pioneers of paediatric migraine, Dr Arthur Prensky, proposed one of the first sets of diagnostic criteria for migraine, which included *abdominal pain* as one of the six key features (Prensky and Sommer 1979). Acceptance of the concept that abdominal pain can be the primary manifestation of migraine in children has been slow.

TABLE 16.3
Criteria for abdominal migraine

(A) Pain is periumbilical or poorly localised

(B) Pain is described as dull or sore in nature

(C) Each attack lasts for $\geq$1h

(D) Pain is associated with any two of the following:

    (1) Anorexia

    (2) Nausea

    (3) Vomiting

    (4) Pallor

(E) Attacks occur at least twice yearly

(F) There is complete resolution of symptoms between attacks

(G) Pain is severe enough to interfere with normal daily activities

(H) The diagnosis is excluded if any of the following is present:

    (1) Mild symptoms not interfering significantly with daily activities

    (2) Burning pain

    (3) Non-midline abdominal pain

    (4) Symptoms suggestive of food intolerance, malabsorption or other gastrointestinal disease, e.g. diarrhoea or weight loss

    (5) Attacks of <1h duration

(I) Persistence of symptoms between attacks

Compiled from Dignan et al (2001).

In 2001, Dignan et al (2001) proposed a comprehensive definition of abdominal migraine that includes seven elements (Table 16.3). The location of the pain is periumbilical and described vaguely as being 'just sore'. An episode lasts for more than an hour, but typically lasts at least 4 hours up to a full day. Attacks are accompanied by at least two associated symptoms of anorexia, nausea, vomiting and/or pallor, although flushing may be seen in some patients. In order to confirm a recurrent nature, the Dignan criteria require that the attacks occur at least twice yearly and that there is interval wellness with complete resolution of symptoms between attacks. Parenthetically, Dignan keenly commented that these 'children are not sickly or unwell, except during attacks, and do not appear to be experiencing anxiety, stress or other psychological problems. Their parents describe them as 'normal and well adjusted'.

To emphasise the intensely disabling nature of the pain, these criteria require that the pain is severe enough to interfere with normal daily activities, which implies that, during an episode, the child is unable to participate in any usual, even enjoyable, leisure activities and prefers to retire to a quite place and rest. Dignan eloquently describes the child's mood as 'one of intense misery'.

The Dignan criteria include several very important *exclusionary* features. The diagnosis of abdominal migraine is not associated with mild symptoms that fail to significantly interfere with daily activities, a burning quality of pain that would suggest acid reflux or pain which

TABLE 16.4

International Classification of Headache Disorders diagnostic criteria for abdominal migraine

(A) At least five attacks fulfilling criteria B–D

(B) Attacks of abdominal pain lasting 1–72h

(C) Abdominal pain has *all* of the following characteristics:

  (1) Midline location, periumbilical or poorly localised

  (2) Dull or 'just sore' quality

  (3) Moderate or severe intensity

(D) During abdominal pain, at least two of the following:

  (1) Anorexia

  (2) Nausea

  (3) Vomiting

  (4) Pallor

(E) Not attributed to another disorder. History and physical examination do not show signs of gastrointestinal or renal disease or such disease has been ruled out by appropriate investigations

Compiled from Headache Classification Subcommittee of the International Headache Society (2004).

is not midline or periumbilical. Furthermore, if symptoms can be explained by food allergy, malabsorption syndrome or another gastrointestinal disease with diarrhoea or weight loss, a diagnosis of abdominal migraine is not appropriate. The duration of attacks is defined so that for episodes that are too brief (duration <1h) or chronic, persistent pain without interval wellness would also exclude the diagnosis of abdominal migraine.

In 2004, the International Headache Society (IHS) published the International Classification of Headache Disorders, 2nd edn (ICHD-II), placing abdominal migraine among the subset of disorders known as 'periodic syndromes of childhood that are precursors for migraine' along with cyclical vomiting syndrome and benign paroxysmal vertigo (Table 16.4) (Olesen 2004). This robust set of diagnostic criteria for abdominal migraine evolved from the Dignan criteria, but with a few more specific requirements such as a minimum of five attacks and a specified duration of 1 to 72 hours. Otherwise, ICHD-II parallels Dignan with the requirement for a midline or periumbilical location, a dull or 'just sore' quality, moderate or severe intensity and associated symptoms of anorexia, nausea, vomiting or pallor (at least two of the four). The ICHD-II criteria typically adds a disclaimer to all its headache definitions by stating that the disorder is 'not attributed to another disorder' with the specific point that history and physical examination do not show signs of (other) gastrointestinal disorder or renal disease, and that such diseases have been ruled out by appropriate investigations.

Curiously, the IHS criteria make no mention of headache.

In 2006, the paediatric gastroenterology community developed the 'Rome III' criteria for functional gastrointestinal disorders, which includes diagnostic criteria for abdominal migraine (Table 16.5) (Rasquin et al 2006). These diagnostic criteria require an episodic nature with two or more episodes during the preceding 12 months. Similar to the other two sets of criteria, the attacks are paroxysms of intense periumbilical pain that last 1 hour or more, with

TABLE 16.5

Rome III (2006) criteria for functional gastrointestinal disorders

Diagnostic criteria for abdominal migraine includes all of the following, with two or more episodes in the preceding 12 months:

(A) Paroxysmal episode of intense, acute periumbilical pain that lasts ≥1h

(B) Intervening periods of usual health lasting weeks to months

(C) The pain interferes with normal activities

(D) The pain is associated with two or more of the following:

    (1) Anorexia

    (2) Nausea

    (3) Vomiting

    (4) Headache

    (5) Photophobia

    (6) Pallor

(E) No evidence of an inflammatory, anatomical, metabolic or neoplastic process

Compiled from Rasquin et al (2006).

intervening weeks to months of usual health. The pain must interfere with normal activities and be associated with anorexia, nausea, vomiting, *headache*, photophobia and/or pallor (two or more). Furthermore, there must be no evidence of an 'inflammatory, anatomic, metabolic, or neoplastic process'. Ironically, it is the gastroenterology community that first includes headache among its associated symptoms as well as photophobia.

From these three sets of definitions, it can be stated that abdominal migraine is an idiopathic, recurrent disorder characterised by episodes of moderate to severe midline abdominal pain which last between 1 and 72 hours. There must be some associated symptoms such as nausea, vomiting, pallor, anorexia or headache during the episodes. Importantly, the child is healthy and growing well without weight loss, chronic diarrhoea or other systemic symptoms between episodes.

Natural course and prognosis

Abdominal migraine is among the three disorders that are termed 'periodic syndromes of childhood that are precursors to migraine'. This elegant phrase captures the episodic, periodic nature as well as the natural history of the disorder to dissipate and 'grow into' more typical migraine. There is evidence of an evolution of abdominal migraine into more typical migraine headaches through childhood, and abdominal migraine rarely persists into adulthood. In the comments section of ICHD-II, the statement is made that 'most children with abdominal migraine will develop migraine headache later in life' (Olesen 2004). Dignan followed a cohort of 54 children with abdominal migraine and found that 70% developed migraine headaches and 39% still suffered from abdominal pain (Table 16.6). Abdominal migraine tended to disappear over time, but clearly can be seen in adults (Dignan et al 2001).

The pathophysiology of abdominal migraine is unknown, but given our understanding of

TABLE 16.6
Prognosis for abdominal migraine (*n*=54)

Symptoms on follow-up	Per cent of patients
No longer experiencing abdominal pain	61%
Never had migraine headache	22%
Currently having migraine headache	20%
Had migraine at one time, not actively	18.5%
Still experiencing abdominal pain	39%
Never had migraine headache	7.4%
Currently having migraine headache	31%
Total percentage that had abdominal migraine and ever experienced migraine headache	70.4%

Compiled from Dignan et al (2001).

the biology of migraine, which includes activation of brainstem centres in the dorsal raphe and locus coeruleus, stimulation of dopaminergic and serotonergic pathways, coupled with the concepts of central sensitisation and allodynia, a basic construct can be generated. These brainstem centres have a key role in the regulation of autonomic circuitry and may play a role in the generation of the nausea, vomiting and gastroparesis seen in migraine. These centres modulate noradrenergic and serotonergic pathways, which may influence gastrointestinal motility and dysmotility. Sensitisation and allodynia (the phenomenon that seemingly innocuous sensory stimuli are perceived as painful) would explain the disproportionate amount of pain reported by the children, in the perplexing absence of objective signs.

Management

GENERAL PRINCIPLES
With abdominal migraine, the focus must be on prevention of attacks with a blend of behavioural interventions and dietary measures, coupled with the judicious use of preventative medications. Russell et al (2002) recommend the following comprehensive treatment regimen following the diagnosis of abdominal migraine:

- explanation and reassurance
- avoidance of known and potential triggers
- simple dietary management
- few-foods diet
- drug therapy.

As is often the case in children with chronic, unexplained illness, the families of children with abdominal migraine are extremely frustrated, stressed and desperate. They have watched their child suffer and have felt extremely helpless and abandoned by the medical community. Families have become convinced through discussions with well-meaning friends and relatives and hours of Internet searching that the doctors are missing some life-threatening illness or tumour. Therefore, establishing the diagnosis and providing both a confident explanation of the problem and a comprehensive treatment plan affords a huge reassurance and sense of relief to the family.

PREVENTION STRATEGIES AND PROPHYLACTIC TREATMENT

Avoidance of known and potential triggers involves maintaining a log or diary of events and circumstances surrounding attacks to help identify triggers. Common dietary precipitants for migraine include cheeses, processed meats, chocolates, nuts, monosodium glutamate, caffeine-containing drinks and, on occasion, citrus. For the child who suffers from frequent attacks, other more heroic dietary interventions may be considered, such as an oligoantigenic diet, but these may require in-patient initiation with close assistance by an experienced dietitian (Egger et al 1983).

Other possible triggers include stress or anxiety, sleep disturbances or irregularity, missed meals or chaotic eating patterns and lack of exercise (Table 16.7). Once a trigger is identified, efforts must be made to avoid, moderate or eliminate it.

TABLE 16.7
Triggers for abdominal migraine

Stress/anxiety
Sleep disturbances
Inactivity/lack of exercise
Overscheduling
Disruption of schedule (vacation/travel)
Fasting
Dietary
Cheese (aged)
Chocolate and cocoa
Processed meats
Sausages, hot dogs, corned beef and other preserved meats (containing nitrites)
Citrus fruits (oranges, lemons, grapefruits, etc.)
Tomatoes, including soup and ketchup
Caffeine-containing drinks (colas, coffee and tea)
Food colourings, especially in lurid sweets and chewing gum
Food flavourings, especially those used for crisps
Monosodium glutamate
Fried foods
Raisins and grapes
Alcohol (beers and red wine)

Compiled from Russell et al (2002).

Pharmacological preventative treatment should be reserved for the small subset of children who demonstrate a clear sense of disability. Although there are few controlled data to support their use, pizotifen, cyproheptadine and propranolol are usually listed as agents of choice.

There was one double-blind, placebo-controlled, crossover trial of pizotifen which studied 14 children (ages 5–13y). The patients had to have at least two attacks per month for longer than 6 months and the attacks had to last more than 2 hours. The patients were randomised to be treated with 0.25mg of pizotifen or placebo orally twice a day, with the option to go to a three times per day dosing schedule after a month if symptoms had not improved sufficiently. After 2 months, they were switched to the other arm (Symon and Russell 1995). The end points were days of abdominal pain and indices of 'severity' and 'misery'. The results demonstrated 4.3 days of abdominal pain in the pizotifen treated group versus 12.5 days in the placebo group (p=0.005), with both indices showing significantly better responses with the active agent than with the placebo. Individuals reported a mean of 8.21 [95% confidence interval (CI) 2.93–13.48] fewer days of pain while taking the active drug (Symon and Russell 1995). They also reported that the mean difference on an 'index of severity' was –16.21 (95% CI –26.51 to –5.90) and on an 'index of misery' was –56.07 (95% CI –94.07 to –18.07) (Huertas-Celballos et al 2002). Weight gain and sedation were the only reported side effects. The authors concluded that 'pizotifen was clearly superior to placebo in the prophylaxis of childhood abdominal migraine' (Symon and Russell 1995); however, this evidence should be taken with caution because of the small number of patients in this study, and there were no other published studies to support the findings.

Symon and Russell (1986) reported a retrospective review of 40 children, of whom 20 were treated with pizotifen 0.5mg orally twice daily for 2 to 6 months. All patients 'claimed improvement' in their symptoms, with 70% (n=14) reporting complete resolution of symptoms.

In an open retrospective study of 38 patients (ages 3–15y, male–female 2:1), Worawattanakul et al (1999) found that 18 of the 24 patients (75%) treated with propranolol had an 'excellent' response, defined as cessation of attacks. Cyproheptadine produced an excellent response in only 33% (n=12) and a 'fair' response in 50%.

There are no data on the role of vitamins (i.e. riboflavin) or minerals (magnesium).

MANAGEMENT OF ACUTE ATTACKS

Little exists in the literature regarding the acute management of abdominal migraine. However, anecdotal evidence suggests that many of the guidelines used in the treatment of migraine headaches may also be efficacious in the treatment of abdominal migraine.

Traditional acute therapies for migraine such as paracetamol (acetaminophen) and ibuprofen, for which there is good evidence to demonstrate value in migraine with and without aura, have not been studied in abdominal migraine. Several drugs among the class of triptan agents (e.g. almotriptan, zolmitriptan, rizatriptan and sumatriptan) that similarly have shown efficacy in migraine headache have not been studied for abdominal migraine, but deserve consideration and investigation for the acute treatment of abdominal migraine if over-the-counter agents prove ineffective.

Antiemetics (e.g. ondansetron, prochlorperazine, metoclopramide) have a role to play if nausea or vomiting is pronounced. There is no defined role for antispasmodics, promotility agents, antacids, antianxiety agents or sedatives. There is a case report of successful treatment of attacks of abdominal migraine in two patients (ages 12 and 17) who were admitted to the hospital for quite severe attacks unresponsive to multiple agents. The 12-year-old child had significant vomiting and this suggests features of cyclical vomiting syndrome. In both cases, intravenous valproic acid relieved symptoms of abdominal pain and nausea, as well as improving any associated mental status changes, quickly 'once therapeutic levels were reached'. Neither child's case is typical of abdominal migraine, so caution should be exercised before this therapeutic avenue is considered (Tan et al 2006).

Conclusions

Abdominal migraine occurs in about 1% to 2.5% of children, and, among children with idiopathic recurrent abdominal pain, abdominal migraine represents about 4% to 15%.

Despite recognition by the fields of headache and gastroenterology with well-established and validated diagnostic criteria in ICHD-II (2004) and Rome III (Rasquin et al 2006), abdominal migraine is underrecognised and underdiagnosed. Given the spectrum of treatment modalities now available for paediatric migraine, increased awareness of the cardinal features of abdominal migraine by paediatricians and paediatric gastroenterologists may result in improved diagnostic accuracy and early institution of both acute and preventive migraine-specific treatments.

Improved recognition and diagnosis of abdominal migraine as a cause of recurrent abdominal pain in children would also stimulate further investigations into the nature and underlying mechanisms of abdominal migraine, as well as controlled trials of specific treatment options. Future directions call for prospective studies with increased sample sizes, and controlled trials of migraine-specific therapies for children with abdominal migraine.

REFERENCES

American Academy of Pediatrics Subcommittee on Chronic Abdominal Pain (2005) Chronic Abdominal Pain in Children. *Pediatrics* 115: 812–15. http://dx.doi.org/10.1542/peds.2004-2497

Abu-Arafeh I, Russell G (1995) Prevalence and clinical features of abdominal migraine compared with those of migraine headache. *Arch Dis Child* 72: 413–17. http://dx.doi.org/10.1136/adc.72.5.413

Bentley D, Hehely A, al-Bayaty M, Michie CA (1995) Abdominal migraine as a cause of vomiting in children: a clinician's view. *J Pediatr Gastroenterol Nutrition* 21 (Suppl 1): S49–51. http://dx.doi.org/10.1097/00005176-199501001-00014

Brams WA (1922) Abdominal migraine. *JAMA* 78: 26–7. http://dx.doi.org/10.1001/jama.1922.02640540032009

Buchanan JA (1921) The abdominal crises of migraine. *J Nerv Ment Dis* 54: 406–12. http://dx.doi.org/10.1097/00005053-192111000-00002

Carson L, Lewis D, Tsou M et al (2011) Abdominal migraine: an under- diagnosed cause of recurrent abdominal pain in children. *Headache* 51: 707–12. http://dx.doi.org/10.1111/j.1526-4610.2011.01855.x

Dignan F, Abu-Arafeh I, Russell G (2001) The prognosis of childhood abdominalmigraine. *Arch Dis Child* 84: 415–18. http://dx.doi.org/10.1136/adc.84.5.415

Egger J, Carter CM, Wilson J, et al (1983) Is migraine food allergy? A double-blindcontrolled trial of oligoantigenic diet treatment. *Lancet* 2: 865–9. http://dx.doi.org/10.1016/S0140-6736(83)90866-8

Headache Classification Subcommittee of the International Headache Society (2004) The International Classification of Headache Disorders, 2nd edition. *Cephalalgia* 24 (Suppl 1): 9–160.

Huertas-Ceballos A, Macarthur C, Logan S (2002) Pharmacological interventions for recurrent abdominal pain (RAP) in childhood. *Cochrane Database Syst Rev* 1: CD003017.

Liveing E (1873) *On Megrim, Sick-headache and some Allied Disorders*. London: J&A Churchill, p. 213.

Mortimer MJ, Kay J, Jaron A, Good, PA (1992) Does a history of maternal migraine or depression predispose children to headache and stomach-ache? *Headache* 32: 353–5. http://dx.doi.org/10.1111/j.1526-4610.1992. hed3207353.x

Mortimer MJ, Kay J, Jaron A (1993) Clinical epidemiology of childhood abdominal migraine in an urban general practice. *Dev Med Child Neurol* 35: 243–8. http://dx.doi.org/10.1111/j.1469-8749.1993.tb11629.x

Prensky AL, Sommer D (1979) Diagnosis and treatment of migraine in children. *Neurology* 29: 506–10. http:// dx.doi.org/10.1212/WNL.29.4.506

Rasquin A, Di Lorenzo C, Forbes D et al (2006) Childhood functional gastrointestinal disorders: child/adolescent. *Gastroenterology* 130: 1527–37. http://dx.doi.org/10.1053/j.gastro.2005.08.063

Russell G, Abu-Arafeh I, Symon DN (2002) Abdominal migraine: evidence for existence and treatment options. *Paediatr Drugs* 4: 1–8.

Russell G, Symon DN, Abu-Arafeh IA (2007) The child with recurrent abdominal pain: is it abdominal migraine? *Br J Hosp Med (Lond)* 68: M110–13.

Symon D, Russell G (1986) Abdominal migraine; a childhood syndrome defined. *Cephalalgia* 6: 223–8. http:// dx.doi.org/10.1046/j.1468-2982.1986.0604223.x

Symon DN, Russell G (1995) Double blind placebo controlled trial of pizotifen syrup in the treatment of abdominal migraine. *Arch Dis Child* 72: 48–50. http://dx.doi.org/10.1136/adc.72.1.48

Tan V, Sahami AR, Peebles R, Shaw RJ (2006) Abdominal migraine and treatment with intravenous valproic acid. *Psychosomatics* 47: 353–6. http://dx.doi.org/10.1176/appi.psy.47.4.353

Worawattanakul M, Rhoads JM, Lichtman SN, Ulshen MH (1999) Abdominal migraine: prophylactic treatment and follow-up. *J Pediatr Gastroenterol Nutr* 28: 37–40. http://dx.doi.org/10.1097/00005176-199901000-00010

Wyllie W, Schlesinger B (1933) The periodic group of disorders in childhood. *Br J Child Dis* 30: 1–21.

17
BENIGN PAROXYSMAL VERTIGO AND BENIGN PAROXYSMAL TORTICOLLIS

George Russell

Allergists have long been accustomed to describing the allergic march, in which infantile eczema gives way to asthma during childhood, which in turn gives way to allergic rhinitis and other allergies in adult life. This 'march' is a somewhat unreliable sequence but supports the concept that the same disease process can give rise to a variety of different clinical syndromes. In the case of migraine, benign paroxysmal torticollis (BPT) tends to affect infants, benign paroxysmal vertigo (BPV) and cyclical vomiting tend to start in the preschool years, abdominal migraine affects schoolchildren and all have an inconsistent tendency to give way to migraine headaches as the child gets older. This chapter deals with two conditions that may initiate the migrainous march, although in many instances they occur in isolation and the child makes a complete recovery.

Benign paroxysmal vertigo

DEFINITION AND CRITERIA FOR DIAGNOSIS

Benign paroxysmal vertigo is a childhood disorder in which attacks of vertigo, usually very brief but occasionally lasting for several hours or even longer, occur in the absence of any apparent stimulus and in the absence of any detectable neurological or auditory disorder. The attacks are sometimes accompanied by nausea, headache, pallor or nystagmus, but there is never loss of consciousness, and there is complete recovery between attacks.

The International Headache Society (IHS) has proposed diagnostic criteria for BPV (Headache Classification Subcommittee of the International Headache Society 2004a). These criteria are essential for defining cases in research studies, but the numerical criterion of at least five attacks is less useful to the clinician wishing to reassure parents about the benign nature of their child's condition. These criteria are as follows:

(A) at least five attacks fulfilling criterion B
(B) multiple episodes of severe vertigo, occurring without warning and resolving spontaneously after minutes to hours
(C) normal neurological examination and audiometric and vestibular functions between attacks
(D) normal electroencephalogram.

Note: often associated with nystagmus or vomiting, unilateral throbbing headache may occur in some attacks.

EPIDEMIOLOGY

The epidemiology of BPV has attracted little attention, a reflection in part of the benign nature of the condition and in part of the difficulty in making the diagnosis in young children even after a full clinical history and examination. It was clear from Basser's original description of BPV that it was not uncommon; he reported 17 cases seen personally over a period of 7 years (Basser 1964). Among Aberdeen schoolchildren aged 5 to 15 years, the prevalence was 2.7% with a peak age at onset of 12 years (Russell and Abu-Arafeh 1999); the subdivision of BPV into two categories, early onset and late onset, has been supported by the authors of the Aberdeen study (Russell and Abu-Arafeh 2002). In Basser's series (Basser 1964), 60% of the affected individuals were females; most recent reports have indicated a similar slight preponderance of females (Abu-Arafeh and Russell 1995, Al-Twaijri and Shevell 2002).

CLINICAL FEATURES

Derived from the Latin *vertere*, meaning to turn or spin, the term vertigo is used to describe an unreal sensation of rotation of either the affected individual or his or her surroundings. In children, vertigo can be remarkably difficult to diagnose with certainty, because younger children find it difficult to describe and often use vague terms such as dizziness or lightheadedness, which they have learned from adults, or are unable to describe their symptoms more precisely than 'feeling funny'. Another impediment to precise diagnosis is that children with BPV are unlikely to be seen medically during attacks, which are usually brief and infrequent. The first step in the diagnosis is therefore to spend time with the child and the parents, teasing out the precise nature of the symptom(s) and any associated phenomena.

In a typical attack, a child who has previously been healthy is suddenly seized by overwhelmingly severe vertigo, leading to loss of balance and possibly a fall; if able to maintain balance the child commonly remains rooted to the spot or clutches at furniture or at bystanders for support. The parents may observe nystagmus. Although benign in the medical sense, these attacks are far from benign as far as the child is concerned, and he or she is justifiably frightened, especially during the first few attacks; a frightened, even terrified, appearance is therefore commonly reported by the parents.

Generally, the attacks are brief, lasting for less than 5 minutes, but in three of Drigo et al's patients they lasted between 1 and 2 days (Drigo et al 2001).

In addition to these features directly attributable to vertigo, numerous other features may accompany an attack of BPV. Pallor, nausea, vomiting, sweating, phonophobia and photophobia may all occur, lending support to the concept that this condition is related to migraine. Some features accompanying BPV attacks in the Aberdeen schools study (Russell and Abu-Arafeh 1999) are presented in Figure 17.1. The child's previous medical history may include migraine headaches and paroxysmal torticollis; six of Drigo et al's (2001) 19 patients had presented previously with benign paroxysmal torticollis, and in the Aberdeen schools study, more than half of BPV sufferers reported current or previous migraine headaches or other periodic conditions related to migraine (see Fig. 17.2). Motion sickness is common in

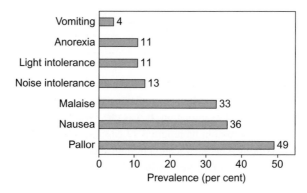

Fig. 17.1 Accompanying symptoms in 45 children during attacks of benign paroxysmal vertigo.

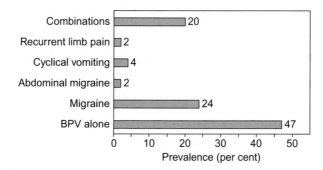

Fig. 17.2 Prevalence of migraine and migraine-related conditions in 45 children with benign paroxysmal vertigo (BPV).

children with BPV (Drigo et al 2001), sometimes to the extent of totally restricting family activities that involve travel.

Because of the links with migraine, it is important to take a detailed family history with emphasis on migraine and migraine-related conditions including motion sickness.

DIFFERENTIAL DIAGNOSIS
In typical cases, the diagnosis of BPV is obvious from the history, from normality between attacks and from the absence of positive findings on neurological examination. However, there are numerous causes of vertigo and dizziness in children, which can usually be differentiated using a systematic approach (Ravid et al 2003). Common causes include ear infections and their complications, previous head trauma, psychiatric problems, vestibular neuritis and benign paroxysmal positional vertigo, in which the attacks do not arise spontaneously but are related to posture or movement (Ralli et al 2009).

INVESTIGATION

Although the IHS diagnostic criteria include negative investigations, most clinicians are content to make the diagnosis clinically, with particular emphasis on total normality between attacks, and would consider such investigations unnecessary in the diagnosis of BPV or restrict their investigations to the minimum needed to reassure the parents. However, in children in whom the diagnosis is in doubt, particularly when it is unclear whether the child is completely well between attacks or the parents are unwilling to accept the diagnosis, any or all of the investigations suggested by the IHS would be appropriate, augmented, where serious pathology such as cerebellar or brainstem tumour is under consideration, by appropriate neuroimaging.

NATURAL COURSE AND PROGNOSIS

The natural course of BPV is extremely varied. In some children there are periods when attacks are frequent, alternating with periods when attacks are few or even disappear completely (Fenichel 1967). In general, however, the tendency is for attacks to diminish in frequency and usually in severity, eventually to disappear over a period ranging from a few months to several years (Lindskog et al 1999). In some cases they give way either to other periodic conditions associated with migraine (Drigo et al 2001, Marcelli et al 2006) or to migraine headaches (Lanzi et al 1994, Lindskog et al 1999, Marcelli et al 2006, Ralli et al 2009).

GENETICS

It is clear from what has already been said that heredity plays a part in the pathogenesis of BPV; parents (especially mothers) and siblings commonly suffer from migraine and migraine-related conditions (Abu-Arafeh and Russell 1995, Drigo et al 2001, Al-Twaijri and Shevell 2002). So far, however, this hereditary tendency has not been related to a specific genetic defect, although a novel abnormality in the *CACNA1A* gene was demonstrated in one patient who progressed from BPT to BPV to familial hemiplegic migraine (Cuenca-Leon et al 2008), a finding that adds further support to the concept that BPV is migraine related, albeit in this instance to one of the rarest forms of migraine.

MANAGEMENT

As in most benign conditions with alarming symptoms, the most important aspect of management is to explain the condition to the parents, and to the child if he or she is old enough. This is not only an important first step in management, but in most children it is the only step.

Attacks of BPV are usually brief and self-limiting, and in such cases drug treatment would be inappropriate. In those few cases in which the attack is more prolonged, it may be justifiable to try drugs such as antiemetics, although there is no objective evidence that they are useful. In children with frequent attacks, it is reasonable to try a favourite migraine prophylactic; the present writer is convinced that pizotifen is useful.

Case report

A 3-year-old female was referred to a general paediatric clinic by her general practitioner, with the request that she be investigated for what appeared to be panic attacks. These were occurring at intervals of 2 or 3 weeks and appeared to be completely unprovoked, and between attacks she was completely well. There was no doubt that the child was having attacks during which she looked extremely frightened – she would turn pale and would clutch at her mother, who quite naturally would pick her up and hug her until the attack passed, usually after only 2 or 3 minutes. The child was, at first, unable to describe what was happening to her, but with some prompting she agreed that the floor was spinning. Because she was hugging the child close to her, the mother had never seen her eyes during an attack, but on one occasion an attack had occurred when the father was at home, and he had seen abnormal eye movements – 'her eyes seemed to be attached to a cog-wheel that was slipping', a good description of nystagmus. This prompted consideration of the diagnosis of BPV, and the mother, who had said previously that her health was normal, revealed that while a student she would get migraines, although she had not had one for several years.

Further enquiry revealed that the child suffered from travel sickness so severe that she could not travel by car to the nearby park without feeling ill. No treatment was recommended and 2 years later the attacks stopped.

Benign paroxysmal torticollis

DEFINITION

Benign paroxysmal torticollis is a disorder of infants and young children characterised by recurrent episodes of head tilt of varying duration, often to the same side, but this may vary. Commonly, the attacks are accompanied by apparent distress but with reversion to complete normality between attacks. The duration of the attacks varies from a few minutes to a few days, and accompanying features may include pallor, irritability, malaise, anorexia and vomiting (Headache Classification Subcommittee of the International Headache Society 2004b). Underlying the head tilt is, unsurprisingly, spasm of the sternocleidomastoid muscle with continuous non-fluctuating electromyographic discharges (Kimura and Nezu 1998).

EPIDEMIOLOGY

There have been no formal studies to determine the population prevalence of BPT, but it is likely that the diagnosis is frequently missed and that the condition is much more common than figures, such as hospital statistics, would suggest. Snyder, who first described the condition in 1969, reported 12 cases from his practice (Snyder 1969), al-Twaijri and Shevell reported the diagnosis in 8 of 5848 patients seen by a single paediatric neurologist over a period of 8 years (Al-Twaijri and Shevell 2002) and Bratt and Menelaus reported four cases seen by a single orthopaedic surgeon over a period of 12 years (Bratt and Menelaus 1992). Reviewing the literature up to 2009, Rosman et al identified 103 cases and added 10 further cases seen in their own practice over a period of 5 years (Rosman et al 2009). Thus, in individual practices, surprisingly large numbers of cases can be collected, but in a series of 700 cases of torticollis only seven were of BPT (Nikolic and Banic 1989), suggesting that BPT is an unusual cause of torticollis.

Attacks begin early, almost always during the first 2 years of life, and persist for a variable period of months to several years. In the background there is frequently a family history of migraine, although its prevalence varies widely in different series (73%, Al-Twaijri and Shevell 2002; 40%, Drigo et al 2000; 14%, Cohen et al 1993). In most series, more females have been affected than males. Otherwise, the background of these children is unremarkable.

CLINICAL FEATURES

Benign paroxysmal torticollis typically starts in the first year of life, with 95% of cases starting within the first 14 months (Rosman et al 2009). During an attack there is rotation and tilting of the head to one side; in some cases the head tilt is always to the same side, but in others the direction varies from attack to attack. Torticollis may be an isolated symptom, but in the majority of cases there are associated symptoms including lethargy, pallor, anorexia and vomiting. In a few cases there is overlap with BPV and there may be ataxia, vertigo or nystagmus (Rosman et al 2009). In some cases, the torticollis is accompanied by postural abnormality involving the trunk (tortipelvis) (Chutorian 1972, Sanner and Bergstrom 1979, Deonna and Martin 1981).

In their review, Rosman et al reported that tortipelvis occurred in about a quarter of all reported cases (Rosman et al 2009).

During an attack, the sternocleidomastoid muscle is hypertonic (Kimura and Nezu 1998) and may be slightly tender on pressure. There is, however, no tumour to be felt and between attacks there is nothing to be found.

The duration and frequency of attacks is highly variable. Rosman et al (2009) cite a range of 10 minutes to 30 days (median 2 days), with the interval between attacks ranging from 1 week to 5 months (median 30 days).

In their review of 103 cases, Rosman et al (2009) found a family history of BPT in six cases and of migraine in 39 cases. Motion sickness was recorded in 13 cases, mostly from a single report (Drigo et al 2000). Although it has long been recognised that the prevalence of motion sickness is higher in migraine sufferers than in healthy individuals, both adults (Graham 1952) and children (Bille 1962), it was not until Barabas et al's (1983) paper that most paediatricians became aware of the strong association between migraine and motion sickness. Even so, motion sickness is seldom reported as a supporting feature for the diagnosis of migraine and migraine-related conditions; among eight series of BPV analysed by Drigo et al (2000), the prevalence of motion sickness was recorded only in their own series of 22 patients, among whom it was 55%.

As in all migraine-related conditions, normality between attacks is at least as important as the features during attacks in making a diagnosis.

DIFFERENTIAL DIAGNOSIS

In a typical case, in which brief attacks are followed by completely symptom-free intervals, there is little doubt as to the correct diagnosis. However, when attacks are prolonged, both the family and their medical advisers become anxious that something is being missed, and investigations are performed. Snyder (1969) found evidence of labyrinthine dysfunction in a high proportion of cases, but this has not been found in subsequent series.

It is tempting in atypical cases to look for anatomical abnormalities, and radiography and other imaging may be performed to exclude spinal and shoulder girdle abnormalities. In children with persistent torticollis, the possibility of posterior fossa tumour will inevitably arise (Extremera et al 2008) and appropriate neuroimaging should be performed.

In the occasional neonate, there may be bizarre dystonic reactions to drugs taken by the mother during pregnancy, including both prescribed drugs and drugs of addiction such as cocaine (Beltran and Coker 1995). Such reactions usually, but by no means always, begin soon after delivery, whereas the earliest that BPT has been reported is at the age of 7 days (Hanukoglu et al 1984) and in most children is much later.

A further source of confusion is Sandifer syndrome (Kinsbourne 1964, Deskin 1995), in which a child with gastro-oesophageal reflux indulges in a variety of contortions of the neck that can amount to torticollis. These head tilts have been shown to improve oesophageal peristalsis (Puntis et al 1989) and to resolve after fundoplication (Deskin 1995), and may occur even in the absence of clinically obvious signs of reflux (Frankel et al 2006). This is probably the only condition that can, on occasion, cause serious diagnostic confusion with BPT.

INVESTIGATION

From what has already been said, it is obvious that investigation plays no part in the diagnosis of clinically typical cases. The principal sources of confusion are Sandifer syndrome, which, if suspected, would justify upper gastrointestinal investigations, and posterior fossa tumour, which would mandate neuroimaging.

NATURAL COURSE AND PROGNOSIS

As the child gets older, the attacks diminish in frequency and severity until eventually they stop. Rosman et al found a range of 35 to 60 months for the age at cessation of attacks; in 95% of children, the attacks had stopped by the age of 4 years (Rosman et al 2009).

There have been few reports of the longer-term prognosis in BPT, but a number of children, almost certainly greater than would be expected by chance, go on to develop migraine and/or other conditions related to migraine.

GENETICS

A history of migraine was reported in the families of 39 of the 103 cases of BPT analysed by Rosman et al (2009), a figure that represents the minimum prevalence, as we cannot be sure that when a family history of migraine was not reported it was not present. It is therefore clear that a family history of migraine is unusually frequent in BPT.

Two patients with BPT have been reported in a kindred with familial hemiplegic migraine and ataxia linked by a mutation of the *CACNA1A* gene (Giffin et al 2002); the implications of this finding for BPT sufferers who come from families with more mundane types of migraine are unclear (see Chapters 3 and 4).

MANAGEMENT

As in BPV, the most important aspect of management in BPT is the making of a firm diagnosis on clinical grounds, followed by an explanation that reassures the family. Although Snyder (1969) tried various drugs in children with BPT, none was successful and it is fair to say that no medication has ever been shown to be effective. Drug treatment is therefore best avoided.

REFERENCES

Abu-Arafeh I, Russell G (1995) Paroxysmal vertigo as a migraine equivalent in children: a population-based study. *Cephalalgia* 15: 22–5. http://dx.doi.org/10.1046/j.1468-2982.1995.1501022.x

Al-Twaijri WA, Shevell MI (2002) Pediatric migraine equivalents: occurrence and clinical features in practice. *Pediatr Neurol* 26: 365–8. http://dx.doi.org/10.1016/S0887-8994(01)00416-7

Barabas G, Matthews WS, Ferrari M (1983) Childhood migraine and motion sickness. *Pediatrics* 72: 188–90.

Basser LS (1964) Benign paroxysmal vertigo of childhood (a variety of vestibular neuronitis). *Brain* 87: 141–52. http://dx.doi.org/10.1093/brain/87.1.141

Beltran RS, Coker SB (1995) Transient dystonia of infancy, a result of intrauterine cocaine exposure? *Pediatr Neurol* 12: 354–6. http://dx.doi.org/10.1016/0887-8994(95)00050-P

Bille BS (1962) Migraine in school children. A study of the incidence and short-term prognosis, and a clinical, psychological and electroencephalographic comparison between children with migraine and matched controls. *Acta Paediatr Scand* 136: 1–151.

Bratt HD, Menelaus MB (1992) Benign paroxysmal torticollis of infancy. *J Bone Joint Surg Br* 74: 449–51.

Chutorian AM (1972) Benign paroxysmal vertigo of childhood. *Dev Med Child Neurol* 14: 513–15. http://dx.doi.org/10.1111/j.1469-8749.1972.tb02627.x

Cohen HA, Nussinovitch M, Ashkenasi A, Straussberg R, Kauschanksy A, Frydman M (1993) Benign paroxysmal torticollis in infancy. *Pediatr Neurol* 9: 488–90. http://dx.doi.org/10.1016/0887-8994(93)90031-7

Cuenca-Leon E, Corominas R, Fernandez-Castillo N et al (2008) Genetic analysis of 27 Spanish patients with hemiplegic migraine, basilartype migraine and childhood periodic syndromes. *Cephalalgia* 28: 1039–47. http://dx.doi.org/10.1111/j.1468-2982.2008.01645.x

Deonna T, Martin D (1981) Benign paroxysmal torticollis in infancy. *Arch Dis Child* 56: 956–9. http://dx.doi.org/10.1136/adc.56.12.956

Deskin RW (1995) Sandifer syndrome: a cause of torticollis in infancy. *Int J Pediatr Otorhinolaryngol* 32: 183–5. http://dx.doi.org/10.1016/0165-5876(95)01130-4

Drigo P, Carli G, Laverda AM (2000) Benign paroxysmal torticollis of infancy. *Brain Dev* 22: 169–72. http://dx.doi.org/10.1016/S0387-7604(00)00099-1

Drigo P, Carli G, Laverda AM (2001) Benign paroxysmal vertigo of childhood. *Brain Dev* 23: 38–41. http://dx.doi.org/10.1016/S0387-7604(01)00175-9

Extremera VC, Alvarez-Coca J, Rodriguez GA, Perez JM, de Villanueva JL, Diaz CP (2008) Torticollis is a usual symptom in posterior fossa tumors. *Eur J Pediatr* 167: 249–50. http://dx.doi.org/10.1007/s00431-007-0453-8

Fenichel GM (1967) Migraine as a cause of benign paroxysmal vertigo of childhood. *J Pediatr* 71: 114–15. http://dx.doi.org/10.1016/S0022-3476(67)80239-7

Frankel EA, Shalaby TM, Orenstein SR (2006) Sandifer syndrome posturing: relation to abdominal wall contractions, gastroesophageal reflux, and fundoplication. *Dig Dis Sci* 51: 635–40. http://dx.doi.org/10.1007/s10620-006-3184-1

Giffin NJ, Benton S, Goadsby PJ (2002) Benign paroxysmal torticollis of infancy: four new cases and linkage to CACNA1A mutation. *Dev Med Child Neurol* 44: 490–3. http://dx.doi.org/10.1111/j.1469-8749.2002.tb00311.x

Graham JR (1952) The natural history of migraine: some observations and a hypothesis. *Trans Am Clin Climatol Assoc* 64: 61–73.

Hanukoglu A, Somekh E, Fried D (1984) Benign paroxysmal torticollis in infancy. *Clin Pediatr (Phila)* 23: 272–4. http://dx.doi.org/10.1177/000992288402300506

Headache Classification Subcommittee of the International Headache Society (2004a) The international classification of headache disorders: 2nd edition. *Cephalalgia* 24(Suppl 1): 31.

Headache Classification Subcommittee of the International Headache Society (2004b) The International Classification of Headache Disorders, 2nd edition. *Cephalalgia* 24(Suppl 1): 140–141.

Kimura S, Nezu A (1998) Electromyographic study in an infant with benign paroxysmal torticollis. *Pediatr Neurol* 19: 236–8. http://dx.doi.org/10.1016/S0887-8994(98)00044-7

Kinsbourne M (1964) Hiatus hernia with contortions of the neck. *Lancet* 1: 1058–61. http://dx.doi.org/10.1016/S0140-6736(64)91264-4

Lanzi G, Balottin U, Fazzi E, Tagliasacchi M, Manfrin M, Mira E (1994) Benign paroxysmal vertigo of childhood: a long-term follow-up. *Cephalalgia* 14: 458–60. http://dx.doi.org/10.1046/j.1468-2982.1994.1406458.x

Lindskog U, Odkvist L, Noaksson L, Wallquist J (1999) Benign paroxysmal vertigo in childhood: a long-term follow-up. *Headache* 39: 33–7. http://dx.doi.org/10.1046/j.1526-4610.1999.3901033.x

Marcelli V, Piazza F, Pisani F, Marciano E (2006) Neuro-otological features of benign paroxysmal vertigo and benign paroxysmal positioning vertigo in children: a follow-up study. *Brain Dev* 28: 80–4. http://dx.doi.org/10.1016/j.braindev.2005.05.003

Nikolic V, Banic M (1989) Paroksizmalni tortikolis u razvojnom dobu. *Med Pregl* 42: 99–101.

Puntis JW, Smith HL, Buick RG, Booth IW (1989) Effect of dystonic movements on oesophageal peristalsis in Sandifer's syndrome. *Arch Dis Child* 64: 1311–13. http://dx.doi.org/10.1136/adc.64.9.1311

Ralli G, Atturo F, de Filippis C (2009) Idiopathic benign paroxysmal vertigo in children, a migraine precursor. *Int J Pediatr Otorhinolaryngol* 73(Suppl 1): S16-18. http://dx.doi.org/10.1016/S0165-5876(09)70004-7

Ravid S, Bienkowski R, Eviatar L (2003) A simplified diagnostic approach to dizziness in children. *Pediatr Neurol* 29: 317–20. http://dx.doi.org/10.1016/S0887-8994(03)00278-9

Rosman NP, Douglass LM, Sharif UM, Paolini J (2009) The neurology of benign paroxysmal torticollis of infancy: report of 10 new cases and review of the literature. *J Child Neurol* 24: 155–60. http://dx.doi.org/10.1177/0883073808322338

Russell G, Abu-Arafeh I (1999) Paroxysmal vertigo in children – an epidemiological study. *Int J Pediatr Otorhinolaryngol* 49(Suppl 1): S105–7. http://dx.doi.org/10.1016/S0165-5876(99)00143-3

Russell G, Abu-Arafeh I (2002) Childhood syndromes related to migraine. In: Abu-Arafeh I, editor. *Childhood Headache*. London: Mac Keith Press, pp. 66–95.

Sanner G, Bergstrom B (1979) Benign paroxysmal torticollis in infancy. *Acta Paediatr Scand* 68: 219–23. http://dx.doi.org/10.1111/j.1651-2227.1979.tb04992.x

Snyder C (1969) Paroxysmal torticollis in infancy; a possible form of labyrinthitis. *Am J Dis Child* 117: 458–60.

18
TENSION-TYPE HEADACHE

Çiçek Wöber-Bingöl

Tension-type headache (TTH) is a frequent problem in children and adolescents but has attracted much less scientific interest than migraine. Searching MEDLINE from 1988 (the year of publication of the first edition of the International Classification of Headache Disorders – ICHD-I) to the present reveals 2511 citations for 'migraine and children' and 3594 citations for 'migraine and adolescents' but only 375 and 601 citations, respectively, for TTH in the two age groups. Regarding treatment, there is not one double-blind, randomised, controlled study on TTH in young patients.

Epidemiology

Tension-type headache is the most common type of primary headache in adults. In epidemiology studies, prevalence of TTH in children have been variable and have ranged from 0.9% (Abu-Arefeh and Russell 1994) to 73% (Barea et al 1996). Studies in Turkey and Norway revealed prevalence rates of 25% and 18%, respectively (Özge et al 2002, Zwart et al 2004). In a Swedish study (Laurell et al 2004), TTH was reported in 9.8% of 7- to 16-year-olds and the prevalence increased to 23% if ICHD-II criteria A and B, i.e. a minimum number of episodes and a minimum duration, were excluded. In a Finnish study (Anttila et al 2002a), 12% of 12-year-olds had TTH. Many of these children had headaches with migrainous features, and, while muscle tenderness was not a characteristic of TTH, it was of migraine (Anttila et al 2002b). In 2004, the International Headache Society criteria were revised (ICHD-II, Headache Classification Subcommittee of the International Headache Society 2004). New epidemiological studies will be necessary to help better characterise the frequency of TTH in children. The latest study coming from South Korea reported a 1-year prevalence of TTH of 13.7% (males 10.7%, females 16.3%) in participants aged 6 to 18 years (Rho et al 2011). In addition, the specificity and sensitivity of these new criteria need to be analysed in terms of their usefulness in childhood TTH.

Pathophysiology

The pathophysiology of TTH in children should be similar to that seen in adults. Myofascial, as well as central, mechanisms have been discussed. Fumal and Schoenen (2008) summarise a model for the pathogenesis of TTH and suggest an interaction between changes in the descending control of trigeminal brainstem nociceptors and peripheral mechanisms, such as myofascial pain sensitivity and strain in the pericranial muscles.

The primary cause of TTH may be physical and/or psychological stress, the first resulting in increased nociception from strained muscles and the latter causing increased muscle tension through the limbic system and reduced tone in the endogenous antinociceptive system. In more frequent TTH, central changes become increasingly important. Long-term potentiation or sensitisation of nociceptive neurons, together with decreased activity in the antinociceptive system, may lead to chronic TTH. The relative importance of peripheral and central factors might vary between patients, and over time in the same patient. Environmental factors seem to be more important in episodic TTH, whereas genetic components may be particularly relevant in chronic TTH.

Clinical features

The clinical features of TTH are similar in children, adolescents and adults. TTH is characterised by a bilateral, pressing tightness occurring anywhere on the cranium or suboccipital region. The pain is mild to moderate in intensity and usually not aggravated by physical activity. Associated symptoms are absent or limited to one out of photophobia and phonophobia in episodic TTH and one out of mild nausea, photophobia and phonophobia in chronic TTH. A cross-sectional study in referral patients showed an increasing headache frequency and duration, an increasing variability of headache location and an increasing frequency of nausea with increasing age. More importantly, the analgesic intake increased markedly from children to adults (Wöber-Bingöl et al 1996).

Diagnosis

Tension-type headache may be hard to differentiate from migraine in children as some of the symptoms overlap (Wöber-Bingöl et al 1995, Kienbacher et al 2006). A headache diary is a useful method for the differentiation of headache types.

Regarding the frequency of TTH, ICHD-II differentiates between infrequent episodic TTH, occurring less than once a month, frequent episodic TTH, present on up to 14 days per month, and chronic TTH, occurring on at least 15 days per month or 180 days per year (Headache Classification Subcommittee of the International Headache Society 2004). The ICHD-II criteria of all types of TTH are given in Table 18.1.

In contrast to the criteria of migraine, the criteria of TTH are identical for all age groups (Headache Classification Subcommittee of the International Headache Society 2004). Regarding criterion E, i.e. that headache is not attributed to another disorder, ICHD-II provides the following rule: history and physical and neurological examinations do not suggest any of the disorders listed in ICHD-II groups 5 to 12, or history and/or physical and/or neurological examinations do suggest such a disorder but it is ruled out by appropriate investigations, or such a disorder is present but headache does not occur for the first time in close temporal relation to the disorder (see Appendix 5.1, Chapter 5, for details of secondary headache disorders).

The international classification of headache disorders allows the classification of headaches not fulfilling all diagnostic criteria. In ICHD-I (Headache Classification Committee of the International Headache Society 1988), the term 'headache of the tension-type not fulfilling the criteria' was used. In ICHD-II this was changed to 'probable tension-type headache' (Headache Classification Subcommittee of the International Headache Society 2004;

TABLE 18.1
ICHD-II criteria for tension-type headache (TTH) (Headache Classification Subcommittee of the International Headache Society 2004)

2.1 Infrequent episodic TTH

(A) At least 10 episodes occurring on <1d/mo on average (<12d/y) and fulfilling criteria B–D

(B) Headache lasting 30min–7d

(C) Headache has at least two of the following characteristics:
    (1) bilateral location
    (2) pressing/tightening (non-pulsating) quality
    (3) mild or moderate intensity
    (4) not aggravated by routine physical activity such as walking or climbing stairs

(D) Headache has both of the following:
    (1) no nausea or vomiting (anorexia may occur)
    (2) no more than one of photophobia or phonophobia

(E) Headache not attributed to another disorder

2.2 Frequent episodic TTH

(A) At least 10 episodes occurring on ≥1 but <15d/mo for ≥3mo (≥12 and <180d/y) and fulfilling criteria B-D

(B–E) As 2.1 Infrequent episodic TTH

2.3 Chronic TTH

(A) Headache occurring on ≥15d/mo on average for >3mo (≥180d/y) and fulfilling criteria B–D

(B) Headache lasts hours or may be continuous

(C) As 2.1 Infrequent episodic TTH

(D) Headache has both of the following:
    (1) no more than one of photophobia, phonophobia or mild nausea
    (2) neither moderate or severe nausea nor vomiting

(E) Headache not attributed to another disorder

2.4.1/2.4.2 Probable infrequent/frequent episodic TTH

(A) Episodes fulfilling all but one of criteria A–D for either
    2.1 Infrequent episodic TTH or
    2.2 Frequent episodic TTH

(B) Episodes do not fulfil criteria for 1.1 Migraine without aura

(C) Headache not attributed to another disorder

2.4.3 Probable chronic TTH

(A) Headache occurring on ≥15d/mo on average for >3mo (≥180d/y) and fulfilling criteria B–D

(B) Headache lasts hours or may be continuous

(C) Headache has at least two of the following characteristics:
    (1) bilateral location
    (2) pressing/tightening (non-pulsating) quality
    (3) mild or moderate intensity
    (4) not aggravated by routine physical activity such as walking or climbing stairs

(D) Both of the following:
    (1) no more than one of photophobia, phonophobia or mild nausea
    (2) neither moderate or severe nausea nor vomiting

(E) Not attributed to another disorder but there is, or has been within the last 2 months, medication overuse fulfilling criterion B for any of the subforms of 8.2 Medication overuse headache

Table 18.1). In children and adolescents, not only may it be difficult to differentiate migraine or probable migraine from tension-type headache or probable tension-type headache, but over time headache may evolve from one diagnosis to the other (Zebenholzer et al 2000, Kienbacher et al 2006).

Stressors in tension-type headache
Stressors should be evaluated in all patients presenting with TTH. In children, a connection seems possible between TTH and psychosocial stress, psychiatric disorders, muscular stress and oromandibular dysfunction. Childhood TTH is associated with a higher rate of divorced parents and fewer peer relations as well as an unhappy family atmosphere. In addition, children with episodic TTH are more likely to report somatic complaints and family problems than those without headache. Children and adolescents with chronic diseases and stressful family events are at increased risk for chronic TTH. Of children with chronic TTH, over 50% have had predisposing physical or emotional stress factors. Compared with children with migraine, children with TTH have greater psychological and temperamental difficulties (Karwautz et al 1999, Abu-Arafeh 2001, Anttila 2002a, Kaynak Key et al 2004).

Management
The general principles of management of TTH in children and adolescents can be summarised as follows (Termine et al 2011):

- Establish the diagnosis.
- Look for possible somatic and psychiatric comorbidities.
- Ask about triggers and assess the degree of disability.
- Educate the child and family about the condition.
- Use a headache calendar to establish the characteristics of headache and associated symptoms.
- Establish realistic expectations and set appropriate goals.
- Discuss the expected benefits of therapy and the time course to achieve them.
- Reduce the emotional mechanisms (on a personal level, within the family and at school) that provoke stress and may favour headache attacks.
- Advise the maintenance of a sound rhythm in daily life, which includes regular meals, sufficient fluid intake, physical exercise and sleep.
- Advise how to cope with trigger factors.

No large-scale treatment studies have been performed in children with TTH and there is not one randomised, controlled study. Treatment covers management of acute attacks as well as prophylaxis. Emphasis should be on non-pharmacological measures such as distraction (in mild TTH) and behavioural treatment (for frequent or chronic TTH).

Behavioural headache treatments include relaxation training, biofeedback training, cognitive–behavioural therapy or combinations of these treatments. Among behavioural headache treatments, the two most common types of biofeedback for headache have been electromyographic biofeedback for TTH and 'handwarming' or thermal biofeedback for migraine (Sarafino and Goehring 2000, Andrasik et al 2003, Larsson et al 2005). A meta-analysis showed that there is very good evidence that psychological treatments, principally relaxation and cognitive–behavioural therapy, are effective in reducing the severity and frequency of chronic headache in children and adolescents (Eccleston et al 2002). The lack of availability and cost of non-pharmacological interventions might diminish the use of some treatment modalities (Antilla 2006).

Small-scale studies have suggested that analgesics and non-steroidal anti-inflammatory drugs (NSAIDs) may be useful in the acute treatment of episodic TTH, while amitriptyline may be useful for prophylaxis of chronic TTH. Analgesics and NSAIDs can be given for more severe, acute tension-type headache, but their use must be restricted, particularly in chronic TTH, in order to prevent medication overuse headache. Paracetamol (acetaminophen) may be used at a dosage of 15mg/kg and ibuprofen at a dosage of 10mg/kg. In children younger than 15 years, aspirin is not recommended because of the concern of Reye syndrome. In patients not sufficiently responding to lifestyle modification and non-pharmacological prophylaxis, amitriptyline may be administered. The treatment with amitriptyline should be started with 0.2mg/kg/day and may be increased slowly to 1mg/kg/day. The most common adverse effects are dry mouth and sedation (Wöber-Bingöl and Hershey 2006, Termine et al 2011). Magnesium may be an effective treatment for paediatric episodic and chronic TTH, but further well-controlled studies are needed (Grazzi et al 2005).

Quality of life

Health-related quality of life (QOL) is an emerging area of headache research with a direct impact on patient adherence, patient satisfaction and treatment effectiveness. On the other hand, the assessment of QOL in children is difficult, as measures must consider children's changing cognitive and social development (Powers et al 2004). Data-based analyses have revealed that children with frequent or severe headaches are significantly more likely than those without frequent or severe headaches to exhibit high levels of emotional, conduct, inattention, hyperactivity and peer problems and be upset or distressed by their difficulties and to have their difficulties interfere with home life, friendships, classroom learning and leisure activities (Strine et al 2006). Headache is the third most common illness-related cause of school absenteeism, and is associated with substantial impairment of quality of life in children (Newacheck and Taylor 1992).

Prognosis

Longitudinal studies in childhood TTH are rare. However, one such study reported that, after 6 years, 38% of children were headache free, 41% still had TTH and in 21% TTH had developed into migraine (Kienbacher et al 2006).

There are few data about the natural history of childhood and adolescent TTH. It is accepted that over 50% of sufferers improve with comprehensive headache management. The most important predictors of prognosis are comorbid medical and psychological conditions and family problems (Karwautz et al 1999).

Implications for future research

Much research is needed for further characterisation of TTHs in children and adolescents; given the mild nature of these headaches, this will require either primary-care involvement or large-scale population-based studies, as most headache specialty centres tend to get a biased component, with headaches being more severe and therefore of the migraine type (Wöber-Bingöl and Hershey 2006).

REFERENCES

Abu-Arafeh I (2001) Chronic tension-type headache in children and adolescents. *Cephalalgia* 21: 830–6. http://dx.doi.org/10.1046/j.0333-1024.2001.00275.x

Abu-Arefeh I, Russell G (1994) Prevalence of headache and migraine in schoolchildren. *BMJ* 309: 765–9. http://dx.doi.org/10.1136/bmj.309.6957.765

Andrasik F, Grazzi L, Usai S, D'Amico D, Leone M, Bussone G (2003) Brief neurologist-administered behavioral treatment of pediatric episodic tension-type headache. *Neurology* 60: 1215–16. http://dx.doi.org/10.1212/01.WNL.0000055922.22637.61

Anttila P (2006) Tension-type headache in childhood and adolescence. *Lancet Neurol* 5: 268–74. http://dx.doi.org/10.1016/S1474-4422(06)70376-3

Anttila P, Metsahonkala L, Aromaa M et al (2002a) Determinants of tension-type headache in children. *Cephalalgia* 22: 401–8. http://dx.doi.org/10.1046/j.1468-2982.2002.00381.x

Anttila P, Metsahonkala L, Mikkelsson M et al (2002b) Muscle tenderness in pericranial and neck-shoulder region in children with headache. A controlled study. *Cephalalgia* 22: 340–4. http://dx.doi.org/10.1046/j.1468-2982.2002.00352.x

Barea JM, Tannhauser M, Rotta NT (1996) An epidemiologic study of headache among children and adolescents of southern Brazil. *Cephalalgia* 16: 545–9. http://dx.doi.org/10.1046/j.1468-2982.1996.1608545.x

Eccleston C, Morley S, Williams A, Yorke L, Mastroyannopoulou K (2002) Systematic review of randomized controlled trials of psychological therapy for chronic pain in children and adolescents, with a subset meta-analysis of pain relief. *Pain* 99: 157–65. http://dx.doi.org/10.1016/S0304-3959(02)00072-6

Grazzi L, Andrasik F, Usai S, Bussone G (2005) Magnesium as a treatment for paediatric tension-type headache: a clinical replication series. *Neurol Sci* 25: 338–41. http://dx.doi.org/10.1007/s10072-004-0367-4

Fumal A, Schoenen J (2008) Tension-type headache: current research and clinical management. *Lancet Neurol* 7: 70–83. http://dx.doi.org/10.1016/S1474-4422(07)70325-3

Headache Classification Committee of the International Headache Society (1988) Classification and diagnostic criteria for headache disorders, cranial neuralgias and facial pain. *Cephalalgia* 8(Suppl 7): 1–96.

Headache Classification Subcommittee of the International Headache Society. (2004) The international classification of headache disorders. *Cephalagia* 24(Suppl 1): 1–160.

Karwautz A, Wöber C, Lang T et al (1999) Psychosocial factors in children and adolescents with migraine and tension-type headache: a controlled study and review of the literature. *Cephalalgia* 19: 32–43. http://dx.doi.org/10.1111/j.1468-2982.1999.1901032.x

Kaynak Key FN, Donmez S, Tuzun U (2004) Epidemiological and clinical characteristics with psychosocial aspects of tension-type headache in Turkish college students. *Cephalalgia* 24: 669–74. http://dx.doi.org/10.1111/j.1468-2982.2004.00736.x

Kienbacher C, Wöber C, Zesch HE et al (2006) Clinical features, classification and prognosis of migraine and tension-type headache in children and adolescents: a long-term follow-up study. *Cephalalgia* 26: 820–30. http://dx.doi.org/10.1111/j.1468-2982.2006.01108.x

Larsson B, Carlsson J, Fichtel A, Melin L (2005) Relaxation treatment of adolescent headache sufferers: results from a school-based replication series. *Headache* 45: 692–704. http://dx.doi.org/10.1111/j.1526-4610.2005.05138.x

Laurell K, Larsson B, Eeg-Olofsson O (2004) Prevalence of headache in Swedish schoolchildren, with a focus on tension-type headache. *Cephalalgia* 24: 380–8. http://dx.doi.org/10.1111/j.1468-2982.2004.00681.x

Newacheck PW, Taylor WR (1992) Childhood chronic illness: prevalence, severity, and impact. *Am J Public Health* 82: 364–71. http://dx.doi.org/10.2105/AJPH.82.3.364

Özge A, Bugdayci R, Sasmaz T et al (2002) The sensitivity and specificity of the case definition criteria in diagnosis of headache: a school-based epidemiological study of 5562 children in Mersin. *Cephalalgia* 22: 791–8. http://dx.doi.org/10.1046/j.1468-2982.2002.00467.x

Powers SW, Patton SR, Hommel KA, Hershey AD (2004) Quality of life in paediatric migraine: characterization of age-related effects using PedsQL 4.0. *Cephalalgia* 24: 120–7. http://dx.doi.org/10.1111/j.1468-2982.2004.00652.x

Rho YI, Chung HJ, Lee KH et al (2011) Prevalence and clinical characteristics of primary headaches among school children in south korea: a nationwide survey. *Headache* Epub ahead of print.

Sarafino EP, Goehring P (2000) Age comparisons in acquiring biofeedback control and success in reduction headache pain. *Ann Behav Med* 22: 10–16. http://dx.doi.org/10.1007/BF02895163

Strine TW, Okoro CA, McGuire LC, Balluz LS (2006) The associations among childhood headaches, emotional and behavioral difficulties, and health care use. *Pediatrics* 117: 1728–35. http://dx.doi.org/10.1542/peds.2005-1024

Termine C, Özge A, Antonaci F, Natriashvili S, Guidetti V, Wöber-Bingöl Ç (2011) Overview of diagnosis and management of paediatric headache. Part II: therapeutic management. *J Headache Pain* 12: 25–34. http://dx.doi.org/10.1007/s10194-010-0256-6

Wöber-Bingöl Ç, Hershey AD (2006) Tension-type headache and other non-migraine primary headaches in the pediatrc population. In: Olesen J, Goadsby PJ, Ramadan NM, Tfelt-hansen P, Welch KMA, editors. *The Headaches*, 3rd edn. Philadelphia: Lippincott, Williams & Wilkins, pp. 1079–81.

Wöber-Bingöl Ç, Wöber C, Karwautz A et al (1995) Diagnosis of headache in childhood and adolescence: a study in 437 patients. *Cephalalgia* 15: 13–21. http://dx.doi.org/10.1046/j.1468-2982.1995.1501013.x

Wöber-Bingöl Ç, Wöber C, Karwautz A et al (1996) Tension-type headache in different age groups at two headache centers. *Pain* 67: 53–8. http://dx.doi.org/10.1016/0304-3959(96)03117-X

Zebenholzer K, Wöber C, Kienbacher C, Wöber-Bingöl Ç (2000) Migrainous disorder and headache of the tension-type not fulfilling the criteria: a follow-up study in children and adolescents. *Cephalalgia* 20: 611–16. http://dx.doi.org/10.1046/j.1468-2982.2000.00090.x

Zwart JA, Dyb G, Holmen TL, Stovner LJ, Sand T (2004) The prevalence of migraine and tension-type headaches among adolescents in Norway. The Nord-Trondelag Health Study (Head-HUNT-Youth), a large population-based epidemiological study. *Cephalalgia* 24: 373–9. http://dx.doi.org/10.1111/j.1468-2982.2004.00680.x

19
CLUSTER HEADACHE AND OTHER TRIGEMINAL AUTONOMIC CEPHALALGIAS

Giorgio Lambru and Manjit Matharu

The trigeminal autonomic cephalalgias are a group of primary headache disorders characterised by unilateral head pain that occurs in association with prominent ipsilateral cranial autonomic features (Headache Classification Subcommittee of the International Headache Society 2004). The trigeminal autonomic cephalalgias include cluster headache, paroxysmal hemicrania and short-lasting unilateral neuralgiform headache attacks with conjunctival injection and tearing (SUNCT). Cluster headache, paroxysmal hemicrania and SUNCT are currently grouped into section 3 of the revised International Classification of Headache Disorders (ICHD-II; Headache Classification Subcommittee of the International Headache Society 2004).

The trigeminal autonomic cephalalgias are relatively rare in the adult population and are considered to be even rarer in the paediatric population. This rarity is likely to be the reason why they are poorly recognised and there is often a delay of several years before the diagnosis is made. While the trigeminal autonomic cephalalgias can be recognised by distinctive short-lasting headaches with autonomic features, they differ in attack duration and frequency. Differentiation between the trigeminal autonomic cephalalgias is essential as the treatments for each are very different. These syndromes are considered to be some of the most painful known to humankind, thereby underlining the importance of early recognition and initiation of the excellent but highly selective treatments.

Cluster headache

Cluster headache is a strictly unilateral headache that occurs in association with cranial autonomic features and, in most patients, has a striking circannual and circadian periodicity. It is an excruciating syndrome and is probably one of the most painful conditions known to humankind, with female patients describing each attack as being worse than childbirth.

Epidemiology

The prevalence of adult cluster headache is estimated to be 0.1% (Tonon et al 2002, Torelli et al 2005). Cluster headache can begin at any age, although onset most commonly occurs in the third or fourth decade of life. The onset of cluster headache in the paediatric population is well reported, although the prevalence seems to be relatively low. A multicentre paediatric study, covering 27 headache centres in Italy and comprising 6629 headache patients younger than 18 years of age, reported the 1-year prevalence of cluster headache to be 0.03% (Gallai et al 2003).

Childhood-onset cluster headache shows a male preponderance with a ratio of 2.5:1, similar to that observed in the adult population (Russell 2004, Antonaci et al 2010). The mean age at onset of cluster headache in childhood and adolescence is 11 to 14 years with a wide range of 3 to 18 years.

CLINICAL FEATURES
Several of the terms relating to cluster headache can be confusing and therefore have been defined here. A *cluster headache* or *attack* is an individual episode of pain that can last from a few minutes to some hours. A *cluster bout* or *period* refers to the duration over which recurrent cluster attacks are occurring; it usually lasts some weeks or months. A *remission* is the pain-free period between two cluster bouts. Cluster headache is a disorder with highly distinctive clinical features. These features are dealt with under two major headings: *the cluster attack* and *the cluster bout*.

The cluster attack
Cluster attacks are strictly unilateral, although the headache may alternate between sides. The headache is centred on the orbital and temporal regions, although any part of the head can be affected. The pain is excruciatingly severe. The duration of headache can range from 15 minutes to 3 hours. The signature feature of cluster headache is the association with cranial autonomic symptoms (see Table 19.1). The autonomic features are transient, lasting only for the duration of the attack, with the exception of partial Horner syndrome. It has been suggested that cranial autonomic features may be less prominent in children than in adults (Del Bene and Poggioni 1987), although the rest of the clinical phenotype seems to be similar in both groups. Migrainous symptoms, such as nausea, vomiting, photophobia and phonophobia, may be seen, as may aura (Silberstein et al 2000, Schurks et al 2006). The vast majority of cluster headache patients report restlessness during the attacks; this often manifests as thrashing around in children and can distract attention from the headache, thereby contributing to a delay in diagnosis (McNabb and Whitehouse 1999). The cluster attack frequency varies between one every alternate day to three daily, although some patients have up to eight daily. The condition can have a striking circadian rhythmicity, with some patients reporting that the attacks occur at the same time each day.

Alcohol, exercise, elevated environmental temperature and the smell of volatile agents are all recognised precipitants of acute cluster attacks. Alcohol induces acute attacks, usually within an hour of intake, in the vast majority of sufferers.

The cluster bout
Cluster headache is classified according to the duration of the bout. About 80% to 90% of patients have *episodic cluster headache*, which is diagnosed by the occurrence of recurrent bouts, each with a duration of more than a week and separated by remissions lasting more than 4 weeks. The bouts typically occur once or twice a year. Often, a striking circannual periodicity is seen with the cluster periods, with the bouts occurring in the same month of the year. The remaining 10% to 20% of patients have *chronic cluster headache*, in which either no remission occurs within 1 year or the remissions last less than 1 month (Headache Classification Subcommittee of the International Headache Society 2004).

TABLE 19.1

**The International Classification of Headache Disorders II diagnostic criteria for cluster headache
(Headache Classification Subcommittee of the International Headache Society 2004)**

Diagnostic criteria

(A) At least five attacks fulfilling B–D

(B) Severe or very severe unilateral orbital, supraorbital and/or temporal pain lasting 15–180min if untreated

(C) Headache is accompanied by at least one of the following:

    (1) ipsilateral conjunctival injection and/or lacrimation

    (2) ipsilateral nasal congestion and/or rhinorrhoea

    (3) ipsilateral eyelid oedema

    (4) ipsilateral forehead and facial sweating

    (5) ipsilateral miosis and/or ptosis

    (6) a sense of restlessness or agitation

(D) Attacks have a frequency from one every other day to eight per day

(E) Not attributed to another disorder

Episodic cluster headache

Description

Occurs in periods lasting 7d–1y separated by pain-free periods lasting 1mo or more

Diagnostic criteria

All fulfilling criteria A–E above

At least two cluster periods lasting 7–365d and separated by pain-free remissions of >1mo

Chronic cluster headache

Description

Attacks occur for more than 1y without remission or with remissions lasting <1mo

Diagnostic criteria

All fulfilling criteria A–E above

Attacks recur over >1y without remission periods or with remission periods <1mo

DIFFERENTIAL DIAGNOSIS

The main differential diagnoses to consider are secondary causes of cluster headache, other trigeminal autonomic cephalalgias and migraine (see Table 19.2). Symptomatic cluster headache has been described with infectious, vascular and neoplastic intracranial lesions. However, the true prevalence of symptomatic causes of cluster headache is unknown as there have been no prospective population-based neuroimaging studies. A review of retrospective case reports published in the medical literature suggested that the trigeminal autonomic cephalalgias may be associated with pituitary tumours, although this most likely reflects a considerable element of publication bias (Cittadini and Matharu 2009).

Differentiating between migraine and cluster headache can be difficult in some cases as unilaterality of pain and the presence of migrainous and autonomic symptoms are features common to both. The features that can be useful in distinguishing cluster headache from

TABLE 19.2
Clinical features of the trigeminal autonomic cephalalgias

Feature	Cluster headache	Paroxysmal hemicrania	SUNCT
Sex F:M	1:2.5–7.2	1:1	1:1.5
Pain			
Type	Sharp, throbbing	Sharp, throbbing	Stabbing, burning
Severity	Very severe	Very severe	Very severe
Site	Orbit, temple	Orbit, temple	Periorbital
Attack frequency	1/alternate day–8/d	1–40/d (>5/d for more than half the time)	3–200/day
Duration of attack	15–180min	2–30min	5–240s
Circadian periodicity	70%	45%	Absent
Autonomic features	Yes	Yes	Yes[a]
Restless or agitated	90%	80%	65%
Migrainous features	Yes	Yes	Rare
Triggers			
Alcohol	++	+	–
Cutaneous	–	–	++
Indometacin effect	–	++	–
Abortive treatment	Sumatriptan injection Sumatriptan nasal spray Zolmitriptan nasal spray Oxygen	Nil	Nil
Prophylactic treatment	Verapamil Methysergide Lithium Topiramate	Indometacin	Lamotrigine Topiramate Gabapentin
Transitional treatment	Corticosteroids GONB	GONB	GONB

[a]Prominent conjunctival injection *and* lacrimation by definition. SUNCT, short-lasting unilateral neuralgiform headache attacks with conjunctival injection and tearing; F, female; M, male; +, moderate response; ++, absolute response to indometacin; –, not present or negative; GONB, greater occipital nerve block.

migraine include a relatively short duration of headache, rapid onset and cessation, circadian periodicity, onset within an hour after taking alcohol, restlessness or agitation during the attack, and clustering of attacks with intervening remissions in episodic cluster headache.

INVESTIGATIONS
The diagnosis of cluster headache is made entirely on the basis of a good clinical history and a detailed neurological examination. Any atypical features in the history or abnormalities on

neurological examination (with the exception of partial Horner syndrome) warrant further investigations to search for organic causes. It remains unclear whether every trigeminal auto- nomic cephalalgia patient requires neuroimaging, although, if it is considered, then magnetic resonance imaging (MRI) is the preferred modality. Given the rarity of cluster headache in childhood and adolescence, it seems reasonable to offer neuroimaging to all paediatric patients to exclude a symptomatic cause.

TREATMENT

Management of paediatric cluster headache (and other trigeminal autonomic cephalalgias) is not well substantiated by appropriate studies and is derived almost exclusively from experience in adult patients. Currently there are both medical and surgical interventions available for these patients. Medical management falls into one of three categories: acute, preventive or transitional therapies. Acute or abortive treatment is given at the onset of an attack and is aimed at aborting the attack itself, whereas the aim of preventive medication is to produce a rapid suppression of attacks and maintain remission while the patient is still in a bout. However, preventive treatments generally need to be titrated to an optimum dose and therefore there can be a delay of a few days to weeks before their beneficial effect emerges. Transitional treatments are therapies that can be used to rapidly suppress the attacks, but are only effective for a few days to weeks and can therefore be very helpful while waiting for the preventive treatments to work. Surgical treatments are generally avoided until the medical treatments are exhausted.

Abortive agents

Because the pain of cluster headache builds up so rapidly, the most efficacious agents are those that involve parenteral or pulmonary administration.

Oxygen

Inhalation of 100% oxygen, at 7 to 12l/minute is rapidly effective in relieving pain in the majority of sufferers (Cohen et al 2009). It should be inhaled continuously for 15 to 30 minutes via a non-rebreathing facial mask. Oxygen has been used successfully in several paediatric cluster headache patients (Del Bene and Poggioni 1987) and, given its good side effect profile, it is the abortive agent of choice for paediatric cluster headache.

Subcutaneous and intranasal triptans

Subcutaneous sumatriptan is the most effective abortive treatment for cluster headache (Ekbom et al 1993). In cluster headache, unlike in migraine, subcutaneous sumatriptan can be prescribed at a frequency of twice daily, on a long-term basis if necessary, without risk of tachyphylaxis or rebound (Ekbom et al 1992, Gobel et al 1998). Sumatriptan and zolmitriptan nasal spray are both more effective than placebo (Van Vliet et al 2003, Cittadini et al 2006, Rapoport et al 2007). Although experience with the use of subcutaneous sumatriptan in the paediatric population is limited, sumatriptan nasal spray at a dose of 20mg has been found, in randomised, placebo-controlled studies, to be well tolerated in children with migraine aged between 12 and 17 years (Winner et al 2000, Lewis et al 2007).

Transitional treatments

Corticosteroids
Corticosteroids are highly efficacious and the most rapid acting of the preventive agents (Couch and Ziegler 1978). Caution has to be exercised in their use because of the potential for serious side effects. Treatment is usually limited to a short intensive course of 2 to 3 weeks in tapering doses because of the potential for side effects (Matharu et al 2002). Unfortunately, relapse almost invariably occurs as the dose is tapered. For this reason, steroids are used as an initial therapy in conjunction with preventives, until the latter are effective.

Greater occipital nerve block
Injection of local anaesthetic and corticosteroid around the greater occipital nerve (GON) on the affected side can abort a bout of cluster headache (Leroux et al 2011). Although there are no reports on the use of GON blocks in paediatric cluster headache, it is an excellent short-term strategy, with only very modest, infrequent side effects.

Preventive treatments
The preventive agents used in the management of cluster headache include verapamil, lithium, topiramate, methysergide, gabapentin, melatonin and valproate. Verapamil is the agent of choice. While the other agents are often used, the evidence base for their use is poor. Table 19.3 provides an overview of the recommendations for cluster headache preventive treatments by the European Federation of Neurological Societies (May et al 2006) and the American Academy of Neurology (Francis et al 2010). The classification of recommendations differs between the two societies and has been fully defined elsewhere (Brainin et al 2004, Francis et al 2010).

Verapamil
Verapamil is the preventive drug of choice in both episodic and chronic cluster headache (Leone et al 2000). There are reports of the efficacy of verapamil in children at doses between 120mg and 240mg (McNabb and Whitehouse 1999, Gallai et al 2003), although this agent is often used at doses of up to 960mg daily in adults. Verapamil can cause heart block by slowing conduction in the atrioventricular node. Observing for PR interval prolongation on electrocardiography can monitor potential development of heart block. There is only one formal guideline in the literature for the titration of the verapamil dose in adults (Matharu et al 2002), which recommends starting patients on 240mg daily and incrementing the dose in steps of 80mg every 2 weeks under electrocardiography guidance. The dose is increased until the cluster attacks are suppressed, side effects intervene or the maximum dose of 960mg daily is achieved. In the paediatric population, we recommend starting at a lower dose of 40 to 80mg daily and titrating the dose in steps of 40mg.

Surgery
In adults, medically intractable chronic cluster headache is rare but a highly disabling disorder and it is therefore appropriate to consider surgical interventions for these patients. There are no

TABLE 19.3
Preventive treatments of cluster headache

Treatment	Level of evidence (EFNS)	Level of evidence (AAN)	Monitoring	Common side effects
Verapamil	A	C	ECG monitoring for cardiac arrhythmias	Hypotension, constipation, peripheral oedema
Lithium	B	C	Lithium levels, renal function, thyroid function	Diarrhoea, tremor, polyuria
Topiramate	B	Not rated		Paraesthesias, weight loss, cognitive dysfunction, fatigue, dizziness, taste alteration
Methysergide	B	Not rated	Annual visceral fibrosis screening: echocardiogram, chest radiography MRI abdomen and pelvis Relevant blood tests	Nausea/vomiting, muscle cramps, abdominal pain, peripheral oedema, retroperitoneal fibrosis (rare)
Gabapentin	Not rated	Not rated		Somnolence, fatigue, dizziness, weight gain, peripheral oedema, ataxia
Melatonin	C	C		Fatigue, sedation
Sodium valproate	C	B	Full blood count, liver function	Weight gain, fatigue, tremor, hair loss, nausea

A, denotes effective; B, denotes probably effective; C, denotes possibly effective.
EFNS, European Federation of Neurological Societies; AAN, American Academy of Neurology; ECG, electrocardiogram; MRI, magnetic resonance imaging.

reports of surgical intervention for the management of paediatric cluster headache, although medically refractory chronic cluster headache cases have been described (Antonaci et al 2010).

Surgery is a last-resort measure in treatment-resistant patients and should be considered only when the pharmacological options have been exploited to the fullest. Historically, destructive procedures involving the trigeminal nerve have been carried out on patients with cluster headache. However, they are associated with considerable morbidity and therefore have been largely abandoned. Most recently, neurostimulation therapies with either hypothalamic deep-brain stimulation or occipital nerve stimulation (ONS) have emerged. These approaches are very promising, and, in particular, ONS offers a more acceptable side effect profile than destructive and invasive approaches.

Paroxysmal hemicrania

Paroxysmal hemicrania, like cluster headache, is characterised by strictly unilateral, brief headaches that occur in association with cranial autonomic features. Paroxysmal hemicrania differs from cluster headache mainly in the higher frequency and shorter duration of individual attacks, although there is a considerable overlap in these characteristics. However, unlike cluster headache, paroxysmal hemicrania responds in a dramatic and absolute fashion to indometacin (Headache Classification Subcommittee of the International Headache Society 2004), thereby underlining the importance of distinguishing it from cluster headache.

EPIDEMIOLOGY

Paroxysmal hemicrania is a very rare syndrome. The prevalence of paroxysmal hemicrania is not known, but the relationship compared with cluster headache is reported to be approximately one to three cases of paroxysmal hemicrania for every 100 cases of cluster headache. The most common age at onset is the second or third decade of life, although there is a wide range (1–68y), with several case reports of onset before the age of 18 years (Kudrow and Kudrow 1989, Gladstein et al 1994, Shabbir and McAbee 1994, Klassen and Dooley 2000, Moorjani and Rothner 2001, de Almeida et al 2004, Talvik et al 2006, Cittadini et al 2008). Paroxysmal hemicrania seems to be equally prevalent in females and males (Cittadini et al 2008).

CLINICAL FEATURES

The clinical phenotype of paroxysmal hemicrania is highly characteristic (Antonaci and Sjaastad 1989, Kudrow and Kudrow 1989, Gladstein et al 1994, Shabbir and McAbee 1994, Klassen and Dooley 2000, Moorjani and Rothner 2001, de Almeida et al 2004, Talvik et al 2006, Cittadini et al 2008). The pain is strictly unilateral and centred on the orbital and temporal regions, although any part of the head can be affected. It is excruciatingly severe. The headache usually lasts 2 to 30 minutes. Attacks of paroxysmal hemicrania invariably occur in association with ipsilateral cranial autonomic features (see Table 19.4). Up to 85% of patients report at least one migrainous feature out of photophobia, nausea or vomiting during an attack. Similar to cluster headache, patients are often restless or agitated during an attack. The attacks occur at a high frequency. Typically, patients have more than five attacks daily, although the frequency of attacks fluctuates considerably, ranging between 1 and 40 daily. The attacks occur randomly throughout the 24-hour period, without a preponderance of nocturnal attacks as in cluster headache. While the majority of attacks are spontaneous, common triggers include stress, release from stress, exercise, alcohol consumption and neck movement.

The classification of paroxysmal hemicrania is dependent on the presence of a remission period. About 35% of patients have *episodic paroxysmal hemicrania*, which is diagnosed when there are clear remission periods between bouts of attacks. The remaining 65% of patients have *chronic paroxysmal hemicrania* (Cittadini et al 2008), which is diagnosed when patients have either no remission within 1 year or the remissions last less than 1 month.

DIFFERENTIAL DIAGNOSIS

The differential diagnoses that need to be considered are secondary causes of paroxysmal hemicrania, other trigeminal autonomic cephalalgias and hemicrania continua. A large number of symptomatic cases of paroxysmal hemicrania, caused by diverse pathological processes at various intracranial sites, have been described, although a causal relationship is difficult to ascertain in most of these cases (Matharu et al 2003a). Paroxysmal hemicrania can be differentiated from cluster headache and SUNCT with a trial of indometacin. Hemicrania

TABLE 19.4

The International Classification of Headache Disorders II diagnostic criteria for paroxysmal hemicrania (Headache Classification Subcommittee of the International Headache Society 2004)

Diagnostic criteria

(A) At least 20 attacks fulfilling criteria B–D

(B) Severe unilateral orbital, supraorbital or temporal pain lasting 2–30min

(C) Headache is accompanied by at least one of the following:

    (1) ipsilateral conjunctival injection and/or lacrimation

    (2) ipsilateral nasal congestion and/or rhinorrhoea

    (3) forehead and facial sweating

    (4) ipsilateral eyelid oedema

    (5) ipsilateral forehead and facial sweating

    (6) ipsilateral miosis and/or ptosis

(D) Attacks have a frequency above five per day for more than half the time, although periods with lower frequency may occur

(E) Attacks are prevented completely by therapeutic doses of indometacin[a]

Episodic paroxysmal headache

Description

Occurs in periods lasting 7d–1y separated by pain-free periods lasting ≥1mo

Chronic paroxysmal headache

Description

Attacks occur for more than 1y without remission or with remissions lasting <1mo

[a]To rule out an incomplete response, indometacin should be used in a dose of >150mg daily orally or rectally, or >100mg by injection. Smaller doses are often sufficient for maintenance.

continua is a strictly unilateral headache that is continuous and associated with ipsilateral cranial autonomic symptoms. Both paroxysmal hemicrania and hemicrania continua are exquisitely responsive to indometacin and can be differentiated on the basis of the clinical phenotype (Matharu et al 2003a).

INVESTIGATIONS

As a relatively high number of symptomatic cases have been reported, MRI of the brain should be routinely performed in all paroxysmal hemicrania patients.

TREATMENT

The treatment of paroxysmal hemicrania is entirely preventive, as attacks are too short and intense for any acute oral treatment to be effective.

Indometacin

Indometacin is the treatment of choice and, in fact, has been deemed the sine qua non for establishing the diagnosis (Headache Classification Subcommittee of the International Headache

Society 2004). Complete resolution of the headache is prompt, usually occurring within 1 to 2 days of initiating the effective dose. The typical maintenance dose ranges from 25 to 100mg daily, but doses up to 300mg daily are occasionally required (Cittadini et al 2008).

Other medications
Patients who cannot tolerate indometacin face a difficult challenge. No other drug is consistently effective in paroxysmal hemicrania. Other drug therapies that have been reported to be effective in paroxysmal hemicrania include cyclooxygenase-2 inhibitors, calcium channel antagonists (verapamil, flunarizine), topiramate or greater occipital nerve blocks (Matharu et al 2003b, Matharu and Goadsby 2007).

SUNCT

SUNCT is a disorder characterised by strictly unilateral, severe, neuralgic attacks, centred on the ophthalmic trigeminal distribution, that are brief in duration and occur in association with both conjunctival injection and lacrimation (Headache Classification Subcommittee of the International Headache Society 2004).

EPIDEMIOLOGY
SUNCT is relatively rare, with a recent study showing a prevalence of 6.6 per 100 000 population (Williams and Broadley 2008). SUNCT has a slight male predominance with a sex ratio of 1.5:1 (Cohen et al 2006). The typical age at onset is between 40 and 70 years, with a mean age at onset at 48 years and a range between 2 and 77 years. Paediatric-onset SUNCT is very rare, with only five case reports in the literature (D'Andrea and Granella 2001, Blattler et al 2003, Sekhara et al 2005, Unalp and Ozturk 2008, Sciruicchio et al 2010).

CLINICAL FEATURES
The attacks are strictly unilateral, but may alternate between sides. The pain is usually maximal in the ophthalmic distribution of the trigeminal nerve, but can radiate to any part of the head. The pain has an excruciating intensity and a neuralgic quality. The individual attacks are relatively brief, lasting between 5 and 240 seconds. Three different types of pain have been described in SUNCT syndrome: single stabs; groups of stabs; and a saw-tooth pattern in which

---

TABLE 19.5

The International Classification of Headache Disorders II (Headache Classification Subcommittee of the International Headache Society 2004) diagnostic criteria for SUNCT

(A) At least 20 attacks fulfilling criteria B–E
(B) Attacks of unilateral orbital, supraorbital or temporal stabbing or pulsating pain lasting 5–240s
(C) Pain is accompanied by ipsilateral conjunctival injection and lacrimation
(D) Attacks occur with a frequency of 3–200/d
(E) Not attributed to another disorder

SUNCT, short-lasting unilateral neuralgiform headache attacks with conjunctival injection and tearing.

repetitive spike-like paroxysms occur without reaching the pain-free baseline between the individual spikes. By definition, all SUNCT patients had both ipsilateral conjunctival injection and lacrimation associated with their attacks (see Table 19.5). Patients are often restless or agitated during the attacks (Cohen et al 2006). The attack frequency during the symptomatic phase varies immensely between sufferers and within an individual sufferer. Attacks may be as infrequent as once a day or less or as frequent as more than 60 per hour.

The majority of patients can precipitate attacks by touching certain trigger zones within the trigeminal innervated distribution and, occasionally, even from an extratrigeminal territory. Precipitants include touching the face or scalp, washing, shaving, eating, chewing, brushing teeth, talking and coughing. Unlike in trigeminal neuralgia, most patients have no refractory period.

The temporal pattern is quite variable, with the symptomatic periods alternating with remissions in an erratic manner. Symptomatic periods generally last from a few days to several months and occur once or twice annually. Remissions typically last a few months but can range from 1 week to 7 years. Symptomatic periods appear to increase in frequency and duration over time (Matharu et al 2003b).

DIFFERENTIAL DIAGNOSIS

Secondary SUNCT is typically seen with either posterior fossa (Blattler et al 2003) or pituitary gland lesions (Matharu et al 2003b). A recent study that systematically looked for trigeminal neurovascular conflict with dedicated trigeminal MRI found a high proportion of ipsilateral vascular loops in contact with the trigeminal nerve in SUNCT (Williams and Broadley 2008).

Differentiating SUNCT from trigeminal neuralgia can be challenging in some cases, as there is a considerable overlap in the clinical phenotypes of the two syndromes.

Table 19.6 outlines the useful differentiating features. Primary stabbing headache refers to a brief, sharp or jabbing pain in the head that occurs either as a single episode or in brief repeated volleys. The pain usually lasts a fraction of a second but can persist for up to 1 minute. These headaches are generally easily distinguished from SUNCT as they differ in several respects: in primary stabbing headache the site and radiation of pain often vary between

TABLE 19.6
Differentiating features of SUNCT and trigeminal neuralgia

Feature	SUNCT	Trigeminal neuralgia
Male–female ratio	1.5:1	1:2
Site of pain	V1	V2/3
Duration (s)	5–240	<5
Autonomic features	Prominent	Sparse or none
Refractory period	Absent	Present

SUNCT, short-lasting unilateral neuralgiform headache attacks with conjunctival injection and tearing.

TABLE 19.7
Management of SUNCT

Preventive treatments	Lamotrigine, topiramate, gabapentin
Transitional treatments	Local blocks (including greater occipital nerve block), intravenous lidocaine
Surgery	Microvascular decompression of the trigeminal nerve, occipital nerve stimulation, hypothalamic deep-brain stimulation

SUNCT, short-lasting unilateral neuralgiform headache attacks with conjunctival injection and tearing.

attacks, the majority of the attacks tend to be spontaneous and cranial autonomic features are absent. Paroxysmal hemicrania can be differentiated from SUNCT with a trial of indometacin.

INVESTIGATIONS

The association of secondary SUNCT with pituitary disorders, posterior fossa abnormalities and trigeminovascular conflict emphasises the need for a cranial MRI, including an adequate view of the pituitary and the trigeminal nerve.

TREATMENT

In view of the rarity of this condition, there are no published placebo-controlled trials of treatments in SUNCT. The management of SUNCT is entirely based on case reports or very small case series. The treatment options are outlined in Table 19.7.

Pathophysiology

Any pathophysiological construct for trigeminal autonomic cephalalgias must account for the three major clinical features characteristic of the various conditions that constitute this group: trigeminal distribution pain, ipsilateral autonomic features and the curious periodicity or regularity that often marks the attack incidence. The pain-producing innervation of the cranium projects through branches of the trigeminal and upper cervical nerves to the trigeminocervical complex, from which nociceptive pathways project to higher centres. This implies an integral role for the ipsilateral trigeminal nociceptive pathways in trigeminal autonomic cephalalgias. The ipsilateral autonomic features suggest cranial parasympathetic activation (lacrimation, rhinorrhoea, nasal congestion and eyelid oedema) and sympathetic hypofunction (ptosis and miosis). It has been suggested that the pathophysiology of the trigeminal autonomic cephalalgias revolves around the trigeminal autonomic reflex (Goadsby and Lipton 1997). There is a considerable amount of experimental animal literature documenting that stimulation of trigeminal afferents can result in cranial autonomic outflow, the trigeminal autonomic reflex (May and Goadsby 1999). In fact, some degree of cranial autonomic symptomatology is a normal physiological response to cranial nociceptive input and patients with other headache syndromes often report these symptoms. The distinction between the trigeminal autonomic cephalalgias and other headache syndromes is the degree of cranial autonomic activation, not its presence (Goadsby et al 2001, Goadsby 2005).

The cranial autonomic symptoms may be prominent in the trigeminal autonomic cephalalgias because of a central disinhibition of the trigeminal autonomic reflex (Leone and Bussone 2009). Supporting evidence is emerging from functional imaging studies: positron emission tomography studies in cluster headache (May et al 1998a) and paroxysmal hemicrania (Matharu et al 2006) and functional MRI studies in SUNCT syndrome (May et al 1999, Cohen et al 2004, Sprenger et al 2005) have demonstrated hypothalamic activation. Importantly, the involvement of posterior hypothalamic structures may account for the rhythmicity or periodicity that is such a hallmark of these conditions. Hypothalamic activation is not seen in experimental trigeminal distribution head pain (May et al 1998b). There are direct hypothalamic–trigeminal connections (Malick and Burstein 1998). There is abundant evidence for a role of the hypothalamus in mediating antinociceptive (Wang et al 1990, Dafny et al 1996) and autonomic responses (Lumb and Lovick 1993). Hence, the trigeminal autonomic cephalalgias are probably due to an abnormality in the hypothalamus with subsequent trigeminovascular and cranial autonomic activation.

Conclusions

The trigeminal autonomic cephalalgias are a group of primary headache disorders characterised by unilateral head pain that occurs in association with ipsilateral cranial autonomic features. The trigeminal autonomic cephalalgias include cluster headache, paroxysmal hemicrania and SUNCT. The underlying pathophysiology is purported to involve a role for neurons in the region of the posterior hypothalamus. Clinically, the syndromes can be distinguished by the frequency of attacks of pain, the length of the attacks and very characteristic responses to medical therapy. The differentiation is important because the treatments are so distinct.

REFERENCES

Antonaci F, Sjaastad O (1989) Chronic paroxysmal hemicrania (CPH): a review of the clinical manifestations. *Headache* 29: 648–56. http://dx.doi.org/10.1111/j.1526-4610.1989.hed2910648.x
Antonaci F, Alfei E, Piazza F, De Cillis I, Balottin U (2010) Therapy-resistant cluster headache in childhood: case report and literature review. *Cephalalgia* 30: 233–8.
Blattler T, Capone Mori A, Boltshauser E, Bassetti C (2003) Symptomatic SUNCT in an eleven-year-old girl. *Neurology* 60: 2012–13. http://dx.doi.org/10.1212/01.WNL.0000068015.58948.D3
Brainin M, Barnes M, Baron JC et al (2004) Guidance for the preparation of neurological management guidelines by EFNS scientific task forces: revised recommendations 2004. *Eur J Neurol* 11: 577–81.
Cittadini E, Matharu MS (2009) Symptomatic trigeminal autonomic cephalalgias. *Neurologist* 15: 305–12. http://dx.doi.org/10.1097/NRL.0b013e3181ad8d67
Cittadini E, May A, Straube A, Evers S, Bussone G, Goadsby PJ (2006) Effectiveness of intranasal zolmitriptan in acute cluster headache: a randomized, placebocontrolled, double-blind crossover study. *Arch Neurol* 63: 1537–42. http://dx.doi.org/10.1001/archneur.63.11.nct60002
Cittadini E, Matharu MS, Goadsby PJ (2008) Paroxysmal hemicrania: a prospective clinical study of 31 cases. *Brain* 131: 1142–55. http://dx.doi.org/10.1093/brain/awn010
Cohen A, Matharu M, Kalisch R, Friston K, Goadsby P (2004) Functional MRI in SUNCT shows differential hypothalamic activation with increasing pain. *Cephalalgia* 24: 1098–9.
Cohen AS, Matharu MS, Goadsby PJ (2006) Short-lasting unilateral neuralgiform headache attacks with conjunctival injection and tearing (SUNCT) or cranial autonomic features (SUNA)-a prospective clinical study of SUNCT and SUNA. *Brain* 129: 2746–60. http://dx.doi.org/10.1093/brain/awl202

Cohen AS, Burns B, Goadsby PJ (2009) High-flow oxygen for treatment of cluster headache: a randomized trial. *JAMA* 302: 2451–7. http://dx.doi.org/10.1001/jama.2009.1855

Couch JR Jr, Ziegler DK (1978) Prednisone therapy for cluster headache. *Headache* 18: 219–21. http://dx.doi.org/10.1111/j.1526-4610.1978.hed1804219.x

Dafny N, Dong WQ, Prieto-Gomez C, Reyes-Vazquez C, Stanford J, Qiao JT (1996) Lateral hypothalamus: site involved in pain modulation. *Neuroscience* 70: 449–60. http://dx.doi.org/10.1016/0306-4522(95)00358-4

D'Andrea G, Granella F (2001) SUNCT syndrome: the first case in childhood. Shortlasting unilateral neuralgiform headache attacks with conjunctival injection and tearing. *Cephalalgia* 21: 701–2. http://dx.doi.org/10.1046/j.1468-2982.2001.00224.x

de Almeida DB, Cunali PA, Santos HL, Brioschi M, Prandini M (2004) Chronic paroxysmal hemicrania in early childhood: case report. *Cephalalgia* 24: 608–9. http://dx.doi.org/10.1111/j.1468-2982.2004.00732.x

Del Bene E, Poggioni M (1987) Typical and atypical cluster headache in childhood. *Cephalalgia* 7(Suppl 6):128–30.

Ekbom K, Waldenlind E, Cole J, Pilgrim A, Kirkham A (1992) Sumatriptan in chronic cluster headache: results of continuous treatment for eleven months. *Cephalalgia* 12: 254–6. http://dx.doi.org/10.1046/j.1468-2982.1992.1204254.x

Ekbom K, Monstad I, Prusinski A, Cole JA, Pilgrim AJ, Noronha D (1993) Subcutaneous sumatriptan in the acute treatment of cluster headache: a dose comparison study. The Sumatriptan Cluster Headache Study Group. *Acta Neurologica Scandinavica* 88: 63–9. http://dx.doi.org/10.1111/j.1600-0404.1993.tb04189.x

Francis GJ, Becker WJ, Pringsheim TM (2010) Acute and preventive pharmacologic treatment of cluster headache. *Neurology* 75: 463–73. http://dx.doi.org/10.1212/WNL.0b013e3181eb58c8

Gallai B, Mazzotta G, Floridi F et al (2003) Cluster headache in childhood and adolescence: one-year prevalence in an out-patient population. *J Headache Pain* 4: 132–7. http://dx.doi.org/10.1007/s10194-003-0047-4

Gladstein J, Holden EW, Peralta L (1994) Chronic paroxysmal hemicrania in a child. *Headache* 34: 519–20. http://dx.doi.org/10.1111/j.1526-4610.1994.hed3409519.x

Goadsby PJ (2005) Trigeminal autonomic cephalalgias: fancy term or constructive change to the IHS classification? *J Neurol Neurosurg Psychiatry* 76: 301–5. http://dx.doi.org/10.1136/jnnp.2004.036012

Goadsby PJ, Lipton RB (1997) A review of paroxysmal hemicranias, SUNCT syndrome and other short-lasting headaches with autonomic feature, including new cases. *Brain* 120: 193–209. http://dx.doi.org/10.1093/brain/120.1.193

Goadsby PJ, Matharu MS, Boes CJ (2001) SUNCT syndrome or trigeminal neuralgia with lacrimation. *Cephalalgia* 21: 82–3. http://dx.doi.org/10.1046/j.1468-2982.2001.00175.x

Gobel H, Lindner V, Heinze A, Ribbat M, Deuschl G (1998) Acute therapy for cluster headache with sumatriptan: findings of a one-year long-term study. *Neurology* 51: 908–11. http://dx.doi.org/10.1212/WNL.51.3.908

Headache Classification Subcommittee of The International Headache Society (2004) The international classification of headache disorders 2nd edition. *Cephalalgia* 24(Suppl 1):1–195.

Klassen BD, Dooley JM (2000) Chronic paroxysmal hemicrania-like headaches in a child: response to a headache diary. *Headache* 40: 853–5. http://dx.doi.org/10.1046/j.1526-4610.2000.00155.x

Kudrow DB, Kudrow L (1989) Successful aspirin prophylaxis in a child with chronic paroxysmal hemicrania. *Headache* 29: 280–1. http://dx.doi.org/10.1111/j.1526-4610.1989.hed2905280.x

Leone M, Bussone G (2009) Pathophysiology of trigeminal autonomic cephalalgias. *Lancet Neurol* 8: 755–64. http://dx.doi.org/10.1016/S1474-4422(09)70133-4

Leone M, D'Amico D, Frediani F e al. (2000). Verapamil in the prophylaxis of episodic cluster headache: a double-blind study versus placebo. *Neurology* 54: 1382–5. http://dx.doi.org/10.1212/WNL.54.6.1382

Leroux E, Valade D, Taifas I et al (2011). Suboccipital steroid injections for transitional treatment of patients with more than two cluster headache attacks per day: a randomised, double-blind, placebocontrolled trial. *Lancet Neurol* 10: 891–7. http://dx.doi.org/10.1016/S1474-4422(11)70186-7

Lewis DW, Winner P, Hershey AD, Wasiewski WW (2007) Efficacy of zolmitriptan nasal spray in adolescent migraine. *Pediatrics* 120: 390–6. http://dx.doi.org/10.1542/peds.2007-0085

Lumb BM, Lovick TA (1993) The rostral hypothalamus: an area for the integration of autonomic and sensory responsiveness. *J Neurophysiol* 70: 1570–7.

McNabb S, Whitehouse W (1999) Cluster headache-like disorder in childhood. *Arch Dis Child* 81: 511–12. http://dx.doi.org/10.1136/adc.81.6.511

Malick A, Burstein R (1998) Cells of origin of the trigeminohypothalamic tract in the rat. *J Comp Neurol* 400: 125–44. http://dx.doi.org/10.1002/(SICI)1096-9861(19981012)400:1<125::AID-CNE9>3.0.CO;2-B

Matharu MS, Goadsby PJ (2002) Trigeminal autonomic cephalgias. *J Neurol Neurosurg Psychiatry* 72(Suppl 2): 19–26.

Matharu M, Goadsby P (2007) Trigeminal autonomic cephalalgias: diagnosis and management. In: Silberstein S, Lipton R, Dodick D, editors. *Wolff's Headache and Other Head Pain*, 8th edn. New York: Oxford University Press, pp. 379–430.

Matharu MS, Boes CJ, Goadsby PJ (2003a) Management of trigeminal autonomic cephalgias and hemicrania continua. *Drugs* 63: 1637–77. http://dx.doi.org/10.2165/00003495-200363160-00002

Matharu MS, Cohen AS, Boes CJ, Goadsby PJ (2003b) Short-lasting unilateral neuralgiform headache with conjunctival injection and tearing syndrome: a review. *Curr Pain Headache Rep* 7: 308–18. http://dx.doi.org/10.1007/s11916-003-0052-y

Matharu MS, Cohen AS, Frackowiak RS, Goadsby PJ (2006) Posterior hypothalamic activation in paroxysmal hemicrania. *Ann Neurol* 59: 535–45. http://dx.doi.org/10.1002/ana.20763

May A, Goadsby PJ (1999) The trigeminovascular system in humans: pathophysiologic implications for primary headache syndromes of the neural influences on the cerebral circulation. *J Cereb Blood Flow Metab* 19: 115–27. http://dx.doi.org/10.1097/00004647-199902000-00001

May A, Bahra A, Buchel C, Frackowiak RS, Goadsby PJ (1998a) Hypothalamic activation in cluster headache attacks. *Lancet* 352: 275–8. http://dx.doi.org/10.1016/S0140-6736(98)02470-2

May A, Kaube H, Buchel C et al (1998b) Experimental cranial pain elicited by capsaicin: a PET study. *Pain* 74: 61–6. http://dx.doi.org/10.1016/S0304-3959(97)00144-9

May A, Bahra A, Buchel C, Turner R, Goadsby PJ (1999) Functional magnetic resonance imaging in spontaneous attacks of SUNCT: short-lasting neuralgiform headache with conjunctival injection and tearing. *Annals of Neurology* 46: 791–4. http://dx.doi.org/10.1002/1531-8249(199911)46:5<791::AID-ANA18>3.0.CO;2-8

May A, Leone M, Afra J et al (2006) EFNS guidelines on the treatment of cluster headache and other trigeminal-autonomic cephalalgias. *Eur J Neurol* 13: 1066–77. http://dx.doi.org/10.1111/j.1468-1331.2006.01566.x

Moorjani BI, Rothner AD (2001) Indomethacin-responsive headaches in children and adolescents. *Semin Pediatr Neurol* 8: 40–5. http://dx.doi.org/10.1053/spen.2001.23328

Rapoport AM, Mathew NT, Silberstein SD et al (2007). Zolmitriptan nasal spray in the acute treatment of cluster headache: a double-blind study. *Neurology* 69: 821–6. http://dx.doi.org/10.1212/01.wnl.0000267886.85210.37

Russell MB (2004) Epidemiology and genetics of cluster headache. *Lancet Neurol* 3: 279–83. http://dx.doi.org/10.1016/S1474-4422(04)00735-5

Schurks M, Kurth T, de Jesus J, Jonjic M, Rosskopf D, Diener HC (2006) Cluster headache: clinical presentation, lifestyle features, and medical treatment. *Headache* 46: 1246–54. http://dx.doi.org/10.1111/j.1526-4610.2006.00534.x

Sciruicchio V, Sardaro M, Gagliardi D, Trabacca A, Galeone D, de Tommaso M (2010) A case of early-onset and monophasic trigeminal autonomic cephalalgia: could it be a SUNCT? *J Headache Pain* 11: 363–5. http://dx.doi.org/10.1007/s10194-010-0219-y

Sekhara T, Pelc K, Mewasingh LD, Boucquey D, Dan B (2005) Pediatric SUNCT Syndrome. *Pediatr Neurol* 33: 206–7. http://dx.doi.org/10.1016/j.pediatrneurol.2005.03.017

Shabbir N, McAbee G (1994) Adolescent chronic paroxysmal hemicrania responsive to verapamil monotherapy. *Headache* 34: 209–10. http://dx.doi.org/10.1111/j.1526-4610.1994.hed3404209.x

Silberstein SD, Niknam R, Rozen TD, Young WB (2000) Cluster headache with aura. *Neurology* 54: 219–21. http://dx.doi.org/10.1212/WNL.54.1.219

Sprenger T, Valet M, Platzer S, Pfaffenrath V, Steude U, Tolle TR (2005) SUNCT: bilateral hypothalamic activation during headache attacks and resolving of symptoms after trigeminal decompression. *Pain* 113: 422–6. http://dx.doi.org/10.1016/j.pain.2004.09.021

Talvik I, Koch K, Kolk A, Talvik T (2006) Chronic paroxysmal hemicrania in a 3- year, 10-month-old female. *Pediatr Neurol* 34: 225–7. http://dx.doi.org/10.1016/j.pediatrneurol.2005.08.026

Tonon C, Guttmann S, Volpini M, Naccarato S, Cortelli P, D'Alessandro R (2002) Prevalence and incidence of cluster headache in the Republic of San Marino. *Neurology* 58: 1407–9. http://dx.doi.org/10.1212/WNL.58.9.1407

Torelli P, Beghi E, Manzoni GC (2005) Cluster headache prevalence in the Italian general population. *Neurology* 64: 469–74. http://dx.doi.org/10.1212/01.WNL.0000150901.47293.BC

Unalp A, Ozturk AA (2008) SUNCT syndrome in a child: a rare cause of paroxysmal headache. *Ann Saudi Med* 28: 386–7. http://dx.doi.org/10.4103/0256-4947.51695

Van Vliet JA, Bahra A, Martin V et al (2003). Intranasal sumatriptan in cluster headache: Randomized placebo-controlled double-blind study. *Neurology* 60: 630–3. http://dx.doi.org/10.1212/01.WNL.0000046589.45855.30

Wang Q, Mao LM, Han JS (1990) Naloxone-reversible analgesia produced by microstimulation of the arcuate nucleus of the hypothalamus in pentobarbital anesthetized rats. *Exp Brain Res* 80: 201–4. http://dx.doi.org/10.1007/BF00228862

Williams MH, Broadley SA (2008) SUNCT and SUNA: clinical features and medical treatment. *J Clin Neurosci* 15: 526–34. http://dx.doi.org/10.1016/j.jocn.2006.09.006

Winner P, Rothner AD, Saper J et al (2000) A randomized, double-blind, placebo-controlled study of sumatriptan nasal spray in the treatment of acute migraine in adolescents. *Pediatrics* 106: 989–97. http://dx.doi.org/10.1542/peds.106.5.989

20
CHRONIC DAILY HEADACHE IN CHILDREN AND ADOLESCENTS

Shashi S Seshia and Ishaq Abu-Arafeh

Introduction

The term 'chronic daily headache' was first used by Mathew and his colleagues to describe headache occurring almost daily in adults (Mathew et al 1982); they found that episodic headache evolved into daily headache in over 75% of patients. They suggested that an overuse of medication and an association with psychiatric symptomatology were likely to have contributed to the transformation (Mathew et al 1982, 1987). These and related seminal observations have been confirmed in adult and paediatric literature. In 1994, Holden et al published the first report of chronic daily headache in children (Holden et al 1994). Since then, the clinical spectrum of symptomatology of chronic daily headache in children (the term will be used to include adolescents) has become increasingly well defined through more than 20 reports worldwide (Seshia et al 2010a). The multifaceted nature of primary chronic daily headache has been reviewed recently (Seshia et al 2010a, Seshia 2012), and is also the thrust of this chapter.

Terminology and classification

The ambiguities and controversies surrounding the terminology and classification of chronic daily headache have been discussed in Chapter 5. In this chapter, all subtypes of chronic daily headache are defined as 'headache occurring on at least 15 days a month for at least 3 months'. The duration of headache attacks can be shorter than 4 hours, as suggested by Welch and Goadsby (2002) and Seshia et al (2010a).

Epidemiology

Precise comparisons between studies cannot be made because of the absence of a universally accepted definition and classification for chronic daily headache (Stovner et al 2007). With these qualifications, the prevalence of chronic daily headache was 0.9% to 7.8% in studies from six countries (Abu-Arafeh and Russell 1994, Laurell et al 2004, Wang et al 2006, Zhang et al 2007, Arruda et al 2010a, Lipton et al 2011). In children, the prevalence of primary chronic daily headache is two to four times greater in females than in males, the difference being greatest in adolescents (Wang et al 2006, Arruda et al 2010b, Lipton et al 2011). The 1-year prevalence of secondary chronic daily headache was 0.04% in Taiwan (Wang et al 2006).

TABLE 20.1

Classification of chronic daily headache

Primary (ICHD-II codes 1–4)

Chronic migraine (1.5.1): (i) solely with migraine features; (ii) with associated tension-type headache features

Chronic tension-type headache (2.3)

Chronic cluster (3.1.2); chronic paroxysmal hemicranias (3.2.2)

Hemicrania continua (4.7); new daily persistent headache (4.8)

Secondary (ICHD-II codes 5–14)

See Chapter 5 and Appendix 5.1

ICHD, International Classification of Headache Disorders.

Subtypes of primary chronic daily headache

Chronic daily headache can be subtyped using the framework and codes of ICHD-II (the International Classification of Headache Disorders) (Table 20.1) (Welch and Goadsby 2002, Headache Classification Subcommittee of the International Headache Society 2004, Seshia et al 2009, 2010a,b, Seshia 2012). A multiaxial classification (see Table 5.2) is ideal for chronic daily headache, because of its multifaceted nature (Seshia et al 2008, 2010b).

Chronic Migraine

The controversies surrounding the current ICHD-II criteria for chronic migraine have been discussed in Chapter 5. The term chronic migraine, rather than transformed migraine, will be used here. The original criteria for the diagnosis of chronic migraine (Code 1.5.1), in which patients report at least 15 days of migraine per month, are favoured over the revised criteria (Code 1.5.1R), which actually describe a mixed type of headache in which tension-type headache has been assimilated into the definition (Headache Classification Committee et al 2006, Seshia et al 2008, 2009, 2010a,b, Seshia 2012).

Thus, the relative frequency of chronic migraine depends upon the definition used. In an adolescent community-based study from Taiwan, the percentage with chronic migraine was 7% with the original ICHD-II criteria, increasing to 23% when the revised criteria were used (Wang et al 2007a).

Auras are uncommon in chronic migraine (personal observation). When these occur, a secondary cause must be excluded, mitochondrial encephalopathy being one consideration.

Our suggested criteria for the diagnosis of chronic migraine in children are in the box below (explanatory comments are in *italics* and parentheses).

Headache fulfilling criteria C and D for 1.1 Migraine without aura, on more than 15 days per month for 3 months or more.

Headache not attributable to another disorder. (*The caveat for the diagnosis of any primary headache disorder in ICHD-II; the clinician needs to exclude secondary causes by history, examination and/or investigations.*)

Headache has at least two of the following characteristics: (1) unilateral or bilateral location; (2) pulsating or equivalent quality; (3) moderate or severe pain intensity (*in chronic migraine the pain intensity can be mild*); and (4) aggravated by or causing avoidance of routine physical activity such as walking, climbing stairs, sports or other recreational activity. (*This may be variable when migraine becomes chronic; however, there may be other reasons for avoiding physical activity.*)

During headache at least one of the following: (1) nausea and/or vomiting; (2) photophobia and phonophobia. (*These features are typically mild once migraine becomes chronic.*)

CHRONIC MIGRAINE WITH TENSION-TYPE HEADACHE ('MIXED')

In children with episodic migraine, there is a tendency for the 'typical migraine' characteristics to become less prominent and tension-type features to predominate as chronic daily headache develops; typical migraine features re-emerge as chronic daily headache improves (Hershey et al 2001, Bigal et al 2005, Wang et al 2007a). It is not clear if this phenomenon can be explained by migraine alone or if tension-type headache also occurs when migraine becomes chronic.

Until there is evidence to the contrary, rather than assimilate tension-type headache into the definition of chronic migraine (in Code 1.5.1R), as the International Headache Society (IHS) proposed (Headache Classification Committee et al 2006), it may be more appropriate to use the term 'chronic migraine with tension-type headache' (Solomon 2007, Seshia et al 2010a,b, Seshia 2012); other descriptors previously employed being comorbid or mixed migraine and tension-type headache. Such a diagnosis (definite or probable) would have accounted for 40% of individuals in the population-based study of chronic daily headache in Taiwan (Wang et al 2007a). In clinical practice, mixed 'chronic migraine with tension-type headache' is the most common subtype of primary chronic daily headache (Seshia et al 2008).

CHRONIC TENSION-TYPE HEADACHE

Chronic tension-type headache is frequently seen in clinical practice but often overlooked as a subtype of chronic daily headache (Abu-Arafeh 2001). Some patients with chronic tension-type headache may experience severe pain intensity (Abu-Arafeh 2001, Seshia et al 2009), rather than the mild or moderate characteristic attributed to chronic tension-type headache in ICHD-II (Headache Classification Subcommittee of the International Headache Society 2004).

CHRONIC TRIGEMINAL AUTONOMIC CEPHALALGIAS AND HEMICRANIA CONTINUA
The defining characteristics of these conditions (see Chapters 5 and 19) are unilateral pain over orbital, supraorbital or temporal regions and prominent cranial autonomic disturbances usually ipsilateral to the pain (conjunctival injection or lacrimation, nasal congestion or discharge, eyelid oedema, forehead or facial sweating, and miosis or ptosis).

Hemicrania continua shares many similarities with chronic cluster headache and chronic paroxysmal hemicranias, including response to indometacin (indomethacin in North America), an essential ICHD-II criterion for diagnosis; for some reason hemicrania continua is coded under 'other primary headaches'. Response to indometacin may not be invariable (Marmura et al 2009). Nevertheless, a trial of indometacin is generally suggested when headache is unilateral (Mack and Gladstein 2008).

These conditions, although uncommon in children, do manifest in the paediatric age group (Tarantino et al 2011), and clinicians should be alert to this possibility. Of 23 patients with unilateral chronic daily headache, two had chronic cluster headache and hemicrania continua and one had chronic paroxysmal hemicrania – response to indometacin was often incomplete (Ji and Mack 2009). Chronic paroxysmal hemicrania can occur as early as 27 months of age (Talvik et al 2009).

NEW DAILY PERSISTENT HEADACHE
New daily persistent headache (NDPH) was included within the concept of chronic daily headache by Silberstein et al (1994), and is currently classified as a primary headache disorder. The controversies surrounding the classification of NDPH are discussed in Chapter 5. NDPH as a clinical entity is discussed in Chapter 21.

Subtypes of secondary chronic daily headache
Many of the secondary causes for chronic daily headache may be associated with red flags (Chapter 9) which prompt the clinician to investigate them. However, these red flags may be subtle or absent.

HEADACHE ATTRIBUTED TO HEAD AND/OR NECK TRAUMA (CODE 5)
Minor concussion related to sports or recreation activity is often a cause of abrupt onset of chronic daily headache (NDPH), but concussion may also cause a transformation from episodic migraine or tension-type headache to chronic daily headache (Seshia 2004, Kirk et al 2008, Seshia et al 2008); hence, a history of concussion should be sought if not forthcoming. Headache characteristics are predominantly of tension type, but may be migrainous if there has been a preceding history of migraine.

HEADACHE ATTRIBUTED TO CRANIAL OR CERVICAL VASCULAR DISORDER (CODE 6)
Most of these disorders will present acutely, and are more often found in adults than in children. However, the author has seen one child with chronic daily headache, localised primarily to the occipital region, who was found to have a basilar aneurysm (Fig. 20.1). In addition, central nervous system angiitis has been occasionally reported in children. Any red flags

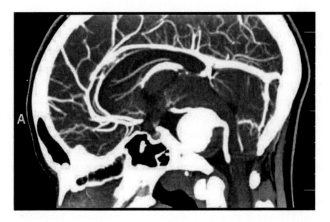

Fig. 20.1 Computed tomographic angiogram showing basilar aneurysm. A, anterior

should prompt investigation. Mitochondrial cytopathies often present in childhood, and the syndrome of mitochondrial encephalopathy, lactic acidosis and stroke-like episodes (MELAS) can present with chronic daily headache in which aura resembling those of migraine can be interspersed. Investigations should be done whenever aura occur with chronic daily headache as this is uncommon in primary chronic daily headache. MELAS is erroneously classified under 'headache attributed to cranial or cervical vascular disorder' in ICHD-II (Headache Classification Subcommittee of the International Headache Society 2004).

HEADACHE ATTRIBUTED TO NON-VASCULAR INTRACRANIAL DISORDER (CODE 7)
Several entities in this category are relevant for paediatric practice. Idiopathic intracranial hypertension can present as chronic daily headache and may have migrainous features. The diagnosis becomes challenging when papilloedema is absent and the patient is not obese (Wang et al 1998, Beri et al 2010).

Hydrocephalus secondary to aqueductal stenosis or a tumour around the aqueductal region may present in later childhood with chronic daily headache as the main symptom. Shunt malfunction may present with headache that may mimic primary chronic daily headache in many respects, and the diagnosis may be overlooked on brain imaging if slit-ventricle syndrome is not recognised (Seshia 1996).

Chiari malformation type 1 may present with chronic daily headache that is typically localised to the occipital region and worsened with physical activity or any Valsalva-like manoeuvre (see Chapter 5 and Fig. 5.1).

Headache attributed to low cerebrospinal fluid pressure secondary to a fistula, leak or idiopathic cause can also occur in children (see Chapter 5 and Fig. 5.2). Postural worsening is characteristic but may not be present. Other red flags may include neck stiffness or discomfort, tinnitus and hyperacusis. The diagnosis should be considered in any child with chronic daily headache that is occipital in location, even when other red flags are absent, especially if there is evidence of an inherited disorder of connective tissue (e.g. Marfan syndrome) in the child or his or her family.

Lupus encephalitis is an extremely rare cause of chronic daily headache, but needs to be considered in children with other suggestive features of lupus. One case was reported from a population-based study of chronic daily headache in adolescents in Taiwan (Wang et al 2006).

HEADACHE ATTRIBUTED TO A SUBSTANCE OR ITS WITHDRAWAL (CODE 8)
Medication overuse headache is the most relevant subform of headaches attributed to substance intake or withdrawal, and analgesia overuse is the most common form of medication overuse in children (Headache Classification Subcommittee of the International Headache Society 2004, Headache Classification Committee et al 2006).

Medication overuse headache is reported in children attending certain clinics but is generally uncommon; there may be regional differences in incidence (Pakalnis et al 2007, Seshia et al 2008, Pakalnis and Kring 2012, Seshia 2012). Common analgesics taken by children, either bought over the counter or prescribed, are paracetamol (acetaminophen), ibuprofen or combination drugs with or without codeine. Codeine is rarely prescribed in childhood headache, but it is probably the most likely to cause medication overuse headache.

The reasons for medication overuse are varied and include the following: (1) teenagers may self-medicate if they experience short-term relief after taking a dose, feeling that additional doses are bound to help; (2) the temptation for parents to give repeated doses, despite absence of sustained relief, because they feel helpless when their child is complaining of constant headache; and (3) physicians may inadvertently contribute to medication overuse by continuing analgesics, some containing codeine, even when these are ineffective. The overuse of medication is a possible contributory factor to the transformation from episodic headache to chronic daily headache (Mathew et al 1982, Bongesebandhu-phubhakdi and Srikiatkhachorn 2012). There is increasing evidence to indicate that medication overuse is likely to be genetically influenced and a reflection of addictive behaviour (Radat et al 2008, Hershey et al 2010).

The criteria for medication overuse headache (ICHD-II) are for adults and their applicability to children is questionable, as discussed in Chapter 5. According to these criteria, chronic daily headache due to analgesia overuse is described as bilateral, tightening (non-pulsating in quality) and mild to moderate in intensity. It is associated with the intake of analgesia on at least 15 days per month for at least 3 months. There is an observed worsening of headache during the period of analgesia overuse followed by resolution of headache or reversion to the previous pattern within 2 months of withdrawal of analgesia. The authors consider the 3-month requirement for diagnosis to be excessive.

In the absence of universally accepted criteria for medication overuse in children, it is not unreasonable to consider a definition, based on clinical experience, as 'the use of analgesics at least once per day on 5 days or more per week for more than 2 weeks' (Seshia 2004). It is now generally agreed that narcotics should not be prescribed and medications that have little or no effect on headache should be withdrawn. Alcohol and other substances may be abused by teenagers, but their contributions to chronic daily headache are not well known.

Carbon monoxide-induced headache is an important cause of chronic daily headache in countries, such as Canada, where natural gas furnaces are used for heating. Constant minor leaks of carbon monoxide due to furnace defects can cause chronic daily headache (personal experience). Clues to aetiology include the appearance of headache during periods when the furnace is on, headaches in other family members and headaches that occur when the child is at home and on awakening in the morning. The headache has tension-type characteristics. A precise diary is invaluable in diagnosing the cause.

Headache or facial pain can result from disorders of the cranium, neck, eyes, ears, nose, sinuses, teeth, mouth or other facial or cranial structures (Code 11). Ocular causes, especially errors of refraction, may present with chronic daily headache mimicking chronic tension-type headache. The prevalence of chronic daily headache due to ocular disorders is not known in children and there is no conclusive evidence for a cause-and-effect association.

Headache attributed to rhinosinusitis frequently enters into the differential diagnosis, with incidental radiological findings often confounding the clinical situation. Consultation with an ear, nose and throat specialist should be sought if there is clinical suspicion. The contributions of dental disorders and temporomandibular joint dysfunction to chronic daily headache are uncertain. Children with rheumatoid arthritis may be predisposed to temporomandibular joint and cervical spine involvement, resulting in chronic daily headache localised mainly to the temporal or cervical regions, respectively.

HEADACHE ATTRIBUTED TO PSYCHIATRIC DISORDER (CODE 12)
There is a strong association between chronic daily headache and psychiatric disorders in community-based and clinical studies, mood (especially depressive) and anxiety disorders being the most common; other associations include high suicidal scores, malingering and possibly adjustment, somatoform and factitious disorders (Pakalnis et al 2007, Wang et al 2007b, Seshia et al 2008, 2010, Fujita et al 2009, da Silva et al 2010, Knook et al 2011). Psychiatric comorbidity is associated with a greater disability and poorer quality of life (Slater et al 2012).

Genetics of primary chronic daily headache
There is strong evidence for genetic factors in primary chronic daily headache, the risk being increased almost 13-fold when the mother has chronic daily headache (Montagna et al 2003, Cevoli et al 2009, Arruda et al 2010c). Of 70 children with chronic daily headache, 7% and 22% had first-degree relatives with anxiety and depressive disorders, respectively (Seshia et al 2008), a possible association that requires further study.

Primary chronic daily headache is a multifaceted syndrome
A number of conditions are intimately linked to and constitute an essential part of chronic daily headache (Fig. 20.2). Their appreciation and recognition is crucial for management (Seshia et al 2010a).

MEDICAL DISORDERS
The association between chronic daily headache and psychiatric disorders in the child and family has been discussed.

Disturbed sleep not related to headache has been reported (Seshia et al 2008), but there is insufficient evidence to determine if the disturbance is due to a sleep disorder, another area requiring further study. The co-occurrence of chronic daily headache with other pain syndromes is well reported and needs further exploration. There is an association between

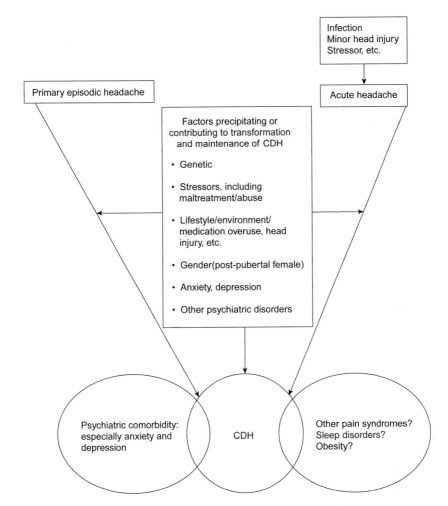

Fig. 20.2 Multifaceted nature of chronic daily headache (CDH). Reproduced with slight modification from Seshia et al (2010a). Permission from the *Canadian Journal of Neurological Sciences* gratefully acknowledged.

obesity and headache in females, but the sex difference has not been studied in chronic daily headache. There are conflicting reports on the association between chronic daily headache and obesity (Seshia et al 2008, Pakalnis and Kring 2012).

STRESSORS (ALSO REFERRED TO AS ADVERSE LIFE EVENTS OR LIFE CHANGES)
There was a significant association between childhood adversity and adolescent chronic daily headache in one study; divorce and physical abuse were the principal events, sexual abuse being difficult to identify (Juang et al 2004). Maltreatment, including sexual, should be considered, especially when chronic daily headache is associated with other pain syndromes,

anxiety and mood disorders (Zafar et al 2011, Seshia 2012). Childhood maltreatment is now recognised as a risk factor for chronic daily headache in adults (Peterlin et al 2007).

Common stressors (see Chapter 8 and Table 8.1) contributing to the transformation and maintenance of chronic daily headache (in at least 50% of patients in several studies) include bereavement (including loss of a pet), chronic illnesses, family, school and peer relationships, teasing, bullying and illnesses in close family members, fear of illness and geographic relocation; stressors may not be readily volunteered (Seshia et al 2010a, 2012). Cyber-bullying is becoming increasingly common (Sourander et al 2010).

OTHER FACTORS
Fluorescent or bright lights, noise (classroom, breaks, school bus), fatigue, caffeine (fizzy drinks), hunger, sleep deprivation and irregular sleep habits are often described as triggers and contributors to chronic daily headache.

Neurobiology of chronic daily headache
A short summary of chronic daily headache neurobiology is given here; readers should refer to cited references for details (Ashina et al 2005, Srikiatkhachorn 2006, Meng and Cao 2007). Central and peripheral sensitisation are considered to be responsible for the transformation to and maintenance of chronic daily headache, chronic migraine being the best example. Central sensitisation refers to a state in which neurons and their connections in the brain and spinal cord, subjected to repeated noxious stimuli (e.g. frequent headache), become more sensitive to subsequent stimuli delivered to the receptive fields. Peripheral sensitisation refers to a similar process involving nociceptors in the skin, muscles and joints (periphery), peripheral nerves and connections to the brain through the spinal cord. The trigeminal system and endogenous analgesic systems are closely involved. The intricate symptom complex of stressors, anxiety and mood disorders, and chronic daily headache can be explained by the concept of the 'limbically augmented pain syndrome' (Rome and Rome 2000), in which corticolimbic connections and sensitisation play an important role. Thus, stress, anxiety and depression are likely to contribute to central sensitisation and enhance pain sensitivity. Medication overuse has been linked to sensitisation (Srikiatkhachorn 2006, Bongsebandhu-phubhakdi and Srikiatkhachorn 2012).

Clinical presentation

Case study
A female first presented at the age of 13 years with a 1-year history of recurrent headache. On occasions, the headaches lasted all day but did not wake her up from sleep. The headache was described as 4/10 to 8/10. The characteristics were those of tension-type headache, but, on some days, there were clear features of migraine without aura. Analgesics had not provided relief, and she had not been overusing them. Several potential adverse psychosocial factors were identified. She had been fostered at 8 months of age because her mother was abusing alcohol and may have been schizophrenic; she was unaware of her natural father. She was of Canadian First Nations heritage but

---

adopted by 'white' foster parents at 4 years of age. The foster parents divorced when she was 10 years of age, and the foster father, with whom she continued to stay, remarried when she was 12 years of age. Her adoptive father had had cardiac bypass surgery a few months prior to her assessment. Her examination was normal. The nature of her headache was discussed, information was provided, the contributory roles of stress were emphasised and analgesia use was discouraged. She was asked to keep a headache diary and given a handout on headache. A referral was made to mental health services in her community with her consent and that of her adoptive father, and a follow-up appointment made. She failed to keep appointments but reappeared 3 years later at the age of 16 years with chronic daily headache of 18 months' duration, subtyped as chronic migraine with tension-type headache. She rated her pain as 8/10 to 9/10, and had not been attending school. She was overusing analgesics with no benefit, often drank alcohol to excess and was using substances such as marijuana. She described challenges with teachers and peers, and had been sexually active. She was admitted to hospital for assessment. In hospital, she volunteered that she was in a lot of emotional pain and that she felt depressed. She readily acknowledged that stressors in her life were playing an important role, and added that there were also conflicts at home. She mentioned that she often exaggerated her headache severity. Her assessment was normal, as was a magnetic resonance image of the head and cervical spine that included magnetic resonance angiography and venography. With informed consent, she was given a course of repetitive dihydroergotamine (DHE) and metoclopramide intravenously (see Table 20.3). Coincidentally or otherwise, headache resolved completely by the third day; treatment was continued for one more day. As she was obese, she was started on a small dose of topiramate and assessed by an adolescent psychiatrist and psychologist. The importance of psychotherapeutic approaches to headache was re-emphasised. She was reassessed 3 months later, at which time she was still headache free; topiramate was gradually discontinued. She was encouraged to continue follow-up with local mental health services and her family physician.

The case study is an extreme example of chronic daily headache, in which psychosocial stressors have probably played an important role in transformation and persistence. A multi-axial approach is ideal in such cases. The cost-beneficial value of the 5-day hospital admission is demonstrated.

Although her adoptive father denied stressors (see discussion on history in Chapter 8), the teenager was more forthcoming. The magnetic resonance imaging (MRI) was carried out to ensure that we were not overlooking an intracranial cause. The response to DHE and metoclopramide may have been a placebo effect. She is at high risk for relapse and alcohol/substance abuse. She was extremely grateful that we had taken her social history, as she had no one she could share the information with.

Several less extreme cases are encountered in clinical practice, in which stressors are denied by the parents but eventually volunteered by the child in a suitable setting. For example, a child with chronic daily headache of the chronic tension type ultimately said that he often faked headaches to get out of chores or when his mother and her partner argued, which they did frequently (stressors were denied by the mother). Another female adolescent in due course volunteered that, after her maternal grandmother had been diagnosed with Alzheimer disease, her mother had been worried about inheriting the condition; the mother's anxiety was not only a significant stressor for the patient, but she also began to worry about inheriting the condition herself. In another situation, the mother of an adolescent with chronic daily headache (chronic migraine and tension-type headache) eventually mentioned that the patient's headaches had stopped after her older sister (with whom she was having frequent arguments, an issue that did not come up earlier) left home. These experiences highlight the importance of interviewing mature minors separately from guardians (see Chapter 8); SSS has only had one situation in which informed consent for such an interview was refused by the mother, although the child was agreeable – significant stressors within this family unit were uncovered in due course. Children feel respected as individuals when such an approach is adopted, and sharing the heavy burden of stressors is itself therapeutic (personal opinion, SSS). Many jurisdictions allow healthcare professionals to exercise their judgement in interviewing mature minors separately from guardians, as long as informed consent is taken.

Clinical assessment and differential diagnosis
Clinical assessment is detailed in Chapter 8. The characteristics of the headache determine the diagnosis of the specific headache disorder. Core steps of management are summarised in Table 20.2. Some of the red flags suggesting a secondary subtype are listed in Tables 9.1 and 9.2.

Investigations
Most children with chronic daily headache have a primary subtype, and will not need specific investigation (Seshia et al 2010a). Investigations are determined by the diagnoses under consideration. For a suspected intracranial cause, MRI of the head including magnetic resonance angiography and venography is the preferred choice, as it does not have the radiation exposure associated with computed tomography and provides a broader range of information; the cervical spine must always be included to identify a Chiari type 1 malformation (Seshia et al 2010a). Continuous cerebrospinal fluid pressure monitoring may be more useful than an isolated measurement if idiopathic intracranial hypertension without papilloedema is suspected (Torbey et al 2004), an investigation that may need to be done after discussion with a paediatric neurosurgeon. The investigations for intracranial hypotension secondary to cerebrospinal fluid leak have been discussed recently – space does not permit further detailing (Harder et al 2012). Sleep studies may need to be done if an associated sleep disorder is suspected.

Management
The multifaceted nature of primary chronic daily headache requires a biopsychosocial and often multidisciplinary approach, drug treatment being only one element (Mack 2010, Seshia et al 2010a, Seshia 2012). Treatment is based on 'expert consensus' (Mack 2010, Seshia et al 2010a, Seshia 2012), extrapolation from adult studies (like much of paediatric practice) and

TABLE 20.2

Steps in management

Core steps

Approach is biopsychosocial

Take history and make an initial (probable) diagnosis

Consider and exclude secondary causes through history and examination (red flags) – always reconsider the diagnosis if chronic daily headache does not improve or red flag symptoms and signs appear

Discuss concept of chronic daily headache (associated conditions, triggers and factors that maintain it) and principles of approach. Written information is essential

Emphasise the importance of prospective headache diaries and identifying triggers, etc.

Warn against medication overuse

Discuss lifestyle issues such as diet, sleep habits, caffeine intake, etc.

Advise the use of ear plugs if noise is a factor

Discuss the use of tinted glasses if bright light is a trigger (no evidence of effectiveness)

Encourage participation in normal routines, but avoid fatigue

Re-assess after a mutually agreed period; make an earlier appointment if there are concerns

Are core steps ineffective?

Reconsider diagnosis? Is a secondary cause being missed?

Explore stressors (including maltreatment) if not being volunteered

Enquire about anxiety, depression and other psychiatric disorders

Discuss a multidisciplinary approach, both psychological and pharmacological

Consider in-patient evaluation

---

pharmacological mechanisms of action. There have not been any randomised, controlled trials. It is also worth emphasising that drugs are often used off-label, dosing is subjective and pharmacogenetic variations have not been studied. Effectiveness is difficult to judge because of the high placebo response rate in children (Lewis et al 2005).

Before embarking on any management, it is worth remembering that chronic daily headache was shown to resolve within 2 years without specific treatment in 72% of 122 children in a community-based study (Wang et al 2007); similar resolution occurred in about 30% to 50% of patients in two clinic-based studies (Seshia 2004, Seshia et al 2008). Thus, in a substantial number of patients, the core steps outlined in Table 20.2 often suffice.

PSYCHOLOGICAL TREATMENT

Many principles used in psychological management can be readily integrated into physicians' practices. It is unclear if chronic daily headache was included in the one Cochrane review on the subject, and the evidence behind the benefit of psychological treatment in chronic daily headache needs critical review (Eccleston et al 2009). Limitations of studies notwithstanding, psychological treatment should be offered as an option or complementary to drug treatment. Psychological therapies become essential in the presence of significant psychosocial stressors, medication overuse, psychiatric disorders, lack of benefit or side effects from drug treatment or when the patient is considered to be at risk for chronicity or relapse. Readers are directed to Chapters 26 and 27 and a recent paper by Sieberg et al (2012) which provide a full review of the subject.

PHARMACOLOGICAL TREATMENT

Pharmacological treatment (Table 20.3) on an outpatient basis should be offered when core measures are ineffective, pain is severe and quality of life is impaired. The choice of drug

TABLE 20.3

Drugs used in the treatment of chronic daily headache in children and adolescents

Drug	Doses (initial)	Remarks
Oral (maintenance)		
Amitriptyline	0.25mg/kg/HS	Doses exceeding 0.5mg/kg/day often associated with troublesome side effects, rarely used
Coenzyme Q10	1–3mg/kg/day	May consider for chronic migraine
Gabapentin	10mg/kg/day	May be increased to 50mg/kg/day; give in three or four divided doses
Riboflavin	Not well established	No data for efficacy or effectiveness
Topiramate	0.25mg/kg/day	Up to 1mg/kg/day; give in two divided doses
Valproic acid	Not well established	Restrict use to males
Intravenous (typically as single dose or a 'course')		
DHE	0.1–0.15mg/dose	Age 6–9y
	0.2mg/dose	Age 9–12y
	0.25mg/dose	Age 12–16y
	0.5mg/dose	Maximum for those ≥70kg. DHE is given as a single dose or as a course every 6h – if tolerated; for a maximum of 48h if no improvement; if headache resolves partially or completely, continue for a further 24h, if tolerated. Metoclopramide is given orally or i.v., 30min before (each) DHE dose
Metoclopramide	0.1–0.2mg/kg	See above; maximum dose 10mg as single dose and 5mg or less as maintenance; dyskinesia can occur at low doses

The doses are from personal practice and expert opinions in cited studies. Readers should consult their local and national formularies and be familiar with the side effects. DHE and metoclopramide doses are slightly modified from Linder (1994) and Seshia (2012). Reproduced with kind permission from Springer Science+Business Media B.V. The evidence for use is based on expert opinion, observational studies, information from adult studies, information on use in intermittent headache (migraine and tension type) and pharmacological mechanisms of action (on pain and headache). To our knowledge, there are no randomised controlled or pragmatic trials on the use of any of the agents in chronic daily headache in children and adolescents (adolescents may have been included in some adult trials, but we are unaware of subgroup analysis by age group). DHE, Dihydroergotamine; HS, at bed time.

is influenced by chronic daily headache subtype, psychiatric comorbidity and associated systemic conditions such as obesity. Once chronic daily headache is established, analgesics are ineffective and should be avoided or withdrawn; also, caffeine, barbiturates and narcotics should not be used (Mack 2008); triptans are also ineffective once chronic daily headache is established. Experimental data strongly suggest that continuing such treatment for chronic daily headache contributes to chronification (Bongsebandhu-phubhakdi and Srikiatkhachorn 2012).

In exceptional situations when the pain is severe and immediate relief of pain is necessary, a single (age- and weight-appropriate) dose of DHE and metoclopramide given intravenously can reduce or abolish the pain of the main subtypes of primary chronic daily headache (this treatment is available only in some countries). DHE, dexamethasone and hydroxyzine, given intravenously once a week for 3 weeks, abolished chronic migraine in seven adolescents (Charles and Jotkowitz 2005). A biopsychosocial approach to management should also be taken in these patients to prevent relapse.

There is a limited role for maintenance treatment with cyproheptadine, flunarizine, pizotifen and propranolol in chronic migraine (personal opinion). Most migraineurs would have tried these drugs earlier. Riboflavin and coenzyme Q10, singly or in combination, may be offered because they are innocuous. The side effects of valproic acid in females limit its use to males.

The most commonly used maintenance drugs for the treatment of primary chronic daily headache (including in those suspected of having chronic trigeminal autonomic cephalalgias or hemicranias unresponsive to more specific treatment) are amitriptyline, gabapentin and topiramate (Mack 2010, Seshia et al 2010a, Seshia 2012). Usage is also based on their beneficial effects on pain (Ashina et al 2005, Colombo et al 2008); relatively low doses are often effective. Increments in dose are generally carried out every week to 3 weeks to minimise side effects, headache charting being essential. The ultimate maintenance dose is the minimum at which maximum benefit is achieved without side effects. Maximum benefit may not be apparent for 1 to 3 months. If successful, treatment is continued for a headache-free period of 3 to 6 months before gradual discontinuation, one of several practices for which there is no high-level evidence.

Amitriptyline is the first choice unless the patient is obese, especially when sleep is disturbed. Once-a-day dosing enhances adherence. Doses exceeding 0.5mg/kg are often accompanied by daytime drowsiness and tiredness; if doses higher than 1mg/kg/day are used, blood levels and electrocardiograms have to be monitored (Mack 2010).

Topiramate is the choice when patients are obese. Gabapentin has to be given three or four times a day, compromising adherence. When pain is severe, as for example with new-onset chronic daily headache secondary to concussion, gabapentin is favoured by the authors, as the dose can be escalated more rapidly than is the case with amitriptyline or topiramate. The authors have used a combination of gabapentin and amitriptyline or topiramate in a few cases with benefit, but placebo effect cannot be excluded. Botulinum toxin type A may also be offered to those who have failed to respond to or experienced side effects with oral medicines (see Chapter 13), another practice based on observational studies (Ahmed et al 2010, Kabbouche et al 2012).

The decision to use selective serotonin reuptake inhibitors should be made by a psychiatrist because of the increased risk of suicidal thinking and behaviour with these drugs. Fluoxetine was not superior to placebo in one small trial (Gherpelli and Esposito 2005).

A trial of indometacin should be considered if headache is primary and unilateral (Mack and Gladstein 2008). However, chronic hemiparoxysmal-like headaches may resolve without specific treatment (Klassen and Dooley 2000).

OTHER TREATMENTS

The role of acupuncture is uncertain; laser acupuncture may be effective in children with headache (Gottschling et al 2008), but data for chronic daily headache are lacking. An observational study on homeopathic treatment showed improvement over two years (Witt et al 2010), but the strength of evidence for the benefits of the drugs we offer is no better.

IN-PATIENT MANAGEMENT

In-patient evaluation is considered after informed discussion with the family for (1) children disabled by chronic daily headache (unable to attend school or participate in their usual extra-curricular activities), (2) those in whom there is a dissociation between their affect and described pain severity or disability, (3) those with clinically significant features of a psychiatric disorder, and (4) those with or suspected of having adverse social factors or significant stressors, particularly maltreatment. The last two are important, but potentially under-recognised, contributors to severe 'intractable' chronic daily headache.

In hospital, the severity of pain and the impact on functioning can be objectively recorded, as can interactions with the family. Children are often more forthcoming with information when guardians are not around (see history taking, Chapter 8). The child participates in the hospital school and child life recreational programmes, and the observations of these professionals are also recorded. Psychiatrists and psychologists can be involved in a more time-effective manner than on an outpatient basis. The appropriate professionals should be consulted if maltreatment is suspected or adverse social factors present.

Secondary causes must be reconsidered and excluded if this has not already been done. In their absence, and with the concurrence of the multidisciplinary team including a psychiatrist and psychologist, in North America, a course of intravenous DHE and metoclopramide (Table 20.3) is often discussed and suggested, a practice that is based on observational studies in children (Linder 1994) and adults. Maintenance treatment that has been ineffective is gradually stopped, and psychological therapies recommended if they are not already in place. If maintenance treatment has not been tried, then either amitriptyline or topiramate, as appropriate, is started and continued along with psychological treatment. A family-centred meeting is held prior to discharge between child, family, school teacher and representatives of healthcare professionals involved in management. The objective is to exchange information, discuss the factors that may have contributed to the chronic daily headache, develop a care plan including resumption of normal routine and address expectations and questions. Strategies to minimise risk of relapse are emphasised. Our goal should be a headache-free state. Patients are usually discharged between 5 and 7 days after admission.

Prognosis

Despite good short-term outcomes, there is compelling information to suggest that chronic daily headache is often not a self-limiting disorder. In a community-based study from Taiwan, of 103 adolescents followed up for 8 years, only 11% were headache free; 11% still had chronic daily headache and 27% continued to have moderate or severe headache (Wang et al 2009). Relapses occurred within 3 years in 10% of 48 individuals in whom chronic daily headache had resolved or was no longer a management problem (Seshia et al 2008). Furthermore, many adults with chronic daily headache recall onset in childhood (Solomon et al 1992, Srikiatkhachorn and Phanthumchinda 1997). The risks of relapse and persistence are higher in females, migraineurs, those with chronic daily headache onset of less than 13 years or chronic daily headache duration of 2 years or more, individuals who abuse medication or have psychiatric disorders, those who are maltreated and possibly those with adverse social factors. These children should be followed up into adult life, ideally in a multidisciplinary manner.

Conclusions

Chronic daily headache is probably the most common chronic pain syndrome in childhood. Most transform from an episodic primary headache. The majority have characteristics of tension-type headache with minimal features of migraine without aura. Stressors are often responsible for transformation and chronicity. Chronic daily headache is often comorbid with psychiatric disorders, especially anxiety and depressive disorders, and may be associated with sleep disorders and other pain syndromes. Management should be biopsychosocial and multidisciplinary.

Chronic daily headache may persist into adult life; hence there has to be a structured transition of care from paediatric to adult. The long-term natural history requires urgent clarification.

Notes

Readers should refer to paediatric drug dosage books specific for their region of practice for doses suitable for their population, and for details on side effects. Any dosages suggested in this chapter are based on our personal practice.

REFERENCES

Abu-Arafeh I (2001) Chronic tension-type headache in children and adolescents. *Cephalalgia* 21: 830–6. http://dx.doi.org/10.1046/j.0333-1024.2001.00275.x

Abu-Arafeh I, Russell G (1994) Prevalence of headache and migraine in schoolchildren. *BMJ* 309: 765–9. http://dx.doi.org/10.1136/bmj.309.6957.765

Ahmed K, Oas KH, Mack KJ, Garza I (2010) Experience with botulinum toxin type A in medically intractable pediatric chronic daily headache. *Pediatr Neurol* 43: 316–19. http://dx.doi.org/10.1016/j.pediatrneurol.2010.06.001

Arruda MA, Guidetti V, Galli F, Albuquerque RC, Bigal ME (2010a) Frequent headaches in the preadolescent pediatric population: a population-based study. *Neurology* 74: 903–8. http://dx.doi.org/10.1212/WNL.0b013e3181d561a2

Arruda MA, Guidetti V, Galli F, Albuquerque RC, Bigal ME (2010b) Primary headaches in childhood – a population-based study. *Cephalalgia* 30: 1056–64. http://dx.doi.org/10.1177/0333102409361214

Arruda MA, Guidetti V, Galli F, Albuquerque RC, Bigal ME (2010c) Frequency of headaches in children is influenced by headache status in the mother. *Headache* 50: 973–80. http://dx.doi.org/10.1111/j.1526-4610.2010.01677.x

Ashina S, Bendtesn L, Ashina M (2005) Pathophysiology of tension-type headache. *Curr Pain Headache Rep* 9: 415–22. http://dx.doi.org/10.1007/s11916-005-0021-8

Beri S, Gosalakkal JA, Hussain N, Balky AP, Parepalli S (2010) Idiopathic intracranial hypertension without papilledema. *Pediatr Neurol* 42: 56–8. http://dx.doi.org/10.1016/j.pediatrneurol.2009.07.021

Bigal ME, Sheftell FD, Tepper SJ, Rapoport AM, Llipton RB (2005) Migraine days decline with duration of illness in adolescents with transformed migraine. *Cephalalgia* 25: 482–7. http://dx.doi.org/10.1111/j.1468-2982.2005.00887.x

Bongsebandhu-phubhakdi S, Srikiatkhacorn A. (2012). Pathophysiology of medication-overuse headache: implications from animal studies. *Curr Pain Headache Rep* 16: 110–15. http://dx.doi.org/10.1007/s11916-011-0234-y

Cevoli S, Sancisi E, Grimaldi D et al (2009) Family history for chronic headache and drug overuse as a risk factor for headache chronification. *Headache* 49: 412–18. http://dx.doi.org/10.1111/j.1526-4610.2008.01257.x

Charles JA, Jotkowitz S (2005) Observations of the 'carry-over effect' following successful termination of chronic migraine in the adolescent with short-term dihydroergotamine, dexamethasone and hydroxyzine: a pilot study. *J Headache Pain* 6: 51–4. http://dx.doi.org/10.1007/s10194-005-0148-3

Colombo B, Dalla Libera D, Annovazzi PO, Comi G (2008) Headache therapy with neuronal stabilising drugs. *Neurol Sci* 29(Suppl 1): S131–6. http://dx.doi.org/10.1007/s10072-008-0904-7

Eccleston C, Palermo TM, Williams AC, Lewandowski A, Morley S (2009) Psychological therapies for the management of chronic and recurrent pain in children and adolescents. *Cochrane Database Syst Rev* 15: CD003968.

Fujita M, Fujiwara J, Maki T, Shibasaki K, Shigeta M, Nii J (2009) Pediatric chronic daily headache associated with school phobia. *Pediatr Int* 51: 621–5. http://dx.doi.org/10.1111/j.1442-200X.2009.02804.x

Gherpelli JL, Esposito SB (2005) A prospective randomized double blind placebo controlled crossover study of fluoxetine efficacy in the prophylaxis of chronic daily headache in children and adolescents. *Arq Neuropsiquiatr* 63: 559–63. http://dx.doi.org/10.1590/S0004-282X2005000400001

Gottschling S, Meyer S, Gribova I et al (2008) Laser acupuncture in children with headache: a double-blind, randomized, bicenter, placebo-controlled trial. *Pain* 137: 405–12. http://dx.doi.org/10.1016/j.pain.2007.10.004

Harder S, Griebel RW, Lemire EG, Kriegler S, Gitlin J, Seshia SS (2012) Spinal CSF leaks: mimicker of primary headache disorder in a child. *Can J Neurol Sci* 39: 388–92.

Headache Classification Committee, Olesen J, Bousser MG et al (2006) New appendix criteria open for a broader concept of chronic migraine. *Cephalalgia* 26: 742–6. http://dx.doi.org/10.1111/j.1468-2982.2006.01172.x

Headache Classification Subcommittee of the International Headache Society (2004) The international classification of headache disorders: 2nd edition. *Cephalalgia* 24(Suppl 1): 9–160.

Hershey AD, Powers SW, Bentti AL, LeCates S, deGrauw TJ (2001) Characterization of chronic daily headaches in children in a multidisciplinary headache center. *Neurology* 56: 1032–7. http://dx.doi.org/10.1212/WNL.56.8.1032

Hershey AD, Burdine D, Kabbouche MA, Power SW (2010) Genomic expression patterns in medication overuse headaches. *Cephalalgia* 31: 161–71. http://dx.doi.org/10.1177/0333102410373155

Holden EW, Gladstein J, Trulsen M, Wall B (1994) Chronic daily headache in children and adolescents. *Headache* 34: 508–14. http://dx.doi.org/10.1111/j.1526-4610.1994.hed3409508.x

Ji T, Mack KJ (2009) Unilateral chronic daily headache in children. *Headache* 49: 1062–5. http://dx.doi.org/10.1111/j.1526-4610.2009.01455.x

Juang KD, Wang SJ, Fuh JL, Lu SR, Chen YS (2004) Association between adolescent chronic daily headache and childhood adversity: a community-based study. *Cephalalgia* 24: 54–9. http://dx.doi.org/10.1111/j.1468-2982.2004.00643.x

Kabbouche M, O'Brien H, Hershey AD (2012) OnabotulinumtoxinA in pediatric chronic daily headache. *Curr Neurol Neurosci Rep* 12: 114–17. http://dx.doi.org/10.1007/s11910-012-0251-1

Kirk C, Nagiub G, Abu-Arafeh I (2008) Chronic post-traumatic headache after head injury in children and adolescents. *Dev Med Child Neurol* 50: 422–5. http://dx.doi.org/10.1111/j.1469-8749.2008.02063.x

Klassen BD, Dooley JM (2000) Chronic paroxysmal hemicrania-like headaches in a child: response to a headache diary, *Headache* 40: 853–5. http://dx.doi.org/10.1046/j.1526-4610.2000.00155.x

Knook LM, Konijnenberg AY, van Der Hoeven J et al (2011) Psychiatric disorders in children and adolescents presenting with unexplained chronic pain: what is the prevalence and clinical relevancy? *Eur Child Adolesc Psychiatry* 20: 39–48. http://dx.doi.org/10.1007/s00787-010-0146-0

Laurell K, Larsson B, Eeg-Olofsson O (2004) Prevalence of headache in Swedish schoolchildren, with a focus on tension-type headache. *Cephalalgia*, 24: 380–8. http://dx.doi.org/10.1111/j.1468-2982.2004.00681.x

Lewis DW, Winner P, Wasiewski W (2005) The placebo responder rate in children and adolescents. *Headache* 45: 232–9. http://dx.doi.org/10.1111/j.1526-4610.2005.05050.x

Linder SL (1994) Treatment of childhood headache with dihydroergotamine mesylate. *Headache* 34: 578–80. http://dx.doi.org/10.1111/j.1526-4610.1994.hed3410578.x

Lipton RB, Manack A, Ricci JA, Chee E, Turkel CC, Winner P (2011) Prevalence and burden of chronic migraine in adolescents: results of the chronic daily headache in adolescents study (CdAS). *Headache* 51: 693–706. http://dx.doi.org/10.1111/j.1526-4610.2011.01885.x

Mack KJ (2010) Management of chronic daily headache in children. *Expert Review Neurother* 10: 1479–86. http://dx.doi.org/10.1586/ern.10.124

Mack KJ, Gladstein J (2008) Management of chronic daily headache in children and adolescents. *Paediatr Drugs* 10: 23–9. http://dx.doi.org/10.2165/00148581-200810010-00003

Marmura MJ, Silberstein SD, Gupta M (2009) Hemicrania continua: who responds to indomethacin? *Cephalalgia* 29: 300–7. http://dx.doi.org/10.1111/j.1468-2982.2008.01719.x

Mathew NT, Stubits E, Nigam MP (1982) Transformation of episodic migraine into daily headache: analysis of factors. *Headache* 22: 66–8. http://dx.doi.org/10.1111/j.1526-4610.1982.hed2202066.x

Mathew NT, Reuveni U, Perez F (1987) Transformed or evolutive migraine. *Headache* 27: 102–6. http://dx.doi.org/10.1111/j.1526-4610.1987.hed2702102.x

Meng ID, Cao L (2007) From migraine to chronic daily headache: the biological basis of headache transformation. *Headache* 47: 1251–8. http://dx.doi.org/10.1111/j.1526-4610.2007.00907.x

Montagna P, Cevoli S, Marzocchi N et al (2003) The genetics of chronic headaches. *Neurol Sci* 24(Suppl 2): S51–6.

Pakalnis A, Butz C, Splaingard D, Kring D, Fong J (2007) Emotional problems and prevalence of medication overuse in pediatric chronic daily headache. *J Child Neurol* 22: 1356–9. http://dx.doi.org/10.1177/0883073807307090

Pakalnis A, Kring D (2012) Chronic daily headache, medication overuse, and obesity in children and adolescents. *J Child Neurol* 27: 577–80. http://dx.doi.org/10.1177/0883073811420869

Peterlin BL, Ward T, Lidicker J, Levin M (2007) A retrospective, comparative study on the frequency of abuse in migraine and chronic daily headache. *Headache* 47: 397–401.

Radat F, Creac'h C, Guegan-Massardier E et al (2008) Behavioral dependence in patients with medication overuse headache: a cross-sectional study in consulting patients using the DSM-IV criteria. *Headache* 48: 1026–36. http://dx.doi.org/10.1111/j.1526-4610.2007.00999.x

Rome HP Jr, Rome JD (2000) Limbically augmented pain syndrome (LAPS): kindling, corticolimbic sensitization, and the convergence of affective and sensory symptoms in chronic pain disorders. *Pain Med* 1: 7–23. http://dx.doi.org/10.1046/j.1526-4637.2000.99105.x

Seshia SS (1996) Specificity of IHS criteria in childhood headache. *Headache* 36: 295–9. http://dx.doi.org/10.1046/j.1526-4610.1996.3605295.x

Seshia SS (2004) Chronic daily headache in children and adolescents. *Can J Neurol Sci* 31: 319–23.

Seshia SS (2012) Chronic daily headache in children and adolescents. *Curr Pain Headache Rep* 16: 60–72. http://dx.doi.org/10.1007/s11916-011-0228-9

Seshia SS, Phillips DF, von Baeyer CL (2008) Childhood chronic daily headache: a biopsychosocial perspective. *Dev Med Child Neurol* 50: 541–5. http://dx.doi.org/10.1111/j.1469-8749.2008.03013.x

Seshia SS, Abu-Arafeh I, Hershey AD (2009) Tension-type headache in children: the Cinderella of headache disorders! *Can J Neurol Sci* 36: 687–95.

Seshia SS, Wang SJ, Abu-Arafeh I et al (2010a) Chronic daily headache in children and adolescents: a multi-faceted syndrome. *Can J Neurol Sci* 37: 769–78.

Seshia SS, Wober-Bingol C, Guidetti V (2010b) The classification of chronic headache: room for further improvement? *Cephalalgia* 30: 1268–70. http://dx.doi.org/10.1177/0333102410374143

Silberstein SD, Lipton RB, Solomon S, Mathew NT (1994) Classification of daily and near-daily headaches: proposed revisions to the IHS criteria. *Headache* 34: 1–7. http://dx.doi.org/10.1111/j.1526-4610.1994.hed3401001.x

da Silva A Jr, Costa EC, Gomes JB et al (2010) Chronic headache and comorbities: a two-phase, population-based, cross-sectional study. *Headache* 50: 1306–12. http://dx.doi.org/10.1111/j.1526-4610.2010.01620.x

Sieberg CB, Huguet A, von Baeyer CL, Seshia SS (2012) Psychological interventions for headache in children and adolescents. *Can J Neurol Sci.* 39: 26–34.

Slater SK, Kashikar-Zuck SM, Allen JR et al (2012) Psychiatric co-morbidity in pediatric chronic daily headache. *Cephalalgia* 32: 1116–22. http://dx.doi.org/10.1177/0333102412460776

Solomon S (2007) New appendix criteria open for a broader concept of chronic migraine. *Cephalalgia* 27: 469; author reply 469–70 http://dx.doi.org/10.1111/j.1468-2982.2007.01292_1.x

Solomon S, Lipton RB, Newman LC (1992) Clinical features of chronic daily headache. *Headache* 32: 325–9. http://dx.doi.org/10.1111/j.1526-4610.1992.hed3207325.x

Sourander A, Brunstein Klomek A, Ikonen M et al (2010) Psychosocial risk factors associated with cyber-bullying among adolescents: a population-based study. *Arch Gen Psychiatry* 67: 720–8. http://dx.doi.org/10.1001/archgenpsychiatry.2010.79

Srikiatkhachorn A (2006) Towards the better understanding about pathogenesis of chronic daily headache. *J Med Assoc Thai* 89(Suppl 3): S234–43.

Srikiatkhachorn A, Phanthumchinda K (1997) Prevalence and clinical features of chronic daily headache in a headache clinic. *Headache* 37: 277–80. http://dx.doi.org/10.1046/j.1526-4610.1997.3705277.x

Stovner L, Hagen K, Jensen R et al (2007) The global burden of headache: a documentation of headache prevalence and disability worldwide. *Cephalalgia* 27: 193–210. http://dx.doi.org/10.1111/j.1468-2982.2007.01288.x

Talvik I, Peet A, Talvik T (2009) Three-year follow-up of a girl with chronic paroxysmal hemicrania. *Pediatr Neurol* 40: 68–9. http://dx.doi.org/10.1016/j.pediatrneurol.2008.10.002

Tarantino S, Vollono C, Capuano A, Vigevano F, Valeriani M (2011) Chronic paroxysmal hemicrania in paediatric age: report of two cases. *J Headache Pain* 12: 263–7. http://dx.doi.org/10.1007/s10194-011-0315-7

Torbey MT, Geocadin RG, Razumovsky AY, Rigamonti D, Williams MA (2004) Utility of CSF pressure monitoring to identify idiopathic intracranial hypertension without papilledema in patients with chronic daily headache. *Cephalalgia* 24: 495–502. http://dx.doi.org/10.1111/j.1468-2982.2004.00688.x

Wang SJ, Silberstein SD, Patterson S, Young WB (1998) Idiopathic intracranial hypertension without papilledema: a case–control study in a headache center. *Neurology* 51: 245–9. http://dx.doi.org/10.1212/WNL.51.1.245

Wang SJ, Fuh JL, Lu SR, Juang KD (2006) Chronic daily headache in adolescents: prevalence, impact, and medication overuse. *Neurology* 66: 193–7. http://dx.doi.org/10.1212/01.wnl.0000183555.54305.fd

Wang SJ, Fuh JL, Lu SR, Juang KD.(2007a) Outcomes and predictors of chronic daily headache in adolescents: a 2-year longitudinal study. *Neurology* 68: 591–6. http://dx.doi.org/10.1212/01.wnl.0000252800.82704.62

Wang SJ, Juang KD, Fuh JL, Lu SR (2007b) Psychiatric comorbidity and suicide risk in adolescents with chronic daily headache. *Neurology* 68: 1468–73. http://dx.doi.org/10.1212/01.wnl.0000260607.90634.d6

Wang SJ, Fuh JL, Lu SR (2009) Chronic daily headache in adolescents: an 8-year follow-up study. *Neurology* 73: 416–22. http://dx.doi.org/10.1212/WNL.0b013e3181ae2377

Welch KM, Goadsby PJ (2002) Chronic daily headache: nosology and pathophysiology. *Curr Opin Neurol* 15: 287–95. http://dx.doi.org/10.1097/00019052-200206000-00011

Witt CM, Ludtke R, Willich SN (2010) Homeopathic treatment of patients with migraine: a prospective observational study with a 2-year follow-up period. *J Altern Complement Med* 16: 347–55. http://dx.doi.org/10.1089/acm.2009.0376

Zafar M, Kashikar-Zuck SM, Slater Sk et al (2012) Childhood abuse in pediatric patients with chronic daily headache. *Clin Pediatr (Phila)* 51: 590–3. http://dx.doi.org/10.1177/0009922811407181

Zhang LM, Zhou SZ, Chai YM, Yang JD, Xue J, Liang J (2007) Prevalence of chronic headache in Shanghai children and adolescents: a questionnaire-based study. *Zhonghua Er Ke Za Zhi* 45: 262–6.

21
NEW DAILY PERSISTENT HEADACHE IN CHILDREN

Kenneth J Mack

New daily persistent headache (NDPH) is frequently seen in young patients with chronic daily headache. NDPH begins with a sudden onset, often associated with an infection or other physical stress. This headache syndrome is difficult to treat, and may persist for years. This chapter discusses the epidemiology, comorbid symptoms, evaluation and treatment of this disorder.

New daily persistent headache is a unique form of chronic daily headache

NDPH was first described in 1986 (Silberstein et al 1994). According to the criteria of the International Headache Society, the defining characteristic of an NDPH is a daily, unremitting headache beginning very soon after the onset of the headache (within 3 days at most). The pain is typically bilateral, pressing or tightening, and of mild to moderate intensity. This condition occurs in patients with no significant prior headache history. Patients with NDPH may describe their headaches as having either migrainous or tension-type features (ICHS 2003, Robbins et al 2010, Peng et al 2011).

New daily persistent headache occurs more frequently in young patients

NDPH is a more frequent diagnosis in children than in adults. In studies looking primarily at adult patients, the frequency of NDPH has been estimated to be 1.7% to 10.8% of patients with chronic daily headache (Bigal et al 2004). In contrast, studies in children have found NDPH to occur more frequently, with a frequency of 13% to 35% (Mack 2004).

From a patient's perspective, the abrupt onset is quite remarkable. In the author's experience, most patients will remember the day (and sometimes the specific hour) in which the headaches began. With such a dramatic onset to the headaches, it is difficult for both the patient and the practitioner to accept that there is frequently no definable abnormality on either neuroimaging studies or other laboratory testing to explain the headaches.

How are new daily persistent headaches triggered?

The pathophysiology of NDPH is unknown. Li and Rozen (2002) identified viral infections, extracranial surgery and stressful life events as triggers for the new-onset headache, primarily in adult patients. However, in up to 40% of their patients there was no known trigger. In addition to the risk factors mentioned above, the transformation of an episodic headache into a chronic headache (or the onset of NDPH) has also been associated with hypothyroidism, hypertension, consumption of alcohol more than three times per week, analgesic overuse, daily consumption of caffeine, multiple types of infections, surgery and stressful life events (Stewart et al 2001, Bigal et al 2002, Mack 2004).

Infections are the factor most frequently associated with NDPH. Diaz-Mitoma et al (1987) noted that 84% of patients with NDPH had evidence of 'active' Epstein–Barr virus infection. However, other infections can provoke an NDPH as well, and 43% of the patients in the childhood NDPH study reported some type of infection at the onset of symptoms (Mack 2004). Taken together, these data suggest that NDPH is not the result of a specific infectious agent but may reflect a non-specific response to infection or physical stress.

Rozen and Swidan (2007) have found that NDPH patients, as well as those with chronic migraine, have elevated levels of tumour necrosis factor alpha (TNF-α) in their cerebrospinal fluid. TNF-α is a proinflammatory cytokine, potentially involved in both inflammation and pain. The presence or absence of a precipitating infection, however, did not affect the TNF-α levels. This is a fascinating finding, but the significance of it remains to be determined.

The same phenomenon of an abrupt onset of a chronic daily headache may also occur in patients with episodic migraine. The author found that 30% of chronic migraine patients reported an abrupt onset of their chronic migraine, reminiscent of an NDPH. These patients would often show similar inciting factors, such as infection, to patients with NDPH.

The exact pathophysiology of how these events result in an NDPH is unknown. The temporal relationship of a seroconversion on viral titres, or head trauma with the onset of headache, is often impressive and striking, but certainly that close temporal relationship does not prove causation. Indeed, these factors may not 'cause' the headache, but rather they may aggravate an underlying predisposition to headaches. The author speculates that these physiological stressors result in the initiation of the headache in a predisposed individual. Unanswered questions include why is there such a persistence of the headache, even after the inciting factor has resolved? And why do only certain individuals develop NDPH? These phenomena may relate to as yet unidentified host factors.

What could be the potential host factors? Rozen et al (2006) reported that cervical joint hypermobility may be a predisposing factor for NDPH. Similar observations have been hypothesised in other childhood pain syndromes. In the author's anecdotal experience, patients with NDPH seem to frequently have a family history of migraine. It is possible that we are dealing with a combination of host factors related to the immune system, connective tissue structure and the familial nature of migraine.

Headache symptoms in new daily persistent headache

Li and Rozen (2002) reported that most (79%) patients had a continuous headache, often with symptoms of nausea (68%), photophobia (66%) and phonophobia (61%). Lightheadedness was also seen in 55% of patients. This was a female-predominant disorder. Gladstein and Holden (1996) reported that many of the children that they diagnosed with NDPH had a pattern of severe intermittent migraines with an underlying continuous tension-type headache. Migrainous features of this disorder have also been commonly found in recent studies of adult patients (Robbins et al 2010, Peng et al 2011).

Comorbid symptoms in new daily persistent headache

Mack and Terrell (2003) have found that the frequency of comorbid symptoms is similar in paediatric patients with NDPH and paediatric patients with chronic or transformed migraine. Sleep is disrupted in at least two-thirds of the patients who have NDPH. A common sleep disturbance is a delayed onset of sleep, and oftentimes these individuals will not be able to fall asleep for several hours after they have gone to bed. In these patients, it is unclear whether the poor sleep is causing chronic headaches, or whether the headaches are not allowing the patients to get good sleep. It is the opinion of the author that, at the start of the chronic daily headache cycle, the poor sleep is often due to the severe headache pain.

However, as the chronic daily headaches persist, usually the sleep problem becomes multifactorial and may include pain issues, poor sleep hygiene and a natural tendency for adolescents to want to be 'night owls'. Improvement in sleep is seen after better headache control, improved sleep hygiene and avoidance of caffeine. The use of some preventatives, such as amitriptyline, may help sleep. Melatonin, given prior to sleep, can also be helpful.

Many chronic daily headache patients have symptoms of dizziness. Often the dizziness occurs during times when the headaches are more severe. The dizziness is associated with feeling weak and unsteady, and with changes (blurring or loss of) in vision. When the dizziness is primarily related to the severe headache, then improvement will occur once the headache control is improved.

At times, however, patients may notice dizziness between the episodes of severe headaches. This dizziness is often positional, and patients will complain of syncope or near-syncope after standing. The dizziness is particularly prominent in the morning after they first get up. The patient often experiences mild symptoms of this dizziness if asked to stand for several minutes in the office. One may see either a significant tachycardia with standing (postural orthostatic tachycardia syndrome; POTS) and/or a decrease in the blood pressure. A tilt-table test will help confirm these findings. Some patients will have developed the sudden onset of both POTS and a chronic (NDPH) headache at the same time. In children, these orthostatic symptoms can be treated by increasing the child's fluid and salt intake, or, when necessary, with the use of beta blockers (such as metoprolol) when there is a significant orthostatic tachycardia, and/or pressors (such as midodrine) when there is an orthostatic drop in blood pressure (Mack et al 2010).

How should patients with new daily persistent headache be evaluated?

The evaluation of a patient with NDPH should include a thorough history and physical examination, as well as consideration of a neuroimaging study and, in the occasional patient, a lumbar puncture. In selected patients, tilt-table testing or sleep studies may also be of value.

In children, the most useful role of the neuroimaging study in chronic daily headache is to reassure the patient and family. An imaging study is most likely to be significantly abnormal if there are focal deficits on examination, or if there is a history of seizures in the patient (Lewis et al 2002). Occasionally, white matter abnormalities, arachnoid cysts or pineal cysts will be seen that are generally believed to be of no clinical significance to the chronic daily headache (Schwedt et al 2006). If a patient has had a significant history of head or neck trauma, particularly at the onset of the chronic daily headache, then magnetic resonance angiography of the neck should also be considered to rule out a possible carotid dissection. When pseudo-tumour cerebri is a strong consideration, then magnetic resonance venography should also be considered as sinus thrombosis can cause elevated intracranial pressure.

As many patients will transition from a headache-free period or from episodic migraines to chronic migraines during an infection, physicians should consider testing for infection as indicated by the clinical features of the presenting illness and the infections prevalent in the local community at the time. Although for some of the viral aetiologies there are no specific treatments, many patients and their families appreciate knowing there was a physiological underpinning for the transition to a chronic headache.

Practical implications for therapy

Expert opinion suggests that NDPH is a very treatment-refractory headache disorder (Meineri et al 2004, Takase et al 2004, Rozen 2011). Comments by the International Headache Society (2003) note that NDPH may take either of two subforms: a self-limiting subform that typically resolves without therapy within several months and a refractory subform that is resistant to aggressive treatment programmes. In the original paper describing NDPH by Vanast (1986), it was noted that 86% of patients were headache free at 24 months.

The author tends to use amitriptyline, propranolol or topiramate as an initial medication in the treatment of chronic daily headache, including NDPH. Amitriptyline is helpful for many of the author's patients with sleep difficulties, and the starting dose is typically 0.5mg/kg/day (25mg in an adolescent), increasing to 1 to 3mg/kg/day (50–150mg/day in a typical adolescent or adult) as a target dose. Nortriptyline seems to be better tolerated by adult patients. Sleep seems to improve first, followed by a reduction in the severe headaches, followed by an improvement in the '24/7' continuous headaches. If that is ineffective or poorly tolerated, then the author tries propranolol at 1mg/kg/day. For adolescents, this comes in a once a day, sustained-released form at 60 or 80mg. In younger children, the author will use atenolol at 25 or 50mg tablet, also given once daily. A typical adult dose will be between 60 and 120mg a day of propranolol. Finally, one can consider topiramate. This could be started at 25mg every evening (0.5mg/kg/day) and titrated weekly upwards by 25mg per week. A typical target dose would be between 50 and 200mg/day topiramate (Mack 2010).

It is important to state the expectations of preventative therapy to the patient and the family. Preventative therapy may improve the headaches, but it will not eliminate the headaches in the short term. After 1 month of an effective therapy, a reasonable expectation would be a reduction in the frequency of severe headache episodes and a decrease in the intensity of the continuous 24/7 headache.

It is rare to see complete resolution of the headaches after a short period of time.

It is usually the 'severe' headaches that keep children out of school, rather than the 24/7 headache. Improvement of the severe headaches usually allows the patient to return to school. In the author's experience, when the continuous 24/7 headache is rated as less than a '5' (on a 10-point scale), the patients are able to become more functional in all of their activities. Once a trend towards improvement is seen, the dose of medication is adjusted for optimal control of the headaches, and the patient is continued on the preventative treatment for at least 6 months of good (but rarely complete) symptom control.

These patients' symptoms are indeed a challenge, and some patients will not respond to medications. In such a situation, one should consider alternative approaches, including the use of biobehavioural strategies, physiotherapy, trigger point injections and botulinum toxin (Mack 2010).

Conclusion

Paediatric patients with no history of headache can abruptly develop a chronic daily headache syndrome. Treating physicians should be aware of the multiple factors that are associated with this transition and offer appropriate counselling and therapies to their patients.

REFERENCES

Bigal ME, Sheftell FD, Rapoport AM, Tepper SJ, Lipton RB (2002) Chronic daily headache: Identification of factors associated with induction and transformation. *Headache* 42: 575–81. http://dx.doi. org/10.1046/j.1526-4610.2002.02143.x

Bigal ME, Lipton RB, Tepper SJ, Rapoport AM, Sheftell, FD (2004) Primary chronic daily headache and its subtypes in adolescents and adults. *Neurology* 63: 843–7. http://dx.doi.org/10.1212/01. WNL.0000137039.08724.18

Diaz-Mitoma F, Vanast WJ, Tyrrell DL (1987) Increased frequency of Epstein–Barr virus excretion in patients with new daily persistent headaches. *Lancet* 21: 411–15. http://dx.doi.org/10.1016/S0140-6736(87)90119-X

Gladstein J, Holden EW (1996) Chronic daily headache in children and adolescents: a 2-year prospective study. *Headache* 36: 349–51. http://dx.doi.org/10.1046/j.1526-4610.1996.3606349.x

Headache Classification Subcommittee of the International Headace Society (2003) The international classification of headache disorders, 2nd ed. *Cephalalgia* 24(Suppl 1): 52–3.

Lewis DW, Ashwal S, Dahl G et al (2002). Practice parameter: evaluation of children and adolescents with recurrent headaches: report of the Quality Standards Subcommittee of the American Academy of Neurology and the Practice Committee of the Child Neurology Society. *Neurology* 59: 490–8. http://dx.doi. org/10.1212/WNL.59.4.490

Li D, Rozen TD (2002) The clinical characteristics of new daily persistent headache. *Cephalalgia* 22: 66–9. http://dx.doi.org/10.1046/j.1468-2982.2002.00326.x

Mack KJ (2004) What incites new daily persitent headache in children? *Pediatr Neurol* 31: 122–5. http://dx.doi. org/10.1016/j.pediatrneurol.2004.02.006

Mack KJ (2010) Management of chronic daily headache in children. *Expert Rev Neurother* 10: 1479–86. http:// dx.doi.org/10.1586/ern.10.124

Mack KJ, Terrell KW (2003) Chronic daily headache of childhood is a complex of multiple symptoms. American Headache Society. *Headache* 43: 572.

Mack KJ, Johnson JN, Rowe PC (2010) Orthostatic intolerance and the headache patient. *Semin Pediatr Neurol* 17: 109–16. http://dx.doi.org/10.1016/j.spen.2010.04.006

Meineri P, Torre E, Rota E, Grasso E (2004) New dialy persistent headache: clinical and serological characteristics in a retrospective study. *Neurol Sci* 25: S281–2. http://dx.doi.org/10.1007/s10072-004-0310-8

Peng KP, Fuh JL, Yuan HK, Shia BC, Wang SJ (2011) New daily persistent headache: should migrainous features be incorporated? *Cephalalgia* 31: 1561–9. http://dx.doi.org/10.1177/0333102411424620

Robbins MS, Grosberg BM, Napchan U, Crystal SC, Lipton RB (2010) Clinical and prognostic subforms of new daily-persistent headache. *Neurology* 74: 1358–64. http://dx.doi.org/10.1212/WNL.0b013e3181dad5de

Rozen TD (2011) New daily persistent headache: clinical perspective. *Headache* 51: 641–9. http://dx.doi. org/10.1111/j.1526-4610.2011.01871.x

Rozen T, Swidan SZ (2007) Elevation of CSF tumor necrosis factor alpha levels in new daily persistent headache and treatment refractory chronic migraine. *Headache* 47: 1050–5. http://dx.doi. org/10.1111/j.1526-4610.2006.00722.x

Rozen TD, Roth JM, Denenberg N (2006) Cervical spine joint hypermobility: a possible predisposing factor for new daily persistent headache. *Cephaligia* 26: 1182–5. http://dx.doi.org/10.1111/j.1468-2982.2006.01187.x

Schwedt TJ, Guo Y, Rothner AD (2006) "Benign" imaging abnormalities in children and adolescents with headache. *Headache* 46: 387–98. http://dx.doi.org/10.1111/j.1526-4610.2006.00371.x

Silberstein SD, Lipton RB, Solomon S, Mathew NT (1994) Classification of daily and near-daily headaches: proposed revisions to HIS criteria. *Headache* 34: 1–7. http://dx.doi.org/10.1111/j.1526-4610.1994.hed3401001.x

Stewart WF, Scher AI, Lipton RB (2001) Stressful life events and risk of chronic daily headache: results from the frequent headache epidemiology study. *Cephalalgia* 21: 278–80.

Takase Y, Nakano M, Tatsumi C, Matsuyama T (2004) Clinical features, effectiveness of drug-based treatment, and prognosis of new daily persistent headache (NDPH): 30 cases in Japan. *Cephalalgia* 24: 955–9. http://dx.doi.org/10.1111/j.1468-2982.2004.00771.x

Vanast WJ (1986) New daily persistent headaches: definition of a benign syndrome. *Headache* 26: 317–20.

22
HEADACHE, BRAIN TUMOURS AND HYDROCEPHALUS

William P Whitehouse

Introduction

One of the creative tensions that arise from effective multidisciplinary working in paediatric neurology is focused on the child who presents with headache and vomiting. To the paediatric neurosurgeon, this is a child with 'a brain tumour until proved otherwise'; to the general practitioner or primary care paediatrician, the child 'probably has migraine'. Paediatric neurologists working in tertiary centres balance these two extremes and the consequences of missed or delayed diagnosis (the beta error) with their experience or knowledge of a wide differential.

In this chapter the roles of history, examination and investigation in identifying children with symptomatic (secondary) headache and brain tumours will be reviewed.

Paediatric brain tumours

Among childhood cancers, the prevalence of brain tumours is second only to that of leukaemias, accounting for 25% of childhood cancers, and having an annual incidence of about 3 per 100 000 in children aged 0 to 15 years (Kaatsch et al 2001), with about 400 new cases a year in the UK. The mortality is relatively high, accounting for about 100 childhood deaths a year in the UK (HeadSmart Campaign 2011). The diagnosis of brain tumours in children takes, on average, about three times as long in the UK as in North America, and, although it is hard to show an effect on mortality, this delay increases family stress and the risk of complications, e.g. visual impairment (HeadSmart Campaign 2011).

Headache in children with brain tumours

Brain tumours can present in many different ways; symptoms and signs may be related to the site of the tumour or may be non-specific, e.g. related to raised intracranial pressure, as shown in a recent systematic review (Wilne et al 2007).

Older series of children with brain tumours presenting with headache are also informative. Of 74 children with brain tumours reviewed by Edgeworth et al (1996), 24% had had a diagnosis of migraine and in 15% a significant psychological diagnosis had been made. Headache occurred in 64%, and was associated with vomiting in 34% and the early morning in 28%. Personality changes occurred in 47%. The mean duration of symptoms before tumour diagnosis was 5 months, 25% only being diagnosed with the advent of impaired consciousness level. Headache was also a major presenting symptom in 62% of 3291 children with brain tumours reported by the Childhood Brain Tumor Consortium (1991).

Battistella et al (1998) compared headache in 60 children with brain tumours and 50 children with idiopathic headache (migraine without aura or tension-type headache). In 10% of children with tumours, headache was the only symptom, and occurred at presentation with other symptoms in a further 17%. The following were significantly more often observed with tumours: projectile vomiting (51% vs 22%); nocturnal or early-morning headache (47% vs 18%); lack of triggers (73% vs 22%); failure to be relieved by sleep or rest (77% vs 20%); and lack of nausea, photophobia and phonophobia. The delay in diagnosis was longer for supratentorial tumours (17mo) than for infratentorial tumours (3mo). Supratentorial tumours are more likely to cause epileptic seizures with or without a focal neurological deficit, whereas infratentorial tumours more often present with headache, vomiting and ataxia.

The occurrence of acquired torticollis or head tilt was an important clue in five cases reported by Gupta et al (1998). One of the five had no other symptoms and the four others also had headache, nausea or vomiting.

Working from this perspective, Wilne et al (2010) have recently developed a very useful evidence-based guideline. They used a consensus workshop with professional and lay parent stakeholders, and a Delphi process, to produce the guideline and have launched an implementation campaign in the UK, through the Royal College of Paediatrics and Child Health (HeadSmart Campaign 2011).

The aim is to alert general practitioners, paediatricians and emergency department staff, to raise awareness and to prompt doctors to at least consider brain imaging in children with symptoms and signs suggestive of a brain tumour. Particular pointers that may be overlooked include persisting awakening headaches, persisting headaches in children under 4 years of age, headache with confusion, change in the character of established migraine or tension-type headache, vomiting from sleep, persisting (>2wk) nausea or vomiting without other signs of infection, deterioration in vision, papilloedema, optic atrophy, new nystagmus, visual field restriction, proptosis and new paralytic squint. Other pointers include regression in motor skills, focal weakness, abnormal gait/coordination, persisting Bell palsy (4wk without improvement), unexplained swallowing difficulties, impaired growth, precocious or delayed puberty, polyuria and polydipsia or secondary nocturnal enuresis (diabetes insipidus) and lethargy in uncharacteristic situations or personality changes.

Although headache is an important symptom of brain tumours, occurring in 40% at presentation and in about 60% by diagnosis (Wilne et al 2012), we need to remember that because brain tumours are relatively rare, and idiopathic headache is very common, the chance that a child presenting with headache has a brain tumour is still very small, perhaps only 10 to 100 times higher than the incidence of brain tumours in the population.

Brain tumours in children with headache
When looking at children referred to a specialist paediatric headache clinic, only 0.5% to 1% can be expected to have an undiagnosed brain tumour or comparably serious underlying pathology.

A recent UK study, based on a prospective follow-up of children presenting with headache, identified the designation of 'unclassified headache' as a useful pointer and key component (together with the traditional additional symptoms and signs) in a draft decision rule of when to image children attending a paediatric outpatient clinic with headache (Ahmed et al 2010). As in the retrospective study by Abu-Arafeh and MacLeod (2005) (see below), Ahmed et al (2010) found significant pathology in children with headache, who were referred to a secondary-care district general hospital outpatient clinic, in 8 out of 729, about 1% [95% confidence interval (CI) 0.6–2.1%], and in 3 out of 709 (0.4%; 95% CI 0.15–1.23%) of those with normal neurological examination. These three all had unclassified headache, compared with 110 out of 706 (15%) who had normal neurological examination and no significant pathology. This is a statistically significant association of the 'unclassified headache' label with significant pathology (p=0.004, two-tailed Fisher's exact test). Even so, only 3 out of 113 (2.7%) children with unclassified headaches and normal neurological examination had significant pathology.

Recently, Rho et al (2011) undertook an ambitious multicentre study to evaluate current imaging practices in the Republic of Korea. The medical notes of 1562 children presenting to paediatric neurology clinics with recurrent headaches were reviewed: 77% had undergone neuroimaging, which is more than the 55% in Ahmed et al's (2010) series, and considerably more than the 18% in Abu-Arafeh and MacLeod's (2005) series. As well as local differences in ease of access to paediatric brain imaging, these differences may also represent a time trend. Of the 1562 patients, 11 (0.7%; 95% CI 0.4–1.2%) underwent neurosurgery for serious underlying lesions found on imaging, including six with space-occupying lesions and one with hydrocephalus and shunt malfunction. Again the rates of significant pathology are similar to those reported in other paediatric headache clinics, and, like Ahmed et al and the American Academy of Neurology and the Practice Committee of the Child Neurology Society (Lewis et al 2002), Rho's group concluded that, in the Republic of Korea, guidelines should be used to help clinicians be more selective in deciding who to image, to reduce the amount of imaging carried out for headache and to increase the yield of significant abnormalities from 0.9% (95% CI 0.5–1.6%).

In a retrospective study of medical notes, 3 of 815 children (0.4%; 95% CI approximately 0.1–1%) attending a paediatric headache clinic had serious intracranial pathology (Abu-Arafeh and MacLeod 2005). In this series, only 142 of 815 (17%) underwent brain imaging, the yield of serious underlying pathology being 3 out of 142 (2%), which is relatively high compared with 3 out of 401 (0.75%) in Ahmed et al's (2010) series or 11 out of 1204 (0.9%) in Rho et al's (2011) series.

The findings of the only prospective *randomised* study of brain imaging in children with headache found by the author are summarised in Table 22.1 (Wober-Bingol et al 1996). In an unselected consecutive series of 462 paediatric headache clinic patients, 429 had idiopathic headache clinically (migraine or tension-type headache), 28 had known clearly symptomatic headache (e.g. post head injury), and two had clinical migraine *and* a known brain lesion. Two (0.4%; 95% CI 0–1%) had previously unknown serious lesions requiring treatment, for which the clinical history led to the suspicion of serious underlying disease. The child with

TABLE 22.1

Published studies on investigations for chronic headache

Author(s)	Year	N	Age group	Setting	Tests	Comments and findings
Chu and Shinnar	1993	104	<9y	Neurology, retrospective	MRI/ CT	None had significant lesions; none of those who were not imaged showed evidence of serious disease or needed interventions at follow-up (95% CI 0–3.7%)
Frishberg	1994	1825		Literature review, retrospective	MRI/ CT	3.2% abnormalities and 1.4% serious abnormalities
Akpek et al	1995	592		Radiology, retrospective	CT	46 were abnormal, none with serious abnormalities
Maytal et al	1995	133	Children	Neurology, retrospective	MRI/ CT	Imaging was indicated or requested for 78 patients. Four were abnormal (3%; 95% CI 0–4.9%). None needed surgical interventions
Demaerel	1996	363		Radiology, retrospective	CT/ MRI	42 had abnormalities, 11 were serious abnormalities (3%; 95% CI 1–5%), five had tumours (1.4%; 95% CI 0.01–2.6%)
Evans	1996	3026		Literature review, retrospective	MRI/ CT	1.6% had serious abnormalities (95% CI 1–2%), of which 0.8% were brain tumour, 0.3% were vascular malformation, 0.3% were hydrocephalus, 0.2% were SDH. In 1440 children with migraine, 0.4% had serious abnormalities (95% CI 0.07–0.7%) (0.3% brain tumour)
Wober-Bingol et al	1996	429	Children	Headache clinic, prospective	MRI	96 patients with migraine or TTH were imaged; 17 had incidental abnormalities, but none needed surgical interventions. 333/429 attended follow-up (3–30mo, no imaging). None changed diagnosis
Medina et al	1997	315	Children	Radiology, retrospective	MRI/ CT	13 had surgical lesions (4%; 95% CI 2-6%)
Kan et al	2000	130	Children	Emergency room, retrospective	CT	53 were imaged, five were abnormal (9%; 95% CI 2–17%), two acute hydrocephalus, 1 SDH, 1 EDH and 1 skull fracture
Jordan et al	2000	1233		Radiology, retrospect	MRI	328 imaged, 165 were abnormal and five had significant abnormalities (1.5%; 95% CI 0.2–2.8%)
						Cost of MRI was USD 517 (1998); cost for each clinically significant abnormal MRI was USD 34 535

TABLE 22.1

(Continued)

Author(s)	Year	*N*	Age group	Setting	Tests	Comments and findings
Lewis and Dorbad	2000	137	Children	Neurology, retrospective	MRI/ CT	54/107 with migraine imaged; four had abnormalities. None needed surgical intervention
						25/30 with chronic daily headache imaged, 5/25 abnormalities; none needed surgical interventions
						Together 0/137: 95% CI 0–2.8%
Lewis and Qureshi	2000	150	Children	Emergency room, prospective	MRI	Nine had serious causes, but also had clear abnormal neurological signs, 6% (95% CI 2–10%).
Abu-Arafeh and MacLeod	2005	815	5–16y	Retrospective	MRI/ CT	142/815 (17%) underwent brain imaging; three children (0.4%; 95% CI 0.1-1%) had serious intracranial pathology
Ahmed et al	2010	709	Children	Prospective	MRI/ CT	Eight children (1%; 95% CI = 0.6–2.1%) had significant pathology; three children (0.4%; 95% CI = 0.15–1.23%) had significant pathology, but normal examination
Rho et al	2011	1562	Children	Retrospective	MRI/ CT	77% had neuroimaging; 11 (0.7%; 95% CI = 0.4-1.2%) had serious underlying lesions (space occupying lesions in six and hydrocephalus and shunt malfunction in one)

Systematic search of PubMed, Cochrane Library, Bandolier, Pediatric Neurology Briefs and hand searches of a selection of paediatric neurology and headache textbooks. MRI, magnetic resonance imaging; CT, computed tomography; CI, confidence interval; TTH, tension-type headache; SDH, subdural haemorrhage; EDH, extradural haemorrhage.

the brain tumour had a normal neurological examination at that time. This is similar to the rates of serious disease in paediatric outpatients presenting with headache in the reports by Abu-Arafeh and MacLeod (2005) and Ahmed et al (2010).

Furthermore, of the 429 with migraine or tension-type headache and no clinical pointers to serious underlying disease (i.e. not 'unclassified headache'), 96 were randomised to undergo MRI; 17 of these 96 patients (18%) had what were considered clinically insignificant abnormalities, similar in quantity and type to a non-headache control group of patients with epilepsies. None of these 96 patients (95% CI 0–4%) was further investigated or received further treatment in light of the MRI results; in particular, none was referred for neurosurgery.

This well-designed study indicates that we might expect previously undiagnosed serious underlying disease in up to 1% of paediatric headache clinic patients but that such cases are likely to be indicated by the history, or history and examination together. This is consistent with the other reported clinical reviews of the yield of neuroimaging in patients without clinical pointers to serious underlying disease attending paediatric clinics.

Combining the series of Lewis and Dorbad (2000), Maytal et al (1995) and Chu and Shinnar (1993), there were no patients with significant lesions (0/319; 95% CI 0–1%). In a series attending emergency departments, 6% to 9% had significant imaging abnormalities, including 2.6% with brain tumours in Lewis and Qureshi's (2000) emergency department series, but all had, at the least, clear neurological signs on examination. Combining the three series reported from departments of diagnostic imaging of patients imaged for headache with no abnormal neurological signs gave significant abnormalities in 16 of 1283 patients (1.2%; 95% CI 0.6%–1.8%).

In these series (Table 22.1), clues that pointed to brain tumours and other serious disease reflected traditional teaching (Tables 22.2 and 22.3): short history (<6mo), worsening headache severity and frequency, headache from sleep, confusion, an abnormal neurological examination, ataxia, hemiparesis and papilloedema.

Hydrocephalus

Table 22.1 also includes cases of hydrocephalus presenting with headache. The importance of routine head circumference measurements in the clinical assessment of children with headache cannot be overemphasised. Compensated hydrocephalus, whether previously diagnosed, shunted or undetected, can decompensate at any time, producing headache and possibly no other suggestive symptoms and signs of raised intracranial pressure.

In children with known hydrocephalus, headache is not always clearly due to high pressure with shunt malfunction or infection. In slit-ventricle syndrome, low pressure, high pressure (Dahlerup et al 1985) or even changes in intracranial pressure that remain within a 'normal' range ($\leq$20cmH$_2$O or 15mmHg) can cause paroxysmal, episodic or continuous chronic daily headache.

The younger child, unable to clearly relay symptoms, may just seem off-colour and non-specifically unwell, perhaps with recurrent bouts of unexplained screaming and/or episodes of aggressive behaviour. Computed tomography (CT) will demonstrate a shunt problem in some but not others. Intracranial pressure monitoring for hours or a few days may be needed to diagnose raised intracranial pressure (Dahlerup et al 1985), even when the CT is normal or shows slit ventricles. Compartmentalised hydrocephalus can be difficult to diagnose, but repeated detailed history and MRI, including of the craniocervical junction, can help.

When raised intracranial pressure and shunt malfunction are excluded and problematic headache continues, other medical, psychological and behavioural strategies should be tried, including a search for emotional and environmental factors, relaxation and standard migraine treatments (James et al 1991).

The role of hindbrain hernia with Chiari type 1 or type 2 malformation in causing headache is controversial, but is probably relevant in cases in which there is a structural shift in the brainstem and/or obstruction to cerebrospinal fluid flow with, perhaps intermittent, raised intracranial pressure. Symptoms such as exertional headache and Valsalva or postural headache, especially occipital or nuchal, have been suggested as clinical pointers and merit imaging of the brain and craniocervical junction with MRI (Kesler and Mendizabal 1999).

TABLE 22.2

Symptoms suggestive of symptomatic (secondary) headache

Past and current history of known

  Brain tumour, tuberous sclerosis, neurofibromatosis type 1, cranial irradiation

  Compensated hydrocephalus, shunted hydrocephalus, hindbrain hernia (Chiari type 1, Chiari type 2 with myelomeningocele), extensive subarachnoid haemorrhage, meningitis, mucopolysaccharidosis

  Head/neck injury

  Potential environmental carbon monoxide

Treatment history of

  Anticoagulation

  Drugs (see Table 22.4)

  Lumbar puncture, neurosurgery

Headache history

  Short history

    Single/first severe headache

    Recurrent severe headache for a few weeks

  Accelerated course

    Every few months, then weeks, then days

    Change in usual headache for worse over weeks or days

Headache timing and posture

  Mainly from sleep[a]

  In the morning before getting up[a]

  Mainly or worse lying down, relieved upright[a]

  Worse with cough, bending over, Valsalva[a]

  Mainly upright, relieved lying down[b]

Associated symptoms

  Vomiting from sleep or in the morning before getting up[a]

  Confusion, impaired conscious level[a,c]

  Altered personality

  Focal weakness, diplopia

  Fever, rigors, seizures

  Snoring and nocturnal arousals

---

[a]Suggestive of raised intracranial pressure e.g. hydrocephalus and/or posterior fossa tumour. [b]Suggestive of low-pressure headache or acute maxillary sinusitis. [c]Never occurs in idiopathic (benign) intracranial hypertension. In addition to symptoms of raised intracranial pressure, brain tumours may present with an accelerated course, seizures, focal neurological deficits and altered personality (see also Table 9.4).

The role of clinical history

Taking the history has several roles: to establish rapport, trust, understanding and confidence; to allow the child and parent or carer to have their say; to establish mutual implicit, or even explicit, expectations, roles and responsibilities; to identify sufficient features to diagnose

TABLE 22.3

Signs suggestive of symptomatic (secondary) headache

Confusion, impaired conscious level[a]

Other signs of raised intracranial pressure

    Large or accelerating head circumference

    Cracked pot sign[b]

    Papilloedema

    VI nerve palsy

    High blood pressure with low heart rate

Other signs of CNS disease

    Cranial nerve palsies/brainstem signs e.g. III, IV, VI nerve pareses, head tilt, upper or lower motor neuron lesions, VII paresis, bulbar or pseudobulbar paresis

    Other focal neurological deficit: spasticity/rigidity, upper motor neuron signs, hemiparesis, quadriplegia/diplegia/paraplegia

    Cerebellar signs: nystagmus, dysarthria, upper limb, or gait, or truncal ataxia/titubation, hypotonia

Signs of systemic disease

    Acutely unwell: looks unwell, febrile, rash, hypertension, tachycardia, poor perfusion

    Underlying disease: wasted, palmar erythema, clubbing, signs of vasculitis, tuberous sclerosis, mucopolysaccharidosis

[a]Use the child's Glasgow Coma Score (e.g. Tatman et al 1997). [b]Percuss skull, ± simultaneous skull auscultation. CNS, central nervous system.

idiopathic headache if possible (see Chapters 8 and 9); and to identify or exclude features suggesting symptomatic (secondary) headache. It is also important to identify factors related to the families' *perception* of the symptoms, differential diagnosis, medical contact, in addition to their levels of intellectual sophistication and use of language. The history should catalogue, for children with idiopathic headache, sufficient associated features and lifestyle clues to set medical advice in a realistic context and identify remediable precipitants and stressors, and to catalogue previous drug and other therapies and the dose or degree to which they were applied and their perceived effect. Symptoms of asthma should be noted.

Some of this information can be distilled from the free history, other aspects are gleaned by observation of body language and social dynamics and other data may best be acquired by use of a questionnaire, pro-forma or checklist. Some information will have to be left for another visit, in particular the use of prospective headache diaries (see Chapter 30 and the appendix in same chapter) is highly recommended.

The clues that point to specific symptomatic (secondary) headaches depend on the diagnosis and the mechanism of pain production. Table 22.4 outlines the main categories of symptomatic (secondary) headache and gives examples. Although this kind of list is helpful for training, it is surprisingly unhelpful in the clinic setting. What it lacks is a sense of proportion and how to focus the diagnostic part of history efficiently. Some causes will be excluded immediately, e.g. by a history of paroxysmal headache in an otherwise well child over several years, without trauma. Others will need extensive enquiry.

TABLE 22.4

Main categories of symptomatic (secondary) headache

I Raised intracranial pressure

Hydrocephalus

    Aqueductal stenosis with late decompensation

    Hindbrain hernia, e.g. Chiari type 1 malformation

    Blockage of ventriculoperitoneal shunt

    Tumour obstructing CSF pathways or reabsorption, e.g. giant cell astrocytoma in tuberous sclerosis, craniopharyngioma, diffuse basal infiltration, spinal cord tumour

    Inflammation or infection obstructing CSF flow or reabsorption (acute cerebellitis, neurocysticercosis)

    Post-haemorrhagic obstruction or reabsorption of CSF flow

    Post-meningitic obstruction or reabsorption of CSF flow

    Infiltration, e.g. of meninges in Scheie, Hurler mucopolysaccharidoses

Cerebral oedema

    Inflammation, e.g. aggressive tumour, trauma, stroke, haemorrhage, vasculitis

    Infection, e.g. meningitis, encephalitis, abscess

    Metabolic disease, e.g. OTC deficiency, Reye syndrome, MCAD, DKA

    Carbon dioxide retention, e.g. OSA, ventilatory failure

    Toxicological, e.g. carbon monoxide poisoning

Idiopathic (benign) intracranial hypertension

II Meningeal and intracranial vessels

Subarachnoid haemorrhage, e.g. from AVM

Carotid or vertebral artery dissection

Mechanical distortion or infiltration: high CSF pressure (as above), low CSF pressure (post lumbar puncture)

Cerebral vasculitis, isolated angiitis of the CNS

III Central (thalamic) pain

Trigeminal distribution causalgia with thalamic and/or trigeminal lesion, ± allodynia, ± anaesthesia dolorosa, +/– more extensive complex regional pain syndrome, e.g. affecting ipsilateral trunk or limb

IV Epilepsy

Postictal, e.g. postconvulsive

Ictal, e.g. early-onset benign occipital lobe epilepsy (Panayiotopoulos type)

V Cranial and local pathology

Optic neuritis

Sinusitis

Dental abscess

Otitis externa/otitis media

Acute head or neck trauma

Post-head/neck injury headache

VI Systemic

Extracranial infection

Malignant hypertension

Benign exertional headache

TABLE 22.4
(Continued)

VII Miscellaneous

Mitochondrial encephalopathy with lactic acidosis and stroke-like episodes associated with migraine-like headache

VIII Adverse drug/substance reactions[a]

Cranial vasodilation, e.g. to nitrates, nitrites, calcium channel blockers, caffeine-containing drinks or caffeine withdrawal, monosodium glutamate, alcohol, marijuana, cocaine, amphetamines

Analgesia-associated headache (analgesia misuse/rebound headache)

Aseptic meningitis, e.g. non-steroidal analgesics

IX Psychological[a]

Stress, conflict, anxiety, depression, post-traumatic stress disorder

---

[a]May also act as triggers or contributory factors to idiopathic headache. CSF, cerebrospinal fluid; OTC, ornithine transcarbamylase; MCAD, medium-chain acyl-coenzyme A dehydrogenase deficiency; DKA, diabetic ketoacidosis; OSA, obstructive sleep apnoea; AVM, arteriovenous malformation; CNS, central nervous system.

An adequate history will not only give the most likely diagnosis but, more importantly, the most important, less likely but worth considering, diagnoses. This differential will inform the examination and choice of management, including investigations.

The risk or probability of a diagnosis varies with the clinical setting and referral pattern, and as the history, examination, investigations and follow-up unfold. This is best modelled by Bayesian statistics, but is 'instinctive' to gifted and experienced physicians.

Symptoms that should alert the physician to the possibility that the child has a symptomatic (secondary) headache are given in Table 22.2.

It is the combination of two or more pointers, from history or examination, that is most informative, especially, but not only, when a specific diagnosis of, for example, 'migraine without aura', 'migraine with aura' or 'paroxysmal hemicrania' cannot be made.

Brain tumours are associated with any kind of headache, including headache otherwise fulfilling diagnostic features for migraine (notably in children who have pre-existing migraine), but it is children with 'unclassified' or 'non-specific' headaches who are probably at an increased risk of harbouring a brain tumour, and who will eventually develop additional symptoms and signs (Ahmed et al 2010).

The role of the clinical examination

Examination will be directed by the history and the clinical context and referral pattern. A thorough neurological examination has been claimed to be therapeutic by adult patients and the worried parents of some children, but is not feasible in younger children, who quickly become restless or unhappy. A focussed and playful examination is required, particularly in preschool and prepubertal children. Nevertheless, the physical examination should include the elements in Figure 22.1, unless recently and reliably undertaken by a colleague, e.g. it would be unnecessary to struggle to clearly view the optic discs by direct fundoscopy in an

Blood pressure	Weight	Height	Head circumference		
Systolic	kg	cm	cm		
Diastolic	Centile	Centile	Centile		
Alert and conscious	Yes	Level of consciousness	Eyes / 4	Verbal / 5	Motor / 6
	No				

	Normal	Abnormal	Details
General examination			
Gait			
Fundi			
Appearance			
Mental state			
Fogs			
ENT and sinuses			
	Yes	No	Details
Alert and cooperative			
Sensory deficit			
Motor deficit			
UMN signs			
Ataxia			
Cranial bruits			
Others			
Handedness*			
Writing and drawing			
Sample of writing			

*R right; L left; B both or unclear.

Fig. 22.1 Summary sheet for examination of children with headache. Under level of consciousness, eyes, verbal and motor are eye opening, verbal and motor components, respectively, of the child's Glasgow Coma Scale (Tatman et al 1997). UMN, upper motor neuron; ENT, ear, nose and throat.

upset child who has recently had a thorough ophthalmological assessment including normal direct or indirect fundoscopy. Signs that should alert the physician to the possibility of the child having a symptomatic (secondary) headache are given in Table 22.3.

Investigations

There is a more secure evidence base for investigations than for history and examination. The decision to recommend investigations, and their urgency and sequence, will be determined by the differential diagnosis generated by the history and, in some situations, by local factors such as ease of access and follow-up, waiting times, patient and carer preferences. Pre-eminent is whether to undertake cranial neuroimaging. From the paediatric neurosurgeon's viewpoint any child with acute, recurrent or chronic headache *could* have a brain tumour, and they will once again be asked by devastated parents if it should not have been diagnosed sooner, if the child should not have had brain imaging sooner. From the epidemiologist's viewpoint any child in the population might have a brain tumour, the risk being indicated by the annual incidence. This risk is increased in children referred for headache (see above), and increased further or reduced by the history and examination. Whether brain imaging is appropriate depends on this risk and also the availability and convenience of neuroimaging, and other family factors mentioned in the introduction. Obtaining a normal or negative scan can be very helpful, even therapeutic, even in a child most unlikely to have a tumour, e.g. when parents are embattled over the issue and a close relative has recently died from a brain tumour whose symptoms were for a long time attributed to migraine. However, obtaining a normal scan can be a source of increased anxiety to children and carers, especially if there is a long waiting list or if incidental, clinically insignificant features are reported. General anaesthesia or sedation may be needed, with their attendant risks, discomfort and inconvenience. Sedation for brain imaging, especially 'failed sedation', can be a particularly traumatic experience for children and their carers (Sammons et al 2011).

Brain imaging is generally best with cranial MRI; however, if delay is to be avoided, cranial CT can be used and can demonstrate haemorrhage more easily and exclude hydrocephalus. Other tests will be indicated by the differential diagnosis or additional possible diagnoses suggested by history and/or examination. Occasionally imaging will need to be repeated, e.g. after 3 or 6 months, because of an unclear scan or a persisting or evolving clinical picture. The opportunity may be taken at that time to administer contrast or undertake non-standard MRI sequences, e.g. magnetic resonance angiography. It is well worth discussing the best imaging approach in a particular case with the local neuroradiologists.

A review of the literature on the investigation of headache and yield of neuroimaging is given in Table 22.1. The 95% confidence intervals were recalculated by the author using standard formulae (Altman et al 2000). These data suggest a low rate of serious intracranial abnormalities, potentially needing treatment, in patients attending children's neurology or headache clinics (0–1%), emergency rooms for headache (6–9%) and diagnostic imaging departments (0–3%, all ages), with risks of 0% to 4% in various studies of headache patients with no neurological deficits on examination.

An original approach was undertaken by Medina et al (2001). They modelled a cost-effectiveness analysis of three hypothetical diagnostic strategies: children were stratified into low risk (headache duration >6mo and no other symptoms and signs, probability of tumour 0.01%), intermediate risk (migraine and normal examination, probability of tumour 0.4%), and high risk (headaches <6mo and additional predictors of tumour, e.g. new abnormal neurological signs, probability of tumour 4%). For those in the low-risk group, clinical follow-up and no imaging were more effective and less costly than imaging. For the high-risk group MRI was the most cost effective [US$ 114 000/quality-adjusted life-year (QALY) (£72 365/QALY) gained compared with no imaging]. For the intermediate-risk group imaging was more effective than not, but was not 'cost-effective' [more than US$ 1 000 000/ QALY (more than £635 000/QALY) gained compared with no imaging], and did not take into account misery and stress in those with non-specific abnormalities or normal scans. This cost-effectiveness analysis supports traditional teaching and the current consensus in the literature reviewed.

Synthesis of history, examination and, when undertaken, investigations

One isolated symptom or sign or investigation result is usually not enough and, when it cannot be made to fit in with the other elements of the clinical picture, it is probably best left out of consideration, at least temporarily.

Often the symptoms and signs and, when appropriate, investigations all fall into place effortlessly to give a confident diagnosis. Sometimes there will be uncertainty. In these circumstances *more* information is needed, e.g. by using a prospective headache diary, arranging an early follow-up, investigating speculatively, or having a period of hospital in-patient observation. The confident exclusion of some underlying diagnoses, feared by the child and/or parent or carer can be therapeutic to all concerned, but the potential advantages and disadvantages outlined above need careful consideration in each case.

Conclusions

Symptomatic headache is usually clearly evident but can be difficult to diagnose. Up to 1% of unselected patients attending a paediatric headache clinic, up to 0.5% of those with a normal neurological examination and up to 10% attending the emergency department may be expected to have a brain tumour or previously undiagnosed serious underlying disease, e.g. presenting with their 'first or worst headache', an accelerating course or an abnormal neurological examination, including head circumference, fundi and gait. However, with a careful history and neurological examination these few cases will generally be identified. Clinical suspicions therefore should prompt brain imaging, especially the accumulation of pointers ('red flags') at presentation or over time, especially in a child with unclassified headache. Brain tumours are rare but often treatable, and delay in diagnosis is best avoided if possible.

However, brain imaging should not be encouraged for all patients with headache or even episodic headache and vomiting, as it carries its own emotional and physical morbidity.

The current Child Neurology Society practice parameter for the evaluation of children and adolescents with recurrent headaches recommends avoiding routine imaging unless there are clinical risk factors in the history or the neurological examination is abnormal (Lewis et al 2002). Sometimes, however, it will be good practice to undertake brain imaging without a clear indication, but only when there is a specific and understandable patient or parental concern.

Thus the traditional medical skills of history, examination, selection of investigations, allaying anxiety and the communication of uncertainty remain the key to the management of headaches and the diagnosis of brain tumours in children.

REFERENCES

Abu-Arafeh I, Macleod S (2005) Serious neurological disorders in children with chronic headache. *Arch Dis Child* 90: 937–40. http://dx.doi.org/10.1136/adc.2004.067256

Ahmed MAS, Martinez A, Cahill D, Chong K, Whitehouse WP (2010) When to image neurologically normal children with headaches: development of a decision rule. *Acta Paediatr* 99: 940–3. http://dx.doi.org/10.1111/j.1651-2227.2010.01728.x

Akpek S, Arac M, Atilla S, Onal B, Yucel C, Isik S (1995) Cost-effectiveness of computed tomography in the evaluation of patients with headache. *Headache* 35: 228–30. http://dx.doi.org/10.1111/j.1526-4610.1995.hed3504228.x

Altman DG, Machin D, Bryant TN, Gardner MJ (2000) *Statistics with Confidence.* Bristol: BMJ Books.

Battistella PA, Naccarella C, Soriani S, Perilongo G (1998) Headache and brain tumours: different features versus primary forms in juvenile patients. *Headache* 9: 245–8.

Childhood Brain Tumor Consortium (1991) The epidemiology of headache among children with brain tumor. Headache in children with brain tumors. *Journal of Neurooncology* 10: 31–46. http://dx.doi.org/10.1007/BF00151245

Chu ML, Shinnar S (1993) Headaches in children younger than 7 years of age. *Arch Neurol* 50: 130–1.

Dahlerup B, Gjerris F, Harmsen A, Sorensen PS (1985) Severe headache as the only symptom of long-standing shunt dysfunction in hydrocephalic children with normal or slit ventricles revealed by computed tomography. *Childs Nerv Syst* 1: 49–52. http://dx.doi.org/10.1007/BF00706731

Demaerel P, Boelaert I, Wilms G, Baert AL (1996) The role of cranial computed tomography in the diagnostic work-up of headache. *Headache* 36: 347–8. http://dx.doi.org/10.1046/j.1526-4610.1996.3606347.x

Edgeworth J, Bullock P, Bailey A, Gallagher A, Crouchman M (1996) Why are brain tumours still being missed? *Arch Dis Child* 74: 148–51.

Evans RW (1996) Diagnostic testing for the evaluation of headaches. *Neurol Clin* 14: 1–26. http://dx.doi.org/10.1016/S0733-8619(05)70240-1

Frishberg BM (1994) The utility of neuroimaging in the evaluation of headache in patients with normal neurologic examinations. *Neurology* 44: 1191–7.

Gupta AK, Roy DR, Conlan ES, Crawford AH (1998) Torticollis secondary to posterior fossa tumours. *J Pediatr Orthop* 18: 415.

HeadSmart Campaign (2011) HeadSmart: Be Brain Tumour Aware. Available at: www.headsmart.org.uk/ (accessed 14 March 2013).

James HE, Nowak TP (1991) Clinical course and diagnosis of migraine headaches in hydrocephalic children. *Pediatr Neurosurg* 17: 310–16. http://dx.doi.org/10.1159/000120616

Jordan JE, Ramirez GF, Bradley WG, Chen DY, Lightfoote JB, Song A (2000) Economic and outcomes assessment of magnetic resonance imaging in the evaluation of headache. *J Natl Med Assoc* 92: 573–8.

Kaatsch P, Rickert CH, Kuhl J, Schuz J, Michaelis J (2001) Population-based epidemiological data on brain tumors in German children. *Cancer* 92: 3155–64. http://dx.doi.org/10.1002/1097-0142(20011215)92:12<3155::AID-CNCR10158>3.0.CO;2-C

Kan L, Nagelberg J, Maytal J (2000) Headaches in a pediatric emergency department: etiology, imaging and treatment. *Headache* 40: 25–9. http://dx.doi.org/10.1046/j.1526-4610.2000.00004.x

Kesler R, Mendizabal JE (1999) Headache in Chiari malformation: a distinct clinical entity? *J Am Osteopath Assoc* 99: 153–6.

Lewis DW, Dorbad D (2000) The utility of neuroimaging in the evaluation of children with migraine or chronic daily headache who have normal neurological examinations. *Headache* 40: 629–32. http://dx.doi.org/10.1046/j.1526-4610.2000.040008629.x

Lewis DW, Qureshi F (2000) Acute headache in children and adolescents presenting to the emergency department. *Headache* 40: 200–3. http://dx.doi.org/10.1046/j.1526-4610.2000.00029.x

Lewis DW, Ashwal S, Dahl G et al (2002) Practice parameter: Evaluation of children and adolescents with recurrent headaches. *Neurology* 59: 490–8. http://dx.doi.org/10.1212/WNL.59.4.490

Maytal J, Bienkowski RS, Patel M, Eviatar L (1995) The value of brain imaging in children with headaches. *Pediatrics* 96: 413–16.

Medina LS, Pinter JD, Zurakowski D, Davis RG, Kuban K, Barnes PD (1997) Children with headache: clinical predictors of surgical space-occupying lesions and the role of neuroimaging. *Radiology* 202: 819–24.

Medina LS, Kuntz KM, Pomery S (2001) Children with headache suspected of having a brain tumour: a cost-effective analysis of diagnostic strategies. *Pediatrics* 108: 255–63.

Rho YI, Cung HE, Suh ES et al (2011) The role of neuroimaging in children and adolescents with recurrent headaches- multicenter study. *Headache* 51: 403–8. http://dx.doi.org/10.1111/j.1526-4610.2011.01845.x

Sammons HM, Edwards J, Rushby R, Picton C, Collier J, Whitehouse WP (2011) General anaesthesia or sedation for paediatric neuroimaging: current practice in a teaching hospital. *Arch Dis Child* 96: 114. http://dx.doi.org/10.1136/adc.2010.185256

Tatman A, Warren A, Williams A, Powell J, Whitehouse W (1997) Development of a paediatric coma scale in intensive care clinical practice. *Arch Dis Child* 77: 519–21. http://dx.doi.org/10.1136/adc.77.6.519

Wilne S, Collier J, Kennedy C, Koller K, Grundy R, Walker D (2007) Presentation of childhood CNS tumours: a systematic review and meta-analysis. *Lancet Oncol* 8 685–95. http://dx.doi.org/10.1016/S1470-2045(07)70207-3

Wilne S, Koller K, Collier J, Kennedy C, Grundy R, Walker D (2010) The diagnosis of brain tumours in children: a guideline to assist healthcare professionals in the assessment of children who may have a brain tumour. *Arch Dis Child* 95 534–9. http://dx.doi.org/10.1136/adc.2009.162057

Wilne S, Collier J, Kennedy C et al (2012) Progression from first symptom to diagnosis in childhood brain tumours. *Eur J Pediatr* 171: 87–93. http://dx.doi.org/10.1007/s00431-011-1485-7

Wober-Bingol C, Wober C, Prayer D et al (1996) Magnetic resonance imaging for recurrent headache in childhood and adolescence. *Headache* 36: 83–90. http://dx.doi.org/10.1046/j.1526-4610.1996.3602083.x

23
IDIOPATHIC INTRACRANIAL HYPERTENSION

William P Whitehouse

Introduction

There have been some helpful reviews of idiopathic intracranial hypertension (IIH), also known as benign intracranial hypertension (BIH) and pseudotumour cerebri, in children (Soler et al 1998, Salman et al 2001, Schexnayder and Chapman 2006). It is much more common in young, obese adult women, with an incidence of up to 19 per 100 000 persons per year (Durcan et al 1988), than in children (0.7 per 100 000 persons per year), in whom there is equal sex distribution, and less association with obesity before adolescence (Matthews et al 2012).

Idiopathic intracranial hypertension not only causes pain and makes children feel ill, but carries a significant, albeit low, risk of permanent visual impairment. Thus, it is vital to diagnose, treat and monitor IIH, especially in children, in whom it is more likely to be atypical in its presentation, and therefore overlooked.

Diagnosis

Operational diagnostic criteria were updated about 10 years ago (Friedman and Jacobson 2002), and can be applied in children and young people, although the threshold for high pressure should be greater than the standard 25cm cerebrospinal fluid (CSF) (19mmHg) applied to adults (see Table 23.1).

Recent research suggests that a normal opening CSF pressure of 28cm is recorded in healthy children and adolescents aged 1 to 18 years as compared with those with optic nerve head oedema (Avery et al 2011), and that for most children and young people between 1 and 18 years of age, opening pressures above 28cmCSF (22mmHg) qualify as elevated (Avery et al 2010).

The diagnosis is often straightforward: papilloedema with or without a VI nerve paresis diplopia and an intact consciousness level in a child with almost any pattern of headache. Headache often has some features of raised intracranial pressure (Table 23.1) and can present as chronic daily headache with or without migraine-like symptoms. Urgent brain imaging – magnetic resonance imaging (MRI) with magnetic resonance venography (MRV) is most efficient (or, if unavailable, computed tomography [CT] with contrast) – is needed to exclude other causes of raised intracranial pressure and any contraindication to lumbar puncture (obstruction to CSF pathway). The opening CSF pressure at lumbar puncture must be measured to confirm the diagnosis. An opening CSF pressure over 28cmCSF

TABLE 23.1

Criteria for diagnosing idiopathic intracranial hypertension

Criteria	Comments
If symptoms present, they may reflect only those of generalised intracranial hypertension or papilloedema	Headache, which may be worse lying down, with coughing or bending, with exercise or awakes the patient from sleep; pulsatile tinnitus; diplopia or transient visual loss or blurring or impaired colour vision or visual field defect; nausea and vomiting; dizziness; ataxia; back or neck pain/stiffness; facial weakness; retro-ocular pain worse with eye movement
If signs present, they may only reflect those of generalised intracranial hypertension or papilloedema	Papilloedema and VI nerve paresis may be unilateral or bilateral; the child may be miserable, tired, quiet and difficult to engage, but will have a normal consciousness level. A reduced consciousness level mandates an urgent alternative diagnosis
Documented elevated ICP measured in the lateral decubitus position	Lumbar puncture in lateral decubitus, or ICP monitoring: over 28cmCSF (22mmHg) in children and young people aged 1 to 18 years (Schexnayder and Chapman 2006, Matthews et al 2012). Remember, if using an intracranial pressure transducer, to check the units of pressure, and to convert mmHg to cmCSF/water by multiplying by 1.3
Normal CSF composition	An atraumatic tap: WBC <6 × 10^6/l; protein <0.4g/l; glucose CSF/plasma ratio >0.5
No evidence of hydrocephalus, mass or structural or vascular lesion on MRI or contrast-enhanced CT, and on MRV or CT venography[a]	Children and young people under 18 years count as atypical so have MRI and MRV or CT venography

[a]Venous sinus thrombosis is excluded; venous sinus narrowing is included. See Table 23.2 for list of other causes of pseudotumour cerebri. ICP, intracranial pressure; CSF, cerebrospinal fluid; WBC, white blood cell count; MRI, magnetic resonance imaging; MRV, magnetic resonance venography; CT, computed tomography.

(28cmH$_2$O, 21mmHg) confirms the diagnosis. However, the distress of the lumbar puncture in children may give erroneous results for opening CSF pressure. Hyperventilation lowers P_{CO_2}, cerebral blood flow, cerebral blood volume and consequently intracranial pressure (ICP). On the other hand, distress and Valsalva raises ICP. Lumbar puncture should, therefore, be performed under sedation and analgesia to avoid distressing the child, if general anaesthesia is necessary, end-tidal CO$_2$ should be monitored, recorded and kept within the normal range. However, the raised pressure in IIH has been shown to fluctuate into the normal range, so a normal opening pressure does not absolutely exclude the diagnosis. In some situations of diagnostic uncertainty, or when treatment does not improve headache, 48 hours of intracranial pressure monitoring can be very useful, especially when linked to a diary recording fluctuations in symptoms (Toma et al 2010, Warden et al 2011). The CSF should be sent for microscopy and culture, protein and glucose estimation with paired blood glucose as routine.

Treatment

Draining CSF at the diagnostic lumbar puncture usually provides headache relief, at least temporarily. The amount of CSF that can be drained safely is not known, but anecdotally it is safe to reduce the pressure from 30cmCSF (22mmHg) to 15cmCSF (11mmHg)and to remove 50 to 60ml without a problem. It may be safe to remove more if the pressure is higher.

IIH can occur without papilloedema, in which case diagnosis is difficult and often delayed. Colour vision disturbances and visual field defects may occur before deterioration of visual acuity and may be suggestive of IIH, especially when the brain scan is normal or demonstrates small ventricles.

Otic hydrocephalus is a condition that has much in common with IIH: the raised intracranial pressure is due to sagittal or sigmoid or lateral sinus thrombosis associated with, often chronic, middle-ear infection. This should be searched for in all cases: MRV is very helpful in this. Other conditions and drugs thought to cause pseudotumour cerebri, which can present similar to IIH, are listed in Tables 23.2 and 23.3. Every effort should be made to identify and treat these contributing conditions, especially obesity (Sinclair et al 2010).

TABLE 23.2

Medical conditions implicated in the differential diagnosis or contributory cause of idiopathic intracranial hypertension

Causes	Comments
Obesity	Especially rapid weight gain, hyperalimentation in nutritional deficiency
Endocrine	Adrenal insufficiency, Cushing syndrome, hypoparathyroidism, hyperparathyroidism, hypothyroidism, hyperthyroidism, menarche, pregnancy, polycystic ovaries
Others	Anaemia (sickle cell, aplastic), Beçhet syndrome, chronic renal failure, HIV/AIDS, iron deficiency, Lyme disease, migraine, otitis media, sarcoidosis, systemic lupus erythematosus, vitamin A deficiency

HIV, human immunodeficiency virus; AIDS, acquired immune deficiency syndrome.

TABLE 23.3

Drugs and toxins implicated in the differential diagnosis or contributory cause of idiopathic intracranial hypertension

Substance	Comments
Hormonal therapy	Antidiuretic hormone (vasopressin), corticosteroid therapy or withdrawal, growth hormone, oral contraceptive pill, thyroxine
Vitamins	Vitamin A excess, etretinate, isotretinoin
Antibiotics	Aminoglycosides, ciclosporin, co-trimoxazole, minocycline, penicillins, nalidixic acid, nitrofurantoin, sulphonamides, tetracyclines
Major tranquillisers	Chlorpromazine, fluoridazine
Others	Amiodarone, ciclosporin, indometacin, lithium carbonate, phenytoin

Once the diagnosis has been confirmed, joint monitoring with an appropriate ophthalmology team interested in children will be needed. Baseline ophthalmological assessment will include well-documented fundoscopy, eye movement assessment, visual acuity, visual fields by formal perimetry if possible, colour vision and contrast sensitivity testing. Review will initially be frequent, e.g. in a week or so, unless vision seems to be immediately at risk, in which case urgent treatment and more frequent assessment may be needed.

In the face of preserved visual acuity, outpatient treatment and follow-up can be arranged (Matthews 2007). If symptoms recur after the lumbar puncture, the following drugs can be tried in turn: frusemide (1–4mg/kg/day, check plasma potassium and supplement if needed), acetazolamide (25mg/kg/d, or 1g/d, increasing to maximum of 100mg/kg/d or 2g/d if tolerated; check plasma potassium and bicarbonate), or both, or topiramate 2 to 15mg/kg/day (may help with weight loss in obese patients, and chronic daily headache and migraine too), with increasing risk of adverse effects. The evidence for drug treatment is derived from open studies and case series reports, but controlled trials are not available.

Urgent treatment can save vision, which can deteriorate over hours or days, including lumboperitoneal shunt, ventriculoperitoneal shunt, subtemporal decompression and optic nerve fenestration. Surgery should also be considered for patients with continuing symptoms or fluctuating visual impairment, or with failed medical treatment. Although the short-term results of shunting are good, shunt failure from blockage, fracture or migration is common by 6 months, especially with lumboperitoneal shunts.

An exciting recent treatment innovation, in cases in which MRV or CT venography has demonstrated a likely stenosis, is endovascular stenting (for a recent review, see Pandey and Steinberg 2010). Having demonstrated a narrowing, a significant pressure gradient should be confirmed before stenting. Results to date are good. Occasionally stenosis reappears adjacent to the stent, but sometimes incapacitating headache will continue even after ICP has returned to the normal range: the pain pathway is 'wound up', and treatment can prove very difficult, although drugs used in chronic pain and migraine can help.

Prognosis

The prognosis for children with IIH appears good; however, the author's personal experience is not so good, with many children pursuing a fluctuating course over years, and some developing continuing headaches even when the ICP is within the normal range. However, the prognosis for vision, with appropriate monitoring and treatment dose, seems good, with very few children suffering long-term visual impairment (Soiberman et al 2011, Matthews et al 2012).

The future

The mechanisms, pathology and causes of IIH are not established. Those cases of pseudotumour cerebri with evident venous thrombosis are excluded from the IIH diagnosis; however, cerebral venous outflow obstruction with stenosis and raised intracranial blood volume does seem to respond to stenting. Of course, venous compression could occur because of raised ICP from any cause, and venous sinus narrowing can improve after therapeutic lumbar puncture. However, IIH could involve a vicious cycle in some patients (Owler et al 2005): fat in the neck or thoracic inlet or even abdominal cavity could lead to a small rise in ICP, but once pressure compresses venous outflow, the rise is likely to increase even more – a small reduction in outflow diameter will have a large effect on outflow rate (Poiseuille's equation related flow to the fourth power of the radius of a pipe, and directly proportional to the pressure gradient). Other causes of obstructed venous flow can also contribute in some cases, for example, giant arachnoid granulations, and indeed any combinations of intrinsic or extrinsic factors. If compliance of the intracranial or spinal CSF compartments is reduced, even a small increase in intracranial blood volume will produce a larger rise in ICP, and intra-abdominal obesity will reduce intraspinal compliance, while surgical shunts of course increase compliance.

Alternative hypotheses include cerebral oedema, which seems unlikely in view of the lack of encephalopathy and MRI diffusion tensor imaging results (Owler et al 2006); CSF obstruction or excess production or insufficient absorption, all of which seem unlikely given the lack of hydrocephalus in IIH; a primary role for leptin (as yet unclear); and the suggestion that IIH itself causes obesity!

Managing IIH in children and young people remains challenging; however, there has been a lot of research in the last 5 years and the author expects the pathophysiology will become clearer and treatments more evidence based in the next 5 years.

REFERENCES

Avery RA, Shah SS, Licht DJ (2010) Reference range for cerebrospinal fluid opening pressure in children. *N Engl J Med* 363: 891–3.

Avery RA, Licht DJ, Shah SS et al (2011) CSF opening pressure in children with optic nerve head edema. *Neurology* 76: 1658–61. http://dx.doi.org/10.1212/WNL.0b013e318219fb80

Durcan FJ, Corbett JJ, Wall M (1988) The incidence of pseudotumour cerebri. Population studies in Iowa and Louisiana. *Arch Neurol* 45: 875–7. http://dx.doi.org/10.1001/archneur.1988.00520320065016

Friedman DI, Jacobson DM (2002) Diagnostic creieria for idiopathic intracranial hypertension. *Neurology* 59: 1492–5. http://dx.doi.org/10.1212/01.WNL.0000029570.69134.1B

Matthews YY (2007) Drugs used in childhood idiopathic or benign intracranial hypertension. *Arch Dis Child Educ Pract Ed* 93: 19–25. http://dx.doi.org/10.1136/adc.2006.107326

Matthews YY, Dean F, Matyka K et al (2012) UK surveillance of childhood Idiopathic Intracranial Hypertension (IIH). *Arch Dis Child* 97(Suppl1): Ab.

Owler BK, Parker G, Halmagyi GM et al (2005) Cranial venous outflow obstruction and pseudotumour cerebri syndrome. *Adv Tech Stand Neurosurg* 30: 107–74. http://dx.doi.org/10.1007/3-211-27208-9_4

Owler BK, Higgins JN, Pena A, Carpenter TA, Pickard JD (2006) Diffusion tensor imaging of benign intracranial hypertension: absence of cerebral oedema. *Br J Neurosurg* 20: 79–81. http://dx.doi.org/10.1080/02688690600682317

Pandey P, Steinberg GK (2010) Endovascular stenting of venous sinus stenosis for idiopathic intracranial hypertension. *World Neurosurg* 75 594–5. http://dx.doi.org/10.1016/j.wneu.2010.12.048

Salman MS, Kirkham FJ, MacGregor DL (2001) Idiopathic "benign" intracranial hypertension: case series and review. *J Child Neurol* 16: 465–70.

Schexnayder LK, Chapman K (2006) Presentation, investigation and management of idiopathic intracranial hypertension in children. *Curr Paediatr* 16: 336–41. http://dx.doi.org/10.1016/j.cupe.2006.07.006

Sinclair AJ, Walker EA, Burdon MA et al (2010) Cerebrospinal fluid corticosteroid levels and cortisol metabolism in patients with idiopathic intracranial hypertension: a link between 11beta-HSD1 and intracranial pressure regulation? *J Clin Endocrinol Metab* 95: 5348–56.

Soiberman U, Stolovitch C, Balcer LJ, Regenbogen M, Constantini S, Kesler A (2011) Idiopathic intracranial hypertension in children: visual outcome and risk of recurrence. *Childs Nerv Syst* 27: 1913–18. http://dx.doi.org/10.1007/s00381-011-1470-5

Soler D, Cox T, Bullock P, Calver DM, Robinson RO (1998) Diagnosis and management of benign intracranial hypertension. *Arch Dis Child* 78: 89–94. http://dx.doi.org/10.1136/adc.78.1.89

Toma AK, Tarnaris A, Kitchen ND, Watkins LD (2010) Continuous intracranial pressure monitoring in pseu-dotumour cerebri: Single centre experience. *Br J Neurosurg* 24: 584–8. http://dx.doi.org/10.3109/02688 697.2010.495169

Warden KF, Alizai AM, Trobe JD, Hoff JT (2011) Short-term continuous intraparenchymal intracranial pressure monitoring in presumed idiopathic intracranial hypertension. *J Neuroophthalmol* 31: 202–5. http://dx.doi.org/10.1097/WNO.0b013e3182183c8d

24
CRANIOFACIAL PAIN: HEADACHE ATTRIBUTED TO DISEASES OF THE PARANASAL SINUSES, THE EYES, THE TEETH AND THE JAWS

Ishaq Abu-Arafeh

Headache attributed to sinusitis

Inflammation and congestion of paranasal sinuses cause a localised pain that may radiate to other areas of the face and head. Acute inflammation of the maxillary and frontal sinuses is often associated with symptoms and signs of upper respiratory tract infections including fever, runny or stuffy nose, sneeze, cough and sore throat. It is also associated with tenderness to touch on the cheek area over the maxillary sinus or the forehead over the frontal sinuses. The illness usually runs a brief course and responds well to treatment with antibiotics, decongestants and simple analgesics.

Acute ethmoid sinusitis is often associated with severe infection, may present with swelling around the eyes and may be complicated with periorbital cellulitis and cavernous sinus thrombosis. It requires urgent investigation and treatment with broad-spectrum antibiotics and close monitoring by paediatricians, ear, nose and throat surgeons, and ophthalmologists.

Chronic sinusitis is rare in the general population and particularly in children and adolescents. The relationship between chronic headache and chronic sinus disease is often exaggerated, especially in children. Chronic sinusitis is defined as persistent mucopurulent nasal discharge for over 30 days (Mellis 2007). Chronic sinusitis is often secondary to other underlying conditions and may follow a prolonged or recurrent upper respiratory tract inflammation, such as seen in allergic rhinitis. Other underlying disorders that cause recurrent or chronic infection of the sinuses may include cystic fibrosis, immune deficiency, primary ciliary dyskinesia or congenital malformation of the facial bones and upper airway.

The prevalence of sinus headache in the general population is not known and is likely to be low. There is a lack of studies on the occurrence of sinus headache in children, although it is frequently reported by patients and misdiagnosed by doctors. A possible reason for the misdiagnosis is the increased use of neuroimaging on children with chronic headache and the incidental findings of thickened sinus mucosa or sinus opacity.

A large study of 214 children (4–16y) with chronic headache (Senbil et al 2008) showed that the majority of children (113; 53%) are investigated by computed tomography or magnetic

TABLE 24.1

Criteria for the diagnosis of headache attributed to rhinosinusitis (Headache Classification Subcommittee of the International Headache Society 2004)

(A) Frontal headache accompanied by pain in one or more regions of the face, ears or teeth fulfilling criteria C and D

(B) Clinical, nasal endoscopic, CT and/or MRI or laboratory evidence of acute or acute-on-chronic rhinosinusitis

(C) Headache and facial pain develop simultaneously with onset of acute exacerbation of rhinosinusitis

(D) Headache and/or facial pain resolves within 7d of remission or successful treatment of acute or acute-on-chronic rhinosinusitis

CT, computed tomography; MRI, magnetic resonance imaging.

resonance imaging of the head. The scans were normal in 57 children (50%), showed sinus opacification in 32 (28%) and showed sinus mucosal thickening in 24 (21%). Clinical history showed that 116 out of the 214 children (54%) had a prior diagnosis of sinusitis, and appropriate treatment with antibiotics and decongestants had no effect on the headache in 70 (60%) children. This study has also shown that 40% of children with migraine and 60% of those with tension-type headache are misdiagnosed with sinus headache. However, a diagnosis of true sinus headache, as defined by the International Headache Society (IHS) criteria (Headache Classification Subcommittee of the International Headache Society 2004) in Table 24.1, was made in 7% of this group of patients as a concomitant headache and in 1% as the only headache, demonstrating the rarity of 'sinus headache' among children with chronic headache (Senbil et al 2008).

The clinical features of chronic sinusitis are usually those of mild and non-specific headache, facial pain, nasal discharge and congestion. The clinical picture may be dominated by symptoms related to those of the underlying disorder of allergic rhinitis, cystic fibrosis or immune deficiency. Headache associated with chronic sinusitis, as defined by the IHS (ICHD-II; Headache Classification Subcommittee of the International Headache Society 2004) (Table 24.1), may be of relevance to older children and adolescents, as sinuses will develop over many years and reach adult sizes by the age of 12 years. The criteria for the diagnosis of headache attributed to chronic sinusitis in adults are used here, despite not having been critically appraised in a childhood population, because they are the only available criteria.

The headache attributed to chronic sinusitis is generally mild and dull in nature and is associated with tenderness to touch on the face in relation to the inflamed sinuses. The headache tends to be constant but has diurnal variation, being worse in the morning and exacerbated by head movement. It is unlikely to be associated with autonomic symptoms, sensory impairment or gastrointestinal upset, but nevertheless it has been often misdiagnosed as migraine. The American Migraine Study showed that 14% of people with headache that fulfil the IHS criteria for the diagnosis of migraine are misdiagnosed as having sinus headache or tension-type headache (Diamond 2002).

TABLE 24.2
Diagnostic criteria for headache attributed to glaucoma (Headache Classification Subcommittee of the International Headache Society 2004)

(A) Pain in the eye and behind or above it fulfilling criteria C and D

(B) Raised intraocular pressure with at least one of the following:

    (1) Conjunctival injection

    (2) Clouding of cornea

    (3) Visual disturbances

(C) Pain develops simultaneously with glaucoma

(D) Pain resolves within 72h of effective treatment of glaucoma

Headache attributed to ocular disorders

GLAUCOMA

Generally, glaucoma is rare in children and can be difficult to diagnose in the paediatric clinic. When suspected, an urgent assessment by an experienced paediatric ophthalmologist is needed. If untreated it may cause progressive visual loss.

Primary congenital glaucoma is a rare disorder and may occur in the course of several syndromes, some of which are genetic in origin and have a familial risk. Symptoms appear during the first 2 years of life with photophobia, tearing and watering of one or both eyes and blepharospasm; pain and discomfort are not uncommon, especially with disease progression. Its diagnosis is confirmed by typical findings on examination and increased intraocular pressure.

Secondary glaucoma may occur in older children because of trauma, following cataract surgery or in association with vascular and ocular malformations such as Sturge–Weber syndrome.

Headache attributed to glaucoma in adult patients is defined by the IHS (Table 24.2), but there are no comparable paediatric criteria.

The treatment of glaucoma is primarily a surgical procedure to allow flow or reduce production of the aqueous fluid.

ERRORS OF REFRACTION

A relationship between headache and errors of refraction has been long suspected but never been established. Patients and parents associate headache with visual impairment, and it is not uncommon for children to visit an optician and have their eyesight checked before seeking medical advice for headache. Therefore, medical practitioners in primary care and hospital practice usually see children who have already attended an optician and have either been found to have normal eyesight or had their eyesight corrected with glasses but continue to have headaches. In a study of the public attitude towards causes of headache, 21% of people with headache consulted an eye care practitioner for advice, whereas 28% consulted a general medical practitioner and only 8% visited a pharmacist (Thomas et al 2004).

TABLE 24.3

**Headache attributed to errors of refraction (Headache Classification
Subcommittee of the International Headache Society 2004)**

(A) Recurrent mild headache, frontal and in the eyes themselves fulfilling criteria C and D

(B) Uncorrected or miscorrected refractive error (hyperopia, astigmatism, presbyopia, wearing incorrect glasses)

(C) Headache and eye pain first develop in close temporal relation to refractive error, are absent on awakening and are aggravated by prolonged visual tasks at the distance or angle where vision is impaired

(D) Headache and eye pain resolve within 7d and do not recur after full correction of the refractive error

Errors of refraction are common in children. In a population-based study in the UK, the prevalence of refractive astigmatism was 24% in children between 6 and 7 years of age and 20% in those between 12 and 13 years. Furthermore, the prevalence of refractive astigmatism was associated with increasing myopia and hyperopia (O'Donoghue et al 2011). Headache is also common in children, as shown in previous chapters, and therefore many children who have errors of refraction may also suffer from primary headache disorders (migraine or tension-type headache). Apart from a temporary relief after starting to wear glasses, the headache disorder may recur and continue for a long time.

In a study of children between 8 and 18 years of age, errors of refraction were significantly more common among a group of 310 children with primary headache (odds ratio 1.57; 95% confidence interval 1.18–2.07) than in a group of 843 healthy control children (Akinci et al 2008). A cross-sectional study of 487 children (aged 11–13y) showed that the prevalence of both habitual errors of refraction and headache complaints is relatively high. Headache was statistically associated with the sphere component of habitual errors of refraction in females and with the cylinder component of habitual errors of refraction in males, but habitual errors of refraction were shown to play only a small part in the causation of headache (Hendricks et al 2007). The correlation between migraine headache and errors of refraction was assessed in young people in a single-blind study. A statistically higher prevalence of uncorrected astigmatism was found in the migraine group than in the group of healthy individuals. Unfortunately, this study, like many others, did not assess the effects of the correction of errors of refraction on migraine severity or frequency (Harle and Evans 2006).

The cause of headache in children with refractive errors is assumed to be increased muscle tension as the child attempts to overcome his or her blurred vision by straining the ocular and pericranial muscles in order to achieve a better focus. The characteristics of headache attributed to errors of refraction are generally those of a mild headache with no associated sensory or gastrointestinal symptoms and the diagnosis is based on the IHS clinical criteria (Table 24.3), which are not specific for children, but serve as a good guide. The clinical features consist of mild headache with diurnal variation that is relieved by eye rest. It responds to or resolves completely following appropriate correction of the vision.

Headache attributed to jaw and dental disorders

Dental caries and infection are common in children. Dental pain is therefore a common occurrence and in most cases presents acutely. Chronic dental pain is less common and may cause referred pain similar to chronic headache. In general, pain due to teeth disorders is a localised toothache or facial pain. It is associated with teeth sensitivity or increased pain on contact with food or hot or cold liquid drinks. The pain resolves after appropriate treatment of the dental disorders. Headache in association with dental disease is usually non-specific, dull in nature and may be associated with nausea and loss of appetite. Headache responds to treatment with simple pain killers and resolves after appropriate treatment of the underlying cause.

The criteria for the diagnosis of headache attributed to dental disorders are presented in Table 24.4.

Headache attributed to temporomandibular joint dysfunction

The epidemiology and prevalence of temporomandibular joint (TMJ) disease in children is not known, but it is generally a rare problem. The most common causes of TMJ dysfunction in the paediatric population are joint trauma and neuromuscular disorders manifesting with joint hypermobility or muscular spasms. The condition can be aggravated by dental malocclusion and excessive chewing (use of chewing gum). Arthritis involving the TMJ is rare in children.

The clinical features of TMJ dysfunction may include localised or referred pain, difficulty in fully opening the mouth, jaw lock or click on mouth opening, and difficulty in chewing. It is associated with tenderness over the TMJ below the ears and the muscles of mastication. The pain is commonly unilateral and does not cross the midline.

The associated or secondary headache is often mild and can be precipitated by jaw movement and chewing. The clinical criteria for the diagnosis are presented in Table 24.5.

Treatment of TMJ dysfunction equates to the treatment of the underlying cause. In the absence of any demonstrable TMJ disease on laboratory and radiological investigations, treatment with simple painkillers is usually sufficient to relieve the TMJ pain and the associated headache. The headache tends to improve, and in the majority of cases the headache is self-limiting.

TABLE 24.4

Criteria for the diagnosis of headache attributed to dental disorders (Headache Classification Subcommittee of the International Headache Society 2004)

(A) Headache accompanied by pain in the teeth and/or jaw and fulfilling criteria C and D

(B) Evidence of disorder of the teeth, jaws or related structure

(C) Headache and pain in teeth and/or jaw develop in close temporal relation to the disorder

(D) Headache and pain in teeth and/or jaw resolve within 3mo of successful treatment of the disorder

TABLE 24.5

IHS clinical criteria for the diagnosis of headache attributed to TMJ dysfunction
(Headache Classification Subcommittee of the International Headache Society 2004)

(A) Recurrent pain in one or more regions of the head and/or face fulfilling criteria C and D

(B) Radiography, MRI and/or bone scintigraphy demonstrate TMJ disorder

(C) Evidence that pain can be attributed to the TMJ disorder based on at least one of the following:

    (1) Pain is precipitated by jaw movement and/or chewing of hard or tough food

    (2) Reduced range of or irregular jaw opening

    (3) Noise from one or both TMJs during jaw movements

    (4) Tenderness of the joint capsule(s) of one or both TMJs

(D) Headache resolves within 3mo and does not recur after successful treatment of the TMJ disorder

IHS, International Headache Society; TMJ, temporomandibular joint.

REFERENCES

Akinci A, Güven A, Degerliyurt A, Kibar E, Mutlu M, Citirik M (2008) The correlation between headache and refractive errors, *J AAPOS* 12: 290–3. http://dx.doi.org/10.1016/j.jaapos.2007.11.018

Diamond ML (2002) The role of concomitant headache types and non-headache co-morbidities in the under-diagnosis of migraine. *Neurology* 58(Suppl 6): S3–9. http://dx.doi.org/10.1212/WNL.58.9_suppl_6.S3

Harle DE, Evans BJW (2006) The correlation between migraine headache and refractive errors. *Optom Vis Sci* 83: 82–7. http://dx.doi.org/10.1097/01.opx.0000200680.95968.3e

Headache Classification Subcommittee of the International Headache Society. (2004) The international classification of headache disorders. 2nd ed. *Cephalalgia* 24(Suppl 1): 1–52.

Hendricks TJW, De Brabander J, Van Der Horst FG, Hendrikse F, Knottenrus JA (2007) Relationship between habitual refractive errors and headache complaints in schoolchildre. *Optom Vis Sci* 84: 137–43. http://dx.doi.org/10.1097/OPX.0b013e318031b649

Mellis C (2007) Rhinitis. In: McIntosh N, Helms P, Smyth R, Logan S, editors. *Forfar and Arneil's Textbook of Pediatrics*, 7th edn. Edinburgh: Churchill Livingstone Elsevier, p. 1193.

O'Donoghue L, Rudnicka AR, McClelland JF, Logan NS, Owen CG, Saunders KJ (2011) Refractive and corneal astigmatism in white school children in northern Ireland. *Invest Ophthalmol Vis Sci* 52: 4048–53. http://dx.doi.org/10.1167/iovs.10-6100

Senbil N, Gurer YYK, Uner C, Barut Y (2008) Sinusitis in children and adolescents with chronic or recurrent headache: a case–control study. *J Headache Pain* 9: 33–6. http://dx.doi.org/10.1007/s10194-008-0007-0

Thomas E, Boardman HF, Ogden H, Millson DS, Croft PR (2004) Advice and care for headaches: who seeks it, who gives it? *Cephalalgia* 24: 740–52. http://dx.doi.org/10.1111/j.1468-2982.2004.00751.x

25
CHRONIC POST-TRAUMATIC HEADACHE

Ishaq Abu-Arafeh

Introduction

Head injuries, regardless of their severity, are major events in a child's life and they stay in parents' memories for a long time. Also, chronic headache is unpleasant, is distressing to the child and provokes anxiety in parents. When the onset of chronic headache is within a short period of time after an injury to the head, it is inevitable that the two events are linked and related to each other. In these situations parents and children are often worried about the possibility of an ongoing brain lesion or the presence of unresolved bleeding, despite the fact that most of these children would have had brain imaging soon after the injury, and their clinical history and examination are normal.

It is not unreasonable in these circumstances to associate the head injury with the development of headache and give the condition a name that would attribute the headache to head trauma. The headache is therefore, by definition, a secondary headache, but commonly it carries all the characteristics of a primary headache, such as those of migraine or tension-type headache. However, the main distinguishing factor for chronic post-traumatic headache (CPTH) is its temporal relationship with head trauma.

Acute post-traumatic (PTH) headache was defined, by the International Headache Society (IHS) in 1988, to start *within 14 days of injury* and resolve completely within 3 months, whereas CPTH continues beyond 3 months from the time of head injury (Headache Classification Committee of the International Headache Society 1988). The onset of PTH was changed to *within 1 week of the head injury* in the second edition of the International Classification of Headache Disorders (ICHD-II; Headache Classification Subcommittee of the International Headache Society 2004).

Moderate to severe head injuries are more likely than minor head injuries to result in neurological and psychological complications and long-term impact. However, there is no evidence to suggest that the prevalence or clinical features of CPTH are influenced by the nature of the injury or its severity.

Classification of head injuries

Mild or minor head injury is often caused by a blunt impact trauma, such as contact sports, low-level falls, playground accidents and assaults. Minor head injuries are not associated with bony fractures, open wounds or scalp laceration. There is a brief (<30min) or no loss

TABLE 25.1

Criteria for the diagnosis of mild and moderate to severe head injury as defined by ICHD-II (Headache Classification Subcommittee of the International Headache Society 2004)

Head injury is considered mild in the presence of the following:

    No loss of consciousness or loss of consciousness for ≤30min

    Glasgow Coma Scale score 13–15

    No post-traumatic amnesia of >24h in duration

    No altered level of awareness of >24h in duration

    Normal brain imaging (if done)

    At least one of the following as evidence of brain injury

        Transient confusion, disorientation or impaired consciousness

        Transient loss of memory for events immediately before or after injury

        Other transient neurological deficits such as focal weakness, numbness, ataxia, dysphasia

Head injury is considered moderate to severe in the presence of at least one of the following:

    Loss of consciousness >30min

    Glasgow Coma Scale score <13

    Post-traumatic amnesia lasting >24h

    Alteration in level of awareness >24h

    Imaging evidence for a traumatic head injury (e.g. bony fracture, intracranial haemorrhage, brain contusion)

of consciousness. Patients may have symptoms of mild concussion and usually make a full recovery (Table 25.1).

Moderate and severe head injuries are often caused by falls from height, road traffic accidents and blast injuries. Patients often lose consciousness for more than 30 minutes and have a prolonged period of amnesia. Neuroimaging may show evidence of bony or soft tissue injuries (Table 25.1).

Criteria for the diagnosis of post-traumatic headache

Post-traumatic headache is a recognised category of secondary headache and is fully described in the IHS's classification and diagnosis of headache disorders of 1988 and the second edition, ICHD-II, of 2004. The definition of CPTH will be further developed in the third edition, to be published in the near future. There is no specific definition for PTH in children, but there is no reason to believe that the definition of PTH in adults should not apply equally to children and adolescents. The IHS's criteria for the diagnosis of CPTH are presented in Table 25.2.

Epidemiology of chronic post-traumatic headache

Head injuries are common in children and probably more common than the official statistics show, as many children with minor head injuries may be looked after at home or in primary care and do not reach hospital departments from which most statistics are collected. In the UK, around 280 in every 100 000 children are admitted to a hospital emergency department

TABLE 25.2

Criteria for the diagnosis of chronic post-traumatic headache due to minor head injury

(A) Headache of any type, fulfilling criteria C and D

(B) Definition of mild head injury as given in Table 25.1

(C) Evidence of causation is shown by headache that is reported to have developed

  (1) Within 7d of head trauma or

  (2) After regaining consciousness or

  (3) After discontinuation of medications that impair the ability of the patient to report or sense headache

(D) Headache persists for >3mo after head trauma

(E) Headache is not better accounted for by another headache diagnosis

every year with head injury, of which the vast majority (>80%) are minor head injuries, 10% moderate, 6% severe and less than 1% fatal. Males are more prone to head injuries than females in a 2:1 ratio (Hawley et al 2003).

The risk of CPTH, as defined by the IHS, in children and adolescents after head injury was shown in a recent prospective observational study of children, who were admitted to a paediatric unit in Scotland with head injury, to be 6.8% (95% confidence interval 3.0–13.0%) (Kirk et al 2008). It has also been shown that the incidence of head injury in the same childhood population is around 300 per 100 000 per year; thus, the estimated incidence of CPTH in the childhood population is around 20.4 per 100 000 children.

A lower prevalence (3.2%) of CPTH was noted in a large multicentre study in Italy of 1656 children after mild to moderate head injury (Moscato et al 2005). The study used the same definition of CPTH, but excluded children with severe head injuries. A higher prevalence was reported in an earlier study of 129 children, in which CPTH was reported in 18.6% of children immediately after the head injury, in 13.5% 2 months after the injury, in 22.6% 6 months after injury, and in 23.2% 1 year after injury (Lanser et al 1988). The findings in this study, although interesting, are difficult to interpret as they are not consistent with the current IHS definition of CPTH.

Aetiology and pathophysiology of chronic post-traumatic headache

The majority of children do not develop chronic headache after head injury. It is therefore very likely that those who do develop headache after head trauma have a genetic predisposition and the head injury serves as a trigger factor. This hypothesis is further supported by the nature of CPTH, which would fit with the clinical diagnosis of tension-type headache or migraine. It is likely that mild head trauma in predisposed individuals sets off a pathophysiological process that leads to initiation of repeated attacks of headache.

The exact cause of PTH remains unknown. Several neuroimaging techniques and functional brain studies have been described to illustrate the anatomical and biochemical changes in the brain after severe as well as minor head injuries, which may help in better understanding the mechanisms that lead to headache.

Following severe and mild head injuries, shearing forces and direct brain injuries may result in diffuse axonal disruption. Other changes may follow axonal injury, including abnormal cerebral haemodynamics, abnormal release of neurotransmitters such as glutamate, increase in extracellular potassium or intracellular sodium or calcium, and accumulation of serotonin (Packard and Ham 1997, Ramadan and Lainez 2006). These mechanisms of initiation of pain are similar but not exclusive to changes seen in primary headaches.

The cause of the chronicity of the headache after head injury is also unknown. It may be related to the above-described pathophysiological processes, but it may also be a consequence of a change in a patient's lifestyle following injury and possibly due to analgesia overuse.

Clinical presentation of chronic post-traumatic headache

Case study

Omar is a 10-year-old male who attended the clinic because of headache. His headaches started 3 months earlier after he sustained a head injury while playing rugby at school. He did not lose consciousness, but a skull radiograph showed a linear non-depressed fracture. He did not require any treatment and was discharged home after observation on the children's ward for 24 hours. A few days after the injury, he started to complain of headaches. The headaches occurred almost every day for 6 to 8 weeks before reducing in frequency to 2 or 3 times per week. Each attack lasted for about 2 hours. The pain was maximal over the forehead and felt dull in quality. The pain was severe enough to stop some but not all activities. During attacks he felt off his food, but there was no nausea, vomiting or light intolerance. He complained of noise intolerance during some attacks. Between headache attacks he was back to his normal self.

Omar's parents are separated. His father suffers from migraine, but his mother and his two sisters do not.

A diagnosis of post-traumatic, frequent, episodic, tension-type headache was made. Omar and his family were given reassurances regarding the benign nature of the condition. He was advised to take paracetamol (acetaminophen) at a dose of 500mg as required, but to avoid taking it on more than 2 days per week.

Omar responded well to treatment and his headache reduced further in frequency. On review 6 months later his headaches were occurring only occasionally and he did not need to take paracetamol (acetaminophen) for a few months.

Chronic post-traumatic headache is more common in males than in females, which is probably a reflection of the higher prevalence of head trauma and other accidental injuries in males than in females, rather than the likelihood of developing CPTH after injury. In addition, the age at onset of CPTH is consistent with the age at which children are active and most prone to accidents.

Patients with CPTH usually present several months after the head injury. Patients and parents, seemingly, do not find it unusual to have headache immediately after head trauma, but they become alarmed when the headache has not resolved after a few months, and that is when they seek medical advice. In more than 80% of cases the head injury is mild and the headache starts within a week of the injury, as per definition. The frequency and duration of attacks are variable and the clinical picture is often that of migraine without aura or tension-type headache, but other types of primary headache may also be present. In a series of 21 children seen in an outpatient clinic, 13 children had tension-type headache (seven chronic and six episodic), five children had migraine (four without and one with aura) and three children had mixed types of headache (Callaghan and Abu-Arafeh 2001).

The cause of the relatively high prevalence of chronic tension-type headache (CTTH; headache occurring ≥15d/mo for ≥3mo) among children with CPTH is not clear. It may be related to the post-traumatic pathophysiological changes in the brain, but it could also be a result of analgesia overuse following trauma. Children with CTTH may pose a special concern to parents and clinicians because of the high frequency of attacks, almost daily, and further investigations may be carried out, including repeat neuroimaging. However, once the clinical diagnosis of CPTH is made, the clinician will be able to reassure the child and his or her parents about the benign nature of the condition.

Although in some children the course of the headache disorder may become protracted over several years, it is not unusual for headaches to resolve completely within 6 months, as seen in a prospective study recently (Kirk et al 2008).

In some patients, CPTH may be part of a wider clinical presentation of post-traumatic stress syndrome, and other symptoms such as dizziness, fatigue, reduced ability to concentrate, psychomotor slowing, mild memory problems, insomnia, anxiety, personality changes and irritability may complicate the picture.

Management of chronic post-traumatic headache

The diagnosis of CPTH is usually made on the basis of the clinical history of a primary headache associated with a normal physical and neurological examination. Only occasionally are investigations necessary, and neuroimaging is unlikely to reveal unexpected abnormalities that may require neurosurgical intervention. However, neuroimaging may be necessary at times to alleviate parental anxiety, and MRI is the investigation of choice, as it has a better resolution than CT and poses no radiation risk. A limiting factor of MRI is the need for the child to lie still for at least 10 minutes in a strange environment, and therefore general anaesthesia may be necessary for young children.

Reassurance about the benign course of the disease is essential in order to help parents and children cope with the distress of headache and also to comply with treatment and advice. Simple analgesia such as paracetamol (acetaminophen) or ibuprofen should be given as necessary and with caution in order to avoid analgesia overuse headache, but when used it should be in appropriate dosages.

The specific management of this type of headache will follow the same lines as in migraine and tension-type headache, described in the relevant chapters, including the need for migraine-preventative medications or pain-modulating agents.

Psychological help and support may be necessary in some patients, especially those who may have also suffered from added symptoms of post-traumatic stress syndrome and those who have lost a large number of school days owing to the headache.

Prognosis

Population-based studies of CPTH suggest a good prognosis. A prospective study of unselected children with head injury for CPTH showed an excellent outcome and prognosis. Headache resolved in all children within 3 to 27 months (mean 13mo) (Kirk et al 2008).

Children seen at specialist clinics may represent a group of children with a severe or prolonged course of CPTH and may have a different prognosis. In a study of 21 children with CPTH, followed up for a period of 5 to 29 months (mean 12.5mo, median 9mo), symptoms resolved completely in only two children. Other children's headaches were well controlled with appropriate advice and treatment (Callaghan and Abu-Arafeh 2001).

REFERENCES

Callaghan M, Abu-Arafeh I (2001) Chronic posttraumatic headache in children and adolescents. *Dev Med Child Neurol* 43: 819–22. http://dx.doi.org/10.1017/S0012162201001487

Hawley CA, Ward AB, Long J, Owen DW, Magnay AR (2003) Prevalence of traumatic brain injury amongst children admitted to hospital in one health district: a population-based study. *Injury* 34: 256–60. http://dx.doi.org/10.1016/S0020-1383(02)00193-6

Headache Classification Committee of the International Headache Society (1988) Classification and diagnostic criteria for headache disorders, cranial neuralgias and facial pain. *Cephalalgia* 8(Suppl 7): 1–96.

Headache Classification Subcommittee of the International Headache Society (2004) The international classification of headache disorders. 2nd ed. *Cephalalgia* 24(Suppl 1): 1–52.

Kirk C, Nagiub G, Abu-Arafeh I (2008) Chronic posttraumatic headache in children and adolescents after head injury. *Dev Med Child Neurol* 50: 422–5. http://dx.doi.org/10.1111/j.1469-8749.2008.02063.x

Lanser JBK, Jennekens-Schinkel A, Peters ACB (1988) Headache after closed head injury in children. *Headache* 28: 176–9. http://dx.doi.org/10.1111/j.1526-4610.1988.hed2803176.x

Moscato D, Peracchi MI, Mazzotta G, Savi L, Battistella PA (2005) Posttraumatic headache from moderate head injury. *J Headache Pain* 6: 284–6. http://dx.doi.org/10.1007/s10194-005-0208-8

Packard RC, Ham LP (1997) Pathogenesis of posttraumatic headache and migraine: a common headache pathway? *Headache* 37: 142–52. http://dx.doi.org/10.1046/j.1526-4610.1997.3703142.x

Ramadan NM, Lainez MJA (2006) Chronic posttraumatic headache. In: Olesen J, Goadsby PJ, Ramadan NM, Tfelt-Hansen P, Welch KMA, editors. *The Headaches, 3rd edition.* Philadelphia: Lippincott Williams & Wilkins, pp. 873–7.

26
PSYCHOLOGICAL ASPECTS OF CHILDHOOD HEADACHE

Amanda Rach and Frank Andrasik

Not only are headaches one of the leading causes of pain in children and adolescents, but their incidence has also increased substantially over the last 30 years (Ozge et al 2011). Researchers attribute the rise to untoward lifestyle changes, especially increasing levels of chronic stress, which are consistently shown to contribute to paediatric headache development (Passchier and Orlebeke 1985, Larsson 1988, Carlsson 1996, Carlsson et al 1996, Bjorling 2009, Ozge et al 2011). For example, an electronic diary study by Connelly and Bickel (2011) found that changes in the intensity level of daily stressors reliably triggered headaches and less than typical sleep quantity predicted headache occurrence. Thus, as child and adolescent environments become more taxing, as a result of school demands, hectic activity schedules and chaotic home situations, incidence rates will probably continue to rise.

The increasing incidence rates are alarming as the negative effects of paediatric headache reach well beyond the immediate pain experience, and unfortunately these associated consequences are often underestimated. Research shows that headaches significantly impair a child's psychosocial adaptation and lead to deteriorated school functioning, increased absenteeism, more school problems, more time needed to finish homework, more after-school exhaustion and reduced participation in leisure activities (Smith et al 1999, Grazzi et al 2004, Kroner-Herwig et al 2007, Karwautz et al 2008). Further, children who experience frequent headaches are at increased risk of developing chronic headaches in adulthood, as discovered by Bille's seminal work, which initially centred on a cohort of 9000 Swedish schoolchildren (Bille 1962). He was able to follow a small subset of these children, all of whom had migraine prior to the age of 6, for several decades and found that the majority of them continued to experience migraines (Bille 1997).

Prevalence rates
Paediatric headache prevalence rates vary by the source, age and sex of the sample, as well as the diagnostic criteria used to classify patients (see Chapter 6).

Longitudinal work with paediatric headache sufferers found that, after four decades, 60% of children continued to experience migraine headaches well into adulthood (Bille 1962, 1997). Additional studies suggest that a considerable proportion of children experience different types of headaches over time, with others concluding that children may experience complete remission with increasing age (Dooley and Bagnell 1995, Guidetti and Galli 1998, Mazzotta et al 1999). For example, Guidetti and Galli (1998) found that, after 8 years' follow-up, 45% of their sample had improved, with 34% being headache free. Some researchers believe that the high transition rates between headache types – in 25% of children, migraine will evolve into tension-type headache (TTH) and in 10% TTH will evolve into migraine – suggest that the diagnoses are related or are extremes of the same disease spectrum (Featherstone 1985, Dooley and Bagnell 1995, Guidetti and Galli 1998). Unfortunately, information regarding the factors that influence the headache trajectory is sparse. A 20-year follow-up study found that those diagnosed with TTH were more likely to be headache free at follow-up (Brna et al 2005). In contrast, two studies spanning 3 and 8 years found that children initially diagnosed with TTH were less likely to experience a remission and more likely to switch headache type to migraine (Guidetti and Galli 1998, Laurell et al 2006). The same study found vomiting and a headache frequency of at least once per week to be the most persisting symptoms, with few children suffering from these symptoms becoming headache free (Laurell et al 2006). Finally, researchers suggest that the initial headache diagnosis is less important in predicting adult headache than headache severity. Research by Brna and colleagues found that patients with mild headaches were more likely to be headache free in adulthood than those with moderate or severe headache (Brna et al 2005). This is also similar to what Bille found when he compared a group of average with severe migraine sufferers. Although after 6 years 51% of the group who suffered migraine of average severity and 34% of those with pronounced migraine had been headache free for at least 1 year, after 16 years 22% of children with pronounced migraine relapsed after an average of 6 migraine-free years (Bille 1962).

The presence of comorbid conditions has been shown to increase the likelihood of headaches continuing over time. Guidetti et al (1998) followed 100 headache patients (migraine and TTH), first seen in late adolescence, for 8 years, to determine if comorbid conditions had a bearing on headache course. At the start of the investigation, patients were divided into two groups: those who had headache alone and those whose headaches were accompanied by two or more comorbid conditions. At the 8-year follow-up, patients were classified into one of three groups: headaches the same or worse, headaches improved or headache free. As Table 26.1 shows, headache sufferers with multiple comorbid conditions fared poorly over the intervening period. Recent studies with adult headache sufferers reveal that experiencing any of a number of adverse events during childhood (e.g. emotional, physical or sexual abuse, witnessing domestic violence, substance use) increases the frequency of headaches in adulthood (Anda et al 2010, Tietjen and Peterlin 2011).

Although prevalence rates of paediatric headaches are high, the presence of headaches does not automatically imply a high level of suffering as a result (Kroner-Herwig 2011).

TABLE 26.1
Eight-year follow-up of late-adolescent headache sufferers (from Guidetti et al 1998)

Comorbid disorder	Same or worse	Improved	Headache free
Two or more	57%	29%	14%
None	7%	53%	40%

Epidemiological studies suggest that only approximately 5% of children and adolescents are moderately or severely impaired by their headaches (Kroner-Herwig 2011). However, the degree of suffering varies significantly depending on where the data were collected. For example, Hershey and colleagues (2004) found that nearly 50% of children from a clinical sample reported being moderately or severely disabled as a result of their headaches. Thus, in the population at large, few children experience significant consequences, but nearly half of all children whose headaches are severe enough to seek healthcare services suffer significantly.

Psychological factors associated with paediatric headache
Different risk factors are responsible for paediatric migraine and TTH development. Migraine attacks are associated with academic stressors, such as amount of homework or examinations (Larsson 1988, Bener et al 2000), whereas TTHs are more often associated with interpersonal difficulties, such as hostile relationships and increased levels of social stress (Battistutta et al 2009, Ozge et al 2011). Children and adolescents with fewer peer relations, divorced parents or an unhappy family atmosphere are at a greater risk for TTH (Ozge et al 2011). Further, parents of adolescents with chronic TTH report their children to have more peer group diff- iculties than adolescents who do not suffer from TTH (Battistutta et al 2009). With regards to the frequency of paediatric headache, family quarrelling, school stress and a fear of failure, family financial burden and number of friends significantly predict both migraine and TTH in children (Kroner-Herwig et al 2007). Paediatric migraine and TTH also impact upon chil- dren differently. Severe migraine attacks are associated with higher levels of disability, cause greater school absenteeism, and are more socially disabling (Fuh et al 2009, Guidetti et al 2002, Laurell et al 2005). TTHs can cause significant psychosocial consequences, particularly for females (Guidetti et al 2002, Laurell et al 2005).

Compared with children without headaches, children with headaches and their parents report more psychosocial problems, higher levels of psychological disorders (anxiety and depression) and more somatic complaints (Andrasik et al 1988, Just et al 2003, Laurell et al 2005, Mazzone et al 2006, Pakalnis et al 2007, Battistutta et al 2009). Additionally, depression, anxiety and anxiety sensitivity have all been found to predict headache frequency (Kroner-Herwig et al 2007). These findings suggest that the relationship between paediatric headaches and psychological symptoms is bidirectional and most likely reciprocal in nature (Kroner-Herwig et al 2007). Thus, psychological treatments that assist children and adoles- cents to develop more effective ways to deal with everyday life stressors are the ideal treatment approach for this population (Larsson and Stinson 2011). Additionally, research suggests that free time for playing is a robust protective factor when it comes to paediatric headache (Kroner- Herwig et al 2007). Spending time pursuing unstructured play is associated with a lower prob- ability of headache, especially in comparison with time spent doing cognitive/artistic hobbies and physical activities (Kroner-Herwig et al 2007). Moreover, female headache patients report higher levels of anxiety and depression than males (Pakalnis et al 2007).

It is important to note that, although children and adolescents with headache have more psychological symptoms, these levels do not typically fall within the pathological range. Early work in the area by Andrasik and colleagues found that all patient groups scored within normal limits on a range of assessments measuring depression, anxiety, somatic complaints and adjustment (Andrasik et al 1988), as have others (Cunningham et al 1987). These basic findings were replicated years later in a comparison study examining the relationship between migraine and depression and anxiety (Ozge et al 2011). These authors again found slightly higher scores on at least one of the anxiety or depression scales in headache patients than in control groups, but not elevated to a clinically significant degree overall.

Headache assessment

Paediatric headache assessment, like assessment of all individuals presenting with head-aches, should not begin until a complete medical evaluation has ruled out the presence of acute medical conditions or disease states (Andrasik et al 2011). A good clinical interview needs to include both the child and the parents and thoroughly assess medical history, family relationships and lifestyle factors (sleep, diet and eating patterns, exercise, caffeine intake, hydration, school performance and attendance, smoking, and the use of alcohol or illicit drugs) (Lay and Broner 2008). Assessment of psychological factors, such as depression, anxiety and self-esteem, is also important, with scales such as the Child Behaviour Checklist (Ozge et al 2011) or more recent instruments developed by Achenbach (*The Achenbach System of Empirically Based Assessment*, available at: http://www.aseba.org/) useful for this purpose (Ozge et al 2011). Adolescent patients should also be interviewed alone (Lay and Broner 2008). We recommend interviewing the adolescent first, to show the importance of his or her input and to help establish a good working therapeutic relationship, followed by an interview with the parent(s), bringing all back together for a feedback conference and discussion of conflicting reports.

When assessing headache dimensions, headache severity should be quantified using a pain rating scale, visual analogue scale (VAS) or other equivalent scale according to the age and cognitive level of the patient (Ozge et al 2011). When patients are asked to describe the quality of their pain, they may use metaphors or descriptive words, which provide valuable clues regarding headache subtype and aetiology. Sometimes children and adolescents may be better able to express their pain experience through drawings – see Chapter 31 (Unruh et al 1983, Stafstrom et al 2005, Wojaczynska-Stanek et al 2008, Andrasik et al 2011).

As large discrepancies have been found between child and parent interviews and the daily diary report of headache parameters, it is imperative to have patients complete a headache diary for several weeks, and even longer if a clear picture does not emerge (Andrasik et al 1985). This is a simple and useful way to gain a more complete and accurate picture of the patient's health, functioning and quality of life – see the appendix at the end of Chapter 30 (Andrasik et al 2005). Diaries may include headache frequency, severity (rated on a scale from 0 to 10) and duration, presence of aura or focal neurological symptoms and medications taken, associated features, mood ratings, life events, and other potential triggers or exacerbators of interest (Andrasik et al 2011). It may also be useful to include information about diet and sleep patterns (Andrasik et al 2011). Recordings can be made at predetermined points (wake-up/breakfast, lunch, dinner and bedtime) or a single reading can be taken that represents the entire day (Richardson et al 1983, Andrasik et al 2011).

Healthcare providers who work with paediatric headache sufferers should not view children and adolescents simply as small adults (Powers and Andrasik 2005, Andrasik and

Schwartz 2006). Level of cognitive development greatly influences individuals' ability to understand their illness (Marcon and Labbé 1990), and, specific to paediatric headaches, children have a highly limited understanding of the function of pain (Galli et al 2002). Further, one's conceptualisation of pain is known to shift from highly concrete to increasingly abstract with age (Galli et al 2002). These factors have a direct bearing on treatment efforts (McGrath et al 2001). As such, children and adolescents with headaches should receive treatment from healthcare providers with specialised training with this population as they have unique medical, psychological, family and educational presentations and needs (Powers and Andrasik 2005, Andrasik and Schwartz 2006).

Instruments
General pain assessment instruments can be used to measure paediatric headache – see Chapter 7 (Hershey 2011). To date, only one instrument has been designed specifically for this population. The PedMIDAS is an adapted version of the Migraine Disability Assessment Questionnaire (MIDAS) (Hershey et al 2001, 2004), an adult tool used in both research and practice settings. The PedMIDAS is a six-item questionnaire assessing functional impairment and burden in the past 3 months at school, at home and during sport and social activities, the need for preventative medication and the response to treatment.

Quality of life measures are also commonly used to assess paediatric headache. To focus solely on pain intensity fails to capture the various ways headache impacts on an individual's functioning. The Quality of Life in Youth (QoL-Y) is a self-administered questionnaire to assess psychological, physical and social functioning and functional status in children aged 12 to 18 (Langeveld et al 1996). Additionally, the Pediatric Quality of Life 4.0 (PedsQL4.0) is one of the most widely used tools for the assessment of quality of life in children and adolescents and addresses the quality of life in a disease-independent manner (Varni et al 2003, Connelly and Rapoff 2006).

Psychological treatment modalities
Psychological interventions designed to treat paediatric headaches do not differ largely between headache types (Kroner-Herwig 2011). Meta-analytical reviews conclude that psychological treatments effectively reduce both the severity and the frequency of paediatric headaches, even in patients younger than 12 (Eccleston et al 2003, Cvengros et al 2007, Palermo et al 2010), with little evidence for differential efficacy between treatment types (Kroner-Herwig 2011). Between 65% and 100% of children with migraine undergoing biofeedback, relaxation or a combination show clinically significant reductions in headache frequency, and between 50% and 85% of children with TTH are known to achieve significant symptom reduction (Cvengros et al 2007). Meta-analyses to date have shown psychologically based and pharmacologically based treatments to have equivalent effects (Hermann et al 1995, Hermann and Blanchard 2002).

The most efficacious psychological treatments in paediatric headache are biofeedback, relaxation training and cognitive–behavioural therapies, which are discussed in brief below and summarised in Table 26.2.

TABLE 26.2

Main features of common psychological treatments for paediatric headaches

Treatment	Features
Relaxation training	In relaxation training the patient concentrates on feelings of tension and is taught how to relax specific muscle groups (extremities, head, shoulders and back) in a step-by-step manner. Training is designed to improve body awareness, reduce general level of arousal and prevent and alleviate the general stress response, which is believed to contribute to headache. A child-adapted 'progressive relaxation' format is often used (Larsson and Andrasik 2002, Kroner-Herwig 2011)
Biofeedback treatment	In biofeedback training, the patient's biological responses are transformed into perceptible signals (visual or auditory) and the patient is taught to modify their physiological state in a way that prevents or alleviates pain (Andrasik et al 1982, Labbé and Williamson 1984, Fentress et al 1986). Biofeedback for the treatment of paediatric headache is most often temperature or electromyography biofeedback, both of which have the objective of inducing a state of relaxation (Andrasik et al 2002, Kroner-Herwig 2011). In general, biofeedback treatments help patients gain voluntary control over bodily functions and enhancement of self-efficacy in dealing with pain episodes (Nestoriuc et al 2008)
Cognitive–behavioural therapy	Cognitive–behavioural therapy for paediatric headache focuses on teaching patients how to monitor their headaches and headache triggers; restructure dysfunctional cognitions and attitudes (decrease catastrophising, ruminations and depressive thoughts); improve coping skills and how to divert attention from pain; and enhance their assertiveness and self-confidence (Richter et al 1986). Most programmes include problem solving and some even educate parents on how not to reinforce their child's pain behaviour and cope with their child's pain (Richter et al 1986, Kroner-Herwig 2011)

In general, research shows that paediatric headache sufferers benefit significantly more than adults from biofeedback treatment (Sarafino and Goehring 2000). Interestingly, the higher treatment success is not accounted for by better biofeedback performance by children (Herman and Blanchard 2002). A meta-analysis of 10 paediatric studies concluded that biofeedback treatment is more effective than relaxation, monitoring or placebo (Nestoriuc et al 2008). Specifically, temperature biofeedback has been proven to be highly successful in alleviating headache activity in children. Using the criterion of at least 50% symptom reduction, two separate studies were able to classify two-thirds of children as treatment successes (Hermann and Blanchard 2002). In addition, electromyographic biofeedback is often the modality of choice for the treatment of TTHs in children (Hermann and Blanchard 2002).

Unlike pharmacological treatment, psychological approaches are not associated with significant side effects, poor medication adherence and the high costs that plague some pharmacological interventions (McGrath et al 2001). However, psychological interventions when routinely implemented are time intensive, can be expensive and often require specialised equipment and training (e.g. biofeedback) (Andrasik 2012). Burke and Andrasik (1989), Guarnieri and Blanchard (1990) and McGrath et al (1992) were among the first to demonstrate that time spent with a therapist could be measurably trimmed back if children with migraine were provided with supplementary training materials to study at home. All of these investigations found that these treatments with more limited contact yielded findings comparable to the more intensive, office-based approaches. This newer approach has variously been referred to as 'reduced', 'minimal' or 'limited' contact or 'home-based', although Andrasik (2012) prefers the term 'prudent limited office treatment', or PLOT, a term first recommended by Schwartz (personal communication). A more recent study by Connelly and colleagues (2006) found a CD-ROM self-management treatment, termed 'Headstrong', which included education, relaxation, thought changing and pain behaviour modification, resulted in greater reductions in headache frequency, duration and intensity than standard medical care (the prior investigations were limited to comparisons of varied forms for delivering psychological treatments only).

When assessing response to treatment, it is important to consider more than pain intensity, despite the fact that intensity is the main efficacy criterion in paediatric headache studies (Trautmann et al 2006). Essential decreases in headache frequency, duration, symptoms and disability may occur and be missed, as demonstrated in a study by Andrasik and colleagues (1985). By comparing child, parent and neurologist reports of post-treatment improvement, researchers found that all parties' VAS scores greatly underestimated improvement when compared with the child's diary report (Andrasik et al 1985). Further, an often ignored but important outcome is treatment satisfaction, from the perspective of both the child and his or her parents. After psychological treatments, children report an increased responsibility for their headache management as a result of an increased ability to cope (Kroner-Herwig 2011). The child then requires less parental support, which leads to substantial parental relief and reduced feelings of helplessness in dealing with their child's pain (Kroner-Herwig 2011).

Role of parents

Parents significantly influence their child's access to both health care and treatment strategies. Their reactions to their child's pain can also influence its course. Utilisation studies find that, despite the substantial burden, adolescents with chronic daily migraines have lower rates of healthcare utilisation than adults (Bigal et al 2008, Blumenfeld et al 2011). Not only do parents regulate their child's access to health care, they have the potential to positively influence treatment efforts. Actively involving parents in treatment makes it possible for them to provide assistance where the problems most frequently occur and allows for preventative rather than only curative efforts (Burke and Andrasik 1989). Allen and McKeen (1991) found that 87% of children who fully completed a home-based migraine treatment protocol experienced at least a 70% reduction in headaches. However, children whose parents failed to complete the protocol did not maintain gains at follow-up.

In a small-scale investigation, Burke and Andrasik (1989) compared biofeedback delivered by therapists to this same treatment administered by parents, who were trained to do so and who conducted most of the training at home. Although Burke and Andrasik (1989) found no difference in treatment response and maintenance at 1-year follow-up, using a cost-effectiveness index the home-based treatment was approximately three times more efficient than the clinical approach. A recent study comparing a group family training programme with an individualised biofeedback programme found that the intensity of headaches was significantly reduced in both groups; however, the family programme was deemed more advantageous because 8 to 10 children could be treated at once, reducing costs while still producing

TABLE 26.3
Pain behaviour management guidelines for parents

Encourage

Independent management of pain: praise and publicly acknowledge practice of self-regulation skills during pain-free episodes. If pain is reported, issue a single prompt to practise self-regulation skills. Praise and reward normal activity when report of pain has been made

Normal activity during pain episodes: insist upon attendance at school, maintenance of daily chores and responsibilities, participation in regular activities (lessons, practices, clubs)

Eliminate status checks: no questions about whether there is pain or how much it hurts

Reduce

Response to pain behaviour: no effort should be made to assist the child in coping. Do not offer assistance or suggestions for coping. Do not offer medications

Pharmacological dependence: If medication is requested, deliver only as prescribed (i.e. follow direct timetable)

Recruit others to follow same guidelines: school personnel should not send child home; child should be encouraged and permitted to practise self-regulation skills in the classroom; workload should not be modified

Treat pain requiring a reduction in activity as illness: If school, activities, chores or responsibilities are missed, the child should be treated as ill and sent to bed for the remainder of the day, *even if pain is resolved*. Do not permit watching television, playing games or special treatment

Compiled from Allen and Shriver (1998).

clinical improvements on par with the evidence-based biofeedback training (Gerber et al 2010). A main advantage to involving parents in treatment efforts is that parents generally know very little about their child's headaches and how their own behaviour may exacerbate their child's pain, as evidenced by the following final study review.

Allen and Shriver (1998) randomly assigned paediatric migraineurs (aged 7–18y) to one of two conditions: thermal biofeedback or thermal biofeedback combined with parent training in behaviour management or how best to respond during headache attacks. These guidelines were based on principles of operant conditioning developed for pain patients long ago by Fordyce (1976) – reinforce well behaviour and ignore illness behaviour. Thus, parents were instructed to minimise reactions to pain behaviour, insist that the child participate in planned activities, and praise and support biofeedback practice and efforts to cope. Parents were provided with specific guidelines to follow (reproduced in Table 26.3), which were reviewed at each session. As revealed in Figure 26.1, adding very specific training for parents led to better outcomes. Mean weekly headache frequency revealed sizeable reductions immediately upon completion of treatment, which continued through the 3-month follow-up, as revealed by diary records. The authors were able to contact the majority of the participants at a 1-year follow-up, but the headache data were collected via telephone report on this measurement occasion, a method that does not always correspond with what is considered the 'criterion standard' measure – daily headache diaries (Andrasik et al 2005). At this data point, differences between conditions were less noticeable. At this time point, 91% of those treated by biofeedback combined with parent training were determined to meet criteria for clinically significant improvement versus

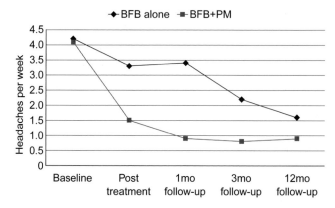

Fig. 26.1 Mean weekly headache frequency for biofeedback alone (BFB alone) versus biofeedback plus parent pain management (BFB+PM) – data from Allen and Shriver (1998).

60% for those receiving biofeedback alone; 45% of those in the combined treatment reported being free of headaches versus 30% for biofeedback alone. Nonetheless, this study illustrates the importance of involving significant others in the psychological management of headaches in children, especially early in the course.

REFERENCES

Allen KD, McKeen LB (1991) Home-based multicomponent treatment of pediatric migraine. *Headache* 31: 467–72. http://dx.doi.org/10.1111/j.1526-4610.1991.hed3107467.x

Allen KD, Shriver MD (1998) Role of parent mediated pain behavior management strategies in biofeedback treatment of childhood migraines. *Behav Ther* 29: 477–90. http://dx.doi.org/10.1016/S0005-7894(98)80044-0

Anda R, Tietjen G, Schulman E, Felitti V, Croft J (2010) Adverse childhood experiences and frequent headaches in adults. *Headache* 50: 1473–81. http://dx.doi.org/10.1111/j.1526-4610.2010.01756.x

Andrasik F (2012) Behavioral treatment of headaches: extending the reach. *Neurol Sci* 33(Suppl 1): 127–30. http://dx.doi.org/10.1007/s10072-012-1073-2

Andrasik F, Schwartz MS (2006) Behavioural assessment and treatment of pediatric headache. *Behav Modif* 30: 91–113. http://dx.doi.org/10.1177/0145445505282164

Andrasik F, Blanchard EB, Edlund SR, Rosenblum EL (1982) Autogenic feedback in the treatment of two children with migraine headache. *Child Fam Behav Ther* 4: 13–23. http://dx.doi.org/10.1300/J019v04n04_02

Andrasik F, Burke EJ, Attanasio V, Rosenblum EL (1985) Child, parent, and physician reports of a child's headache pain: relationships prior to and following treatment. *Headache* 25: 421–5.

Andrasik F, Kabela E, Quinn S, Attanasio V, Blanchard EB, Rosenblum EL (1988) Psychological functioning of children who have recurrent migraine. *Pain* 34: 43–52. http://dx.doi.org/10.1016/0304-3959(88)90180-7

Andrasik F, Larsson B, Grazzi L (2002) Biofeedback treatment of recurrent headaches in children and adolescents. In: Guidetti V, Russell G, Sillanpää M, Winner P , editors. *Headache and Migraine in Childhood and Adolescence*. London: Martin Dunitz Ltd, pp. 317–32.

Andrasik F, Lipchik GL, McCrory DC, Wittrock DA (2005) Outcome measurement in behavioural headache research: headache parameters and psychosocial outcomes. *Headache* 45: 429–37. http://dx.doi.org/10.1111/j.1526-4610.2005.05094.x

Andrasik F, Buse DC, Lettich A (2011) Assessment of headaches. In: Turk D, Melzack R editor. *Handbook of Pain Assessment*. New York: Guilford Press, pp. 354–75.

Battistutta S, Aliverti R, Montico M, Zin R, Carrozzi M (2009) Chronic tension-type headache in adolescents. Clinical and psychological characteristics analyzed through self- and parent-report questionnaires. *J Pediatr Psychol* 34: 697–706. http://dx.doi.org/10.1093/jpepsy/jsn102

Bener A, Uduman SA, Qassimi EM et al (2000) Genetic and environmental factors associated with migraine in schoolchildren. *Headache* 40: 152–7. http://dx.doi.org/10.1046/j.1526-4610.2000.00021.x

Bigal ME, Serrano D, Reed M, Lipton RB (2008) Chronic migraine in the population. Burden, diagnosis, and satisfaction with treatment. *Neurology* 71: 559–66. http://dx.doi.org/10.1212/01.wnl.0000323925.29520.e7

Bille B (1962) Migraine in school children. *Acta Paediatr* 51: 1–151. http://dx.doi.org/10.1111/j.1651-2227.1962.tb06591.x

Bille B (1997) A 40-year follow-up of school children with migraine. *Cephalalgia* 17: 488–91. http://dx.doi.org/10.1046/j.1468-2982.1997.1704488.x

Bjorling EA (2009) The momentary relationship between stress and headaches in adolescent girls. *Headache* 49: 1186–97. http://dx.doi.org/10.1111/j.1526-4610.2009.01406.x

Blumenfeld A, Varon S, Wilcox TK et al (2011) Disability, HRQoL and resource use among chronic and episodic migraineurs: results from the International Burden of Migraine Study (IBMS). *Cephalalgia* 31: 301–15. http://dx.doi.org/10.1177/0333102410381145

Brna P, Dooley J, Gordon K, Dewan T (2005) The prognosis of childhood headache. *Arch Pediatr Adolesc Med* 159: 1157–60. http://dx.doi.org/10.1001/archpedi.159.12.1157

Burke EJ, Andrasik F (1989) Home- vs. clinic-based biofeedback for pediatric migraine: results of treatment through one-year follow-up. *Headache* 29: 434–40. http://dx.doi.org/10.1111/j.1526-4610.1989.hed2907434.x

Carlsson J (1996) Prevalence of headache in schoolchildren: relation to family and school factors. *Acta Pediatr* 85: 692–6. http://dx.doi.org/10.1111/j.1651-2227.1996.tb14128.x

Carlsson J, Larsson B, Marc A (1996) Psychosocial functioning in schoolchildren with recurrent headaches. *Headache* 36: 77–82. http://dx.doi.org/10.1046/j.1526-4610.1996.3602077.x

Connelly M, Bickel J (2011) An electronic daily diary process study of stress and health behavior triggers of primary headaches in children. *J Pediatr Psychol* 36: 852–62. http://dx.doi.org/10.1093/jpepsy/jsr017

Connelly M, Rapoff MA (2006) Assessing health-related quality of life in children with recurrent headache: reliability and validity of the PedsQLTM4.0 in a pediatric headache sample. *J Pediatr Psychol* 31: 698–702. http://dx.doi.org/10.1093/jpepsy/jsj063

Connelly M, Rapoff MA, Thompson N, Connelly W (2006) Headstrong: a pilot study of a CD-ROM intervention for recurrent pediatric headache. *J Pediatr Psychol* 31: 737–47. http://dx.doi.org/10.1093/jpepsy/jsj003

Cunningham SJ, McGrath PJ, Ferguson HB et al (1987) Personality and behavioural characteristics in pediatric migraine. *Headache* 27: 16–20. http://dx.doi.org/10.1111/j.1526-4610.1987.hed2701016.x

Cvengros J, Harper D, Shevell M (2007) Pediatric headache: an examination of process variables in treatment. *J Child Neurol* 22: 1172–81. http://dx.doi.org/10.1177/0883073807305786

Dooley J, Bagnell A (1995) The prognosis and treatment of headaches in children- a ten year follow-up. *Can J Neurol Sci* 22: 47–9.

Eccleston C, Yorke L, Morley S, William AC, Mastroyannopoulou K (2003) Psychological therapies for the management of chronic and recurrent pain in children and adolescents. *Cochrane Database Syst Rev* 1: 1–46.

Featherstone HJ (1985) Migraine and muscle contraction headache: a continuum. *Headache* 25: 194–8. http://dx.doi.org/10.1111/j.1526-4610.1985.hed2504194.x

Fentress DW, Masek BJ, Mehegan JE, Benson H (1986) Biofeedback and relaxation-response training in the treatment of pediatric migraine. *Dev Med Child Neurol* 28: 139–46. http://dx.doi.org/10.1111/j.1469-8749.1986.tb03847.x

Fordyce WE (1976) *Behavioral Methods for Chronic Pain and Illness*. St. Louis: CV Mosby.

Fuh JL, Wang SJ, Lu SR, Laio YC, Chen SP, Yang YC (2009). Headache disability among adolescents: a student population based study. *Headache* 50: 210–18. http://dx.doi.org/10.1111/j.1526-4610.2009.01531.x

Galli F, Guidetti V, Tafa M (2002) Developmental age psychology: elements for general framing of headaches. In Guidetti V, Russell G, Sillanppa M, Winner P, editors. *Headaches and Migraine in Childhood and Adolescence*. London: Martin Dunitz, pp. 445–58.

Gerber WD, Petermann F, Gerber-von Muller G et al (2010). MIPAS-family-evaluation of a new multi-modal behavioral training program for pediatric headaches: clinical effects and the impact on quality of life. *J Headache Pain* 11: 215–25. http://dx.doi.org/10.1007/s10194-010-0192-5

Grazzi L, D'Amico D, Usai S, Solari A, Bussone G (2004) Disability in young patients suffering from primary headaches. *Neurol Sci* 25: 111–22. http://dx.doi.org/10.1007/s10072-004-0265-9

Guarnieri P, Blanchard EB (1990) Evaluation of home-based thermal biofeedback treatment of pediatric migraine headache. *Biofeedback Self Regul* 15: 179–84. http://dx.doi.org/10.1007/BF00999148

Guidetti V, Galli F (1998) Evolution of headache in childhood and adolescence: an 8-year follow-up. *Cephalalgia* 18 : 449–54. http://dx.doi.org/10.1046/j.1468-2982.1998.1807449.x

Guidetti V, Galli F, Fabrizi P et al (1998). Headache and psychiatric comorbidity: clinical aspects and outcome in an 8-year follow-up study. *Cephalalgia* 18, 455–62. http://dx.doi.org/10.1046/j.1468-2982.1998.1807455.x

Guidetti V, Russell G, Sillanpää M, Winner P (2002). *Headache and Migraine in Childhood and Adolescence.* London: Martin Dunitz.

Hermann C, Blanchard EB (2002) Biofeedback in the treatment of headache and other childhood pain. *Appl Psychophysiol Biofeedback* 27: 143–62. http://dx.doi.org/10.1023/A:1016295727345

Hermann C, Kim M, Blanchard EB (1995) Behavioral and prophylactic pharmacological intervention studies of pediatric migraine: an exploratory meta-analysis. *Pain* 60: 239–55. http://dx.doi.org/10.1016/0304-3959(94)00210-6

Hershey A (2011) Current approaches to the diagnosis and management of paediatric migraine. *Lancet* 9: 190–204.

Hershey AD, Powers SW, Vockell AL, LeCates S, Kabbouche MA, Maynard MK (2001) PedMIDAS: development of a questionnaire to assess disability of migraines in children. *Neurology* 57: 2034–9. http://dx.doi.org/10.1212/WNL.57.11.2034

Hershey AD, Powers SW, Vockell AL, LeCates SL, Segers A, Kabbouche MA (2004) Development of a patient-based grading scale for PedMIDAS. *Cephalalgia* 24: 844–9. http://dx.doi.org/10.1111/j.1468-2982.2004.00757.x

Just U, Oelkers R, Bender S et al (2003). Emotional and behavioural problems in children and adolescents with primary headache. *Cephalalgia* 23: 206–13. http://dx.doi.org/10.1046/j.1468-2982.2003.00486.x

Karwautz A, Wober C, Lang T et al (2008). Psychosocial factors in children and adolescents with migraine and tension-type headache: a controlled study and review of the literature. *Cephalalgia* 19: 32–43. http://dx.doi.org/10.1111/j.1468-2982.1999.1901032.x

Kroner-Herwig B (2011) Psychological treatments for pediatric headache. *Expert Rev Neurother* 11: 403–10. http://dx.doi.org/10.1586/ern.11.10

Kroner-Herwig B, Morris L, Heinrich M (2007) Headache in German children and adolescents: a population-based epidemiological study. *Cephalalgia* 27: 519–27. http://dx.doi.org/10.1111/j.1468-2982.2007.01319.x

Labbé EL, Williamson DA (1984) Treatment of childhood migraine using autogenic feedback training. *J Consult Clin Psychol* 52: 968–76. http://dx.doi.org/10.1037/0022-006X.52.6.968

Langeveld JH, Koot HM, Loonen MC, Hazebroek-Kampschreur AA, Passchier J (1996) A quality of life instrument for adolescents with chronic headache. *Cephalalgia* 16: 183–96. http://dx.doi.org/10.1046/j.1468-2982.1996.1603183.x

Larsson B (1988) The role of psychological, health-behavior and medical factors in adolescent headache. *Dev Med Child Neurol* 30: 616–25. http://dx.doi.org/10.1111/j.1469-8749.1988.tb04799.x

Larsson B, Andrasik F (2002) Relaxation treatment of recurrent headaches in children and adolescents. In: Guidetti V, Russell G, Sillanpää M, Winner P, editors. *Headache and Migraine in Childhood and Adolescence.* London: Martin Dunitz Ltd, pp. 307–16.

Larsson B, Stinson J (2011) Commentary: on the importance of using prospective diary data in the assessment of recurrent headaches, stressors, and health behaviours in children and adolescents. *J Pediatr Psychol* 36: 863–7. http://dx.doi.org/10.1093/jpepsy/jsr034

Laurell K, Larsson B, Eeg-Olofsson O (2005) Headache in schoolchildren: association with other pain, family history, and psychosocial factors. *Pain* 119: 150–8. http://dx.doi.org/10.1016/j.pain.2005.09.030

Laurell K, Larsson B, Mattsson P, Eeg-Olofsson O (2006) A 3-year follow-up of headache diagnosis and symptoms in Swedish schoolchildren. *Cephalalgia* 26: 209–15. http://dx.doi.org/10.1111/j.1468-2982.2006.01113.x

Lay CL, Broner SW (2008) Adolescent issues in migraine: a focus on menstrual migraine. *Curr Pain Headache Rep* 12: 384–7. http://dx.doi.org/10.1007/s11916-008-0065-7

Marcon RA, Labbé EE (1990) Assessment and treatment of children's headache from a developmental perspective. *Headache* 30: 586–92. http://dx.doi.org/10.1111/j.1526-4610.1990.hed3009586.x

Mazzone L, Vitiello B, Incorpora G, Mazzone D (2006) Behavioural and temperamental characteristics of children and adolescents suffering from primary headache. *Cephalalgia* 26: 194–201. http://dx.doi.org/10.1111/j.1468-2982.2005.01015.x

Mazzotta G, Carboni F, Guidetti V et al (1999) Outcome of juvenile headache in outpatients attending 23 Italian headache clinics. Italian Collaborative Study Group on Juvenile Headache. *Headache* 39: 737–46. http://dx.doi.org/10.1046/j.1526-4610.1999.3910737.x

McGrath PJ, Humphreys P, Keene D et al (1992) The efficacy and efficiency of a self-administered treatment for adolescent migraine. *Pain* 49: 321–4. http://dx.doi.org/10.1016/0304-3959(92)90238-7

McGrath PS, Stewart D, Koster AL (2001) Nondrug therapies for childhood headache. In: McGrath PA, Hillier LM, editors. *The Child with Headache: Diagnosis and Treatment.* Seattle: IASP Press, pp. 129–58.

Nestoriuc Y, Rief W, Martin A (2008) Meta-analysis of biofeedback for tension-type headache: efficacy, specificity, and treatment moderators. *J Consult Clin Psychol* 76: 379–96. http://dx.doi.org/10.1037/0022-006X.76.3.379

Ozge A, Termine C, Antonaci F, Natriashvili S, Guidetti V, Wober-Bingol C (2011) Overview of diagnosis and management of paediatric headache. Part I: diagnosis. *J Headache Pain* 12: 13–23. http://dx.doi.org/10.1007/s10194-011-0297-5

Pakalnis A, Butz C, Splaingard D, Kring D, Fong J (2007) Emotional problems and prevalence of medication overuse in pediatric chronic daily headache. *J Child Neurol* 22: 1356–9. http://dx.doi.org/10.1177/0883073807307090

Palermo TM, Eccleston C, Lewandowski AS, Williams AC, Morley S (2010) Randomized controlled trials of psychological therapies for management of chronic pain in children and adolescents: an updated meta-analytic review. *Pain* 148: 387–97. http://dx.doi.org/10.1016/j.pain.2009.10.004

Passchier J, Orlebeke JF (1985) Headaches and stress in schoolchildren: an epidemiological study. *Cephalalgia* 5: 167–76. http://dx.doi.org/10.1046/j.1468-2982.1985.0503167.x

Powers SW, Andrasik F (2005) Biobehavioural treatment, disability, and psychological effects of pediatric headache. *Pediatr Ann* 34: 461–5.

Richardson GM, McGrath PJ, Cunningham SJ, Humphreys P (1983) Validity of the headache diary for children. *Headache* 23: 184–7. http://dx.doi.org/10.1111/j.1526-4610.1983.hed2304184.x

Richter IL, McGrath PJ, Humphreys PJ, Goodman JT, Firestone P, Keene D (1986) Cognitive and relaxation treatment of paediatric migraine. *Pain* 25: 195–203. http://dx.doi.org/10.1016/0304-3959(86)90093-X

Sarafino EP, Goehring P (2000) Age comparisons in acquiring biofeedback control and success in reducing headache pain. *Ann Behav Med* 22: 10–16. http://dx.doi.org/10.1007/BF02895163

Smith MS, Martin-Herz SP, Womack WM (1999) Recurrent headache in adolescents: nonreferred versus clinic population. *Headache* 39: 616–24. http://dx.doi.org/10.1046/j.1526-4610.1999.3909616.x

Stafstrom CE, Goldenholz SR, Dulli DA (2005) Serial headache drawings by children with migraine: correlation with clinical headache status. *J Child Neurol* 20: 809–13. http://dx.doi.org/10.1177/08830738050200100501

Tietjen GE, Peterlin BL (2011) Childhood abuse and migraine: epidemiology, sex differences, and potential mechanisms. *Headache* 51: 869–79. http://dx.doi.org/10.1111/j.1526-4610.2011.01906.x

Trautmann E, Lackschewitz H, Kroner-Herwig B (2006) Psychological treatment of migraine. *Semin Neurol* 26: 1411–26.

Unruh A, McGrath P, Cunningham SJ, Humphreys P (1983). Children's drawings of their pain. *Pain* 17: 385–92. http://dx.doi.org/10.1016/0304-3959(83)90170-7

Wojaczynska-Stanek K, Koprowski R, Wrobel Z, Gola M (2008) Headache in children's pain experiences. *Issues Compr Pediatr Nurs* 26: 203–16.

Varni JW, Burwinkle TM, Seid M, Skarr D (2003) The PedsQL™ 4.0 as a pediatric population health measure: feasibility, reliability, and validity. *Ambul Pediatr* 3: 329–41. http://dx.doi.org/10.1367/1539-4409(2003)003<0329:TPAAPP>2.0.CO;2

27
PSYCHOLOGICAL TREATMENT OF HEADACHE IN CHILDREN AND ADOLESCENTS

Susanne Osterhaus

In Chapter 26 the association between headache and psychological factors was established with a full literature review of comorbidity and treatment modalities. In this chapter the aim is to examine the psychological treatment methods with emphasis on their clinical applications.

Psychological treatments, although similar in principles, should be tailored to meet the needs of each individual based on the appropriate collection of all necessary information and clinical history. In planning psychological management, most headache treatment programmes are divided into three phases. During the first (introductory) phase, headache-related factors are monitored using a headache diary. During the second phase, specific treatment is given, and during the final, post-treatment, follow-up phase the headaches are monitored daily and the newly acquired behavioural and cognitive skills are consolidated.

Prospective daily diaries are recorded for 4 to 5 weeks. Analysis of the headache diary will consider the three main headache variables: frequency (number of attacks), duration and intensity of each attack. The therapist will record other qualitative information including children's perceptions of the positive and negative consequences of their pain, positive effects of their contact with their parents, use of medication, probable causative factors, the nature and diversity of their pain-coping strategies and their pain history and pain behaviours. The therapist will need also to explore the parents' own pain histories, the parents' responses during painful periods and stresses in the family.

In this section, a brief description is presented of the therapy elements that have been used in various psychological treatment programmes for young headache patients. Some order in the field of headache treatment techniques will be created to enable the distinction between cognitive and behavioural components of psychological treatment, although the borders may be blurred. Behavioural methods that involve physical relaxation (relaxation training and biofeedback) will be considered separately and may be referred to as a 'physical–behavioural component'. Mechanical or physical non-pharmacological techniques (e.g. pressure, massage, and hot and cold stimulation) will not be included, as they have generally been evaluated and utilised in adults only.

A multistrategy treatment package commonly combines two or more approaches to the psychological treatment of paediatric headache. A patient-administered, self-help, multitreatment method is also available in the form of a workbook for a home-based treatment for young headache patients (McGrath et al 1990). Because the behavioural management element is always included in the psychological treatment programme, it is sometimes used as a synonym for psychological treatment. In this chapter psychological treatment will be used as a term for all possible non-pharmacological methods, whereas behavioural treatment will be used only for this specific component.

The physical–behavioural component

PROGRESSIVE RELAXATION TRAINING
This is the most common technique for assisting children to relax. Children are taught to sequentially tighten and relax muscle groups followed by sequential relaxation of muscle groups without tensing and self-cued relaxation (whereby the children gradually learn to relax by concentrating on the feeling of relaxation that was caused by the progressive muscle relaxation). Many of these procedures used for children are revisions of the technique developed for adults by Jacobson (1938).

Case study 1: chronic daily headache, anxiety management and relaxation

CLINICAL HISTORY AND HYPOTHESES
Sandra, a 14-year-old female, has suffered from mixed tension-type and migraine headaches since she was 10 years of age. She had at least two or three attacks per week, lasting between morning and dinnertime, for an average of 8 hours. The pain was mild to moderate in severity (at times she could ignore the headache) and frontal in location. The headaches were triggered by noise, weather changes, school tests and quarrels at home. There were no symptoms. Occasionally (one or two attacks per month) the headache was severe enough to stop all activities and make her lie in bed. She treated the headaches with ibuprofen. She rarely missed school because of the attacks. Her schoolwork was good, but she was unable to achieve her own standards, a matter that caused her distress.

Sandra lives with her parents and three older sisters. Her father is a salesman and is often away from home. She feels that her father has high expectations of his daughters for academic achievement. Also, he has a volatile personality and becomes very tense and angry in minor incidents. Her mother is a housewife and looks after her own ill mother, who lives on her own. Therefore, Sandra and her sisters take responsibility of the home during her absence.

Because of her headaches Sandra had little autonomy. Her parents decided what was best for her, considering the fact that she could easily experience an attack. Sandra was fearful and anxious about the reasons for her headaches. She was concerned that she would always have them. As she had to work hard at school, she thought she was unintelligent. She had internalised the wishes of her father and was happy about herself only when she achieved A grades at school (which did not happen very often). To compensate for her 'unintelligence', she tried to be 'kind'. She had difficulty expressing

---

her emotions and tried to appear consistently happy and untroubled. She lived under the impression that she could only be loved if she were kind to others, especially her mother, when they had problems. It was clear that there was not enough space in her life for her own feelings and wishes. Because she feared her father's moods, she used to give up her own wishes and try to obtain her mother's love instead. She wanted to become beloved by being kind and social. At the same time, she felt responsible for the well-being of her mother, who could not organise her own life. From this, it is clear that several emotional, situational and familial factors contributed to her recurrent pains.

THE THERAPY

Sandra was interested in learning about pain and headaches, and she and her parents had positive expectations for the pain programme. Sandra was very cooperative at the sessions. She learned relaxation and distraction techniques to reduce her anxiety. She learned how to recognise potential stressful situations so that they did not cause headaches. She learned to gain insight into her thoughts and feelings, and described her worries about school and about the situation at home. She challenged her ideal of being perfect, and found out that it was not enough to think differently about the situation at home – things had to change as well. Assertiveness training helped her to express her feelings about her father spoiling the atmosphere at home, and with her newly acquired problem-solving skills she managed to negotiate with her parents about activities out-side of the home (going to parties, physical activities, etc.).

Within the eight-session programme she learned to identify and modify many head-ache triggers. Her headaches occurred progressively less often and were less strong. She maintained improvement at follow-up 7 months later.

AUTOGENIC RELAXATION TRAINING

Autogenic relaxation procedures for adults were adapted for special use in children (Schultz 1956). In autogenic relaxation training, a deeply relaxed bodily state may be reached when children concentrate on sensations in their body, through self-suggestive remarks and guided imagery. For instance, patients may get 'autogenic instructions' indicating how to imagine their hands becoming warm as well as how to relax. The therapist provides consistent sugg-estions, rather than authoritative commands. After a period of daily practice by means of an audiotape, children will learn how to follow the instructions on their own. By means of autogenic training, children can gradually learn to warm their hands or they may gradually learn to relax the muscles of their head by concentrating on these muscles. It is this aspect of autogenous training that connects it to biofeedback.

SELF-HYPNOSIS

Self-hypnosis is a form of autogenic relaxation with more emphasis on the self-suggestive and the imaginative part. Self-hypnosis has a clear positive influence on pain, even though the manner in which hypnosis reduces pain is not yet fully understood.

BIOFEEDBACK TECHNIQUES

Biofeedback is short for 'biological feedback'. It involves the use of instrumentation to give feedback (or information) about biological processes, which were once thought to be automatic and beyond conscious control. These biological conditions are, for instance, muscle tension, skin temperature, pulse amplitude, brain wave activity, blood pressure and heart rate. Biofeedback has been shown to be very useful in the treatment of pain, which is caused or exacerbated by physiological changes associated with a stressed or tense state. As stress is the most often mentioned trigger of headaches, biofeedback is useful for everybody who suffers from headaches. Children are excellent candidates for self-regulation procedures, because the relaxation response is easier to elicit in them, and because they seem to learn and respond more quickly in treatment than adults (Werder and Sargent 1984). The major contraindication for biofeedback-assisted pain reduction is for children whose pain is related to their high aspiration level in all activities. They may become more stressed by their need to achieve high reductions. Children's relatively brief attention span, their limited understanding and their potential fear of the electronic equipment have been mentioned as potential disadvantages for the use of biofeedback, but these difficulties are not insurmountable (McGrath 1990). The forms of biofeedback most frequently used to treat headaches in children are electromyographic (EMG) biofeedback and skin temperature biofeedback.

Electromyographic biofeedback

Electromyographic biofeedback is a commonly used type of biofeedback in headache, especially tension-type headache. Surface electrodes measure electrical discharges from the frontal muscle fibres. The information about levels of muscle activity is fed back to the patient via visual or auditory display (lights that change colour or audio tones that vary in pitch and frequency). In EMG biofeedback training, headache patients apply relaxation techniques (which they have learnt in earlier sessions) to relax the muscles of the neck, face and head, while they receive feedback about the efficacy of their muscle relaxation by means of a digital or analogue display of electromyogram levels (Fig. 27.1). Thus, by means of the feedback, patients become more aware of their muscle activity and they learn how to reduce it. If the patient succeeds in reducing the muscle tension, EMG levels go down.

Skin temperature biofeedback

Both EMG and skin temperature biofeedback training may be useful for tension-type headache and migraine, as both techniques reduce autonomic activity. Skin temperature biofeedback training has traditionally been used in the treatment of migraine, but only recently have clinicians begun to use the technique for all types of headache.

During a migraine (or other headache) attack, patients usually have an increased blood flow to the head, as a result of extracranial vasodilatation, and a decreased blood flow to the extremities (e.g. the hands), due to peripheral vasoconstriction. Superficial skin temperature is in part a function of blood flow, with increased temperature during the state of vasodilatation and decreased skin temperature associated with a state of vasoconstriction. Thus, during a headache attack, a patient usually has cold hands and feet and a warm head. Most studies on skin temperature demonstrate that headache pain decreases as skin temperature rises.

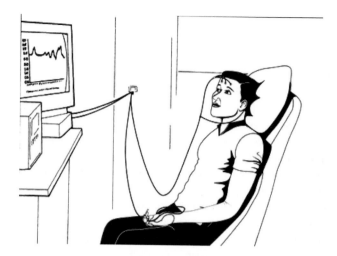

Fig. 27.1 Biofeedback using imagery.

Therefore, if the patient were able to reduce body tension, the skin temperature may rise. This principle has been used in biofeedback training, in which patients use their relaxation skills to raise their hand temperature.

In *skin temperature biofeedback* a surface thermometer is attached to the patient's fingers. Information about vasomotor changes can be fed back via the thermometer, which detects changes in skin temperature and provides the patient with visible or auditory feedback. Other factors influence vasomotor activity (e.g. the external temperature of the environment, dietary factors such as caffeine, stress and medications) by triggering autonomic arousal. For physiological reasons, the 'hand warming technique' is more difficult for children to learn than EMG activity reduction. For that reason thermal training techniques may be taught only after EMG biofeedback control has been achieved.

How are Relaxation and/or Biofeedback Introduced to Young Patients?
The physiological changes associated with a relaxed state, 'the relaxation response', are consistent with a general decrease in sympathetic nervous system response (Richter 1984), which is thought to have a positive effect on headache-related physiological activity.

The specific rationale used to teach children about the pain-reducing effect of relaxation depends on the child's age and cognitive level. In a multistrategy headache programme in which relaxation and/or biofeedback training are included, the children are generally taught the relationship between their thoughts, their emotions and their internal physiological states. In this manner, children can learn to realise that their body is responding to stressful situations, even if they do not recognise these situations as difficult. They also learn that relaxation training will help them to recognise (and later control) bodily tension, so that they can use the technique to prevent physical and mental tension. When biofeedback is part of the treatment, the young patients receive recognisable signals about their internal bodily states. The objective is to reduce the EMG levels (or increase the skin temperature) throughout the session, using relaxation techniques, as well as to reduce (or increase) baseline levels gradually during the entire programme.

Cognitive components in psychological treatment

EDUCATION ON PAIN: A PREREQUISITE FOR PSYCHOLOGICAL HEADACHE TREATMENT

Education on pain can best be considered as a cognitive aspect of the treatment. Knowledge of headache, pain and stress makes young patients change their thoughts about their physical condition. Education on pain and headache is included at the start of most psychological management programmes. In this part of treatment the medical information is intended to give children insight into the nociceptive systems and the factors that modify pain perceptions. Furthermore, the children will be provided with knowledge about the syndrome as well as information about the multiple causal factors of headache and about the relationship between their thoughts, (hidden) stress and the onset of headache attacks. This knowledge helps children to understand why they can expect success from the treatment.

COGNITIVE METHODS THAT ARE CLOSELY RELATED TO RELAXATION TECHNIQUES

Attention focusing (distraction)

Attention focusing or distraction is a common method that parents generally use when their child is in pain. After comforting the child, they try to move the child's attention from the pain to something interesting on which he or she can concentrate. It has recently been recognised that distraction is a very active process that can actually reduce the neuronal responses to a noxious stimulus. However, to be effective, the child must really like the distraction and be enthralled by it. Therefore, the distraction has to be selected according to the child's age and interests. The most interesting distraction will be different for each child.

Imagery (visualisation or imaging)

Imagery can be considered a cognitive extension of the attention focusing method. It requires that children not only move their attention away from the pain but also concentrate on a vivid image in their mind that is linked to positive feelings, relaxation and pain relief. Usually, the positive image is a memory or a fantasy. Some children are able to lose themselves in their imaginations more easily than others. Nonetheless, children who are not very imaginative may also learn the skill of using imagery, if they receive help in making the image as vivid as possible. This can be done, for instance, by helping the child to imagine the specific characteristics and details of the positive image (smell, weather, sounds, etc.). The child will have the opportunity to practise the technique over and over again. Imagery can be used to change people's physical states, although, once again, the mechanism is not yet fully understood.

Behaviour rehearsal

Patients are taught to break a difficult event down into a few steps and to imagine the steps one after another while at the same time trying to relax as deeply as possible by means of newly acquired relaxation skills. When children have mentally 'attacked' stress-producing situations in this manner, they will be able to elicit the relaxation response again, so that they can control feelings of tension in stress-producing situations in the future.

COGNITIVE THERAPY: CHANGING CHILDREN'S AUTOMATIC THOUGHTS
Cognitive therapy is based on the theory that an individual's affect (how he feels) and behaviour are largely determined by how that person perceives events (Spinhoven 1988).

Rational emotive therapy
Rational emotive therapy (RET) is one of several cognitive therapies that have been shown to be effective in making patients aware of basic assumptions or beliefs about themselves or others (Ellis and Harper 1975). The goal of RET is to help individuals to identify and change their irrational beliefs, so that their emotionally dysfunctional behaviour may be altered, thus contributing to a reduction in stress. The concept of RET is illustrated by using the ABC sequence (Dryden and Ellis 1987), in which A stands for the event or situation taking place, B is the thought (based on beliefs) about the event and C represents behaviour and emotions arising from the event and thought.

In cognitive training, ABC schemes are used to help the children to describe their cognition, feelings and behaviour. The impact of irrational thoughts may be explained to the youngsters by emphasising that 'anything that makes you feel bad or act inadequately may be caused by irrational beliefs'. Examples of irrational beliefs may include 'I must be loved and accepted by everyone for everything I do', 'I should be perfect and never make mistakes', 'Life must be fair and should go the way I want (or I cannot stand it)' or 'My unhappiness is caused by circumstances I cannot control'.

The therapist's role is (1) to recognise situations that are stressful by using bodily cues, i.e. muscle tension, nail biting, or cold or sweaty hands; (2) to identify the stress-inducing thoughts/irrational beliefs that accompany the muscle tension; (3) to understand that irrational beliefs influence emotions and behaviour; and (4) to change the irrational beliefs into more realistic ones that are easier to deal with.

Case study 2: successful management with cognitive and relaxation techniques

CLINICAL HISTORY
Roy is a 14-year-old male who has suffered from mixed types of headaches (tension and migraine) since the age of 9 years, but the headaches became worse after starting secondary school. He had at least two attacks per week and the pain was described as mild in nature and could be ignored at times. The attacks usually started in the morning or the afternoon and reached highest intensity late in the day. The attacks lasted for an average of 9 hours.

He had no aura symptoms, but attacks were triggered by food, physical exercise, noise, quarrels with his mother (and feeling guilty about it) and school. The headache was associated with light and noise intolerance and dizziness. A general practitioner

---

and a neurologist prescribed him prophylactic as well as symptomatic medication. Unfortunately, the treatment was unsuccessful and was stopped. He managed 'very severe headache attacks' with paracetamol, rest in a dark room and sleep. He missed an average of one school day per week and thus fell behind in his schoolwork, which worried him very much.

Roy lives with his mother and younger sister. His parents have been divorced for the past 8 years. His mother has a job as well as her housekeeping duties. She is concerned about his ability to organise his own life. In addition, she finds it difficult to discipline him because of the headaches. Roy sees his father once every 3 weeks. Roy told the therapist that he did not talk much about his headache with his father, because he thought he would not understand it.

THE THERAPY

In the group sessions, Roy always came in loud and restless, making a lot of jokes. However, after the relaxation exercises, he became relaxed, intelligent and socially engaged. For the first two individual sessions Roy arrived 10 to 15 minutes late. He apologised and told the therapist how busy he was. As usual, he talked and laughed loudly and it took some time to get him into a state of rest.

Biofeedback helped him to relax and enabled the therapist and Roy to work at his daily-life problems. It was clear that Roy had already benefited from the group sessions. He had been asked to work out the ABC schemes in his workbook, and, although it was difficult for him to label feelings of anger, grief and helplessness, he had made good attempts to describe some debilitating thoughts about himself. The first interventions were to reassure and praise him for his clear schemes, which made him visibly happy. The working relationship between Roy and the therapist had already been established during the group sessions. Their relationship improved further when the therapist ignored his resistance during the first session and only praised the good work he had already done.

IDENTIFICATION OF IRRATIONAL BELIEFS AND NEGATIVE FEELINGS

Roy saw himself as chaotic but funny. Strikingly, he described his father in the same way. He despised his father because of what he labelled as his chaotic life and also adored him because of the creative/funny side of his character. This self-image made life very difficult for him. Negative feelings about himself had a weakening effect, while positive ideas worked as heavy demands upon him. He had to be funny, kind and loved by everybody. His mother could not stop herself from telling him he was like his father when he acted irresponsibly. Further, she gave him the idea that he would end up as a 'loser' if he could not change his ways. It was evident that her remarks could become self-fulfilling. Roy's negative feeling about himself affected all aspects of his daily life. He started his homework just before he had to go to bed at night, which worried him and kept him awake. He woke up late in the morning feeling insecure about his lessons and had to run to school, arriving late, and lacked confidence about his school tests. On coming back home, he often had a headache, sometimes so bad that he had to lie in the dark and keep quiet. When it was mild, he sat down, trying to relax, reading or playing at the computer. Generally he did not tell his mother when he had a mild headache, which made her think that he was lazy and did not want to do his homework. They often quarrelled, which made him feel even worse. Sometimes he came home early from school with a migraine attack. He did not have much time for his friends as he was always behind at school and had to catch up on unfinished work. At school, he tried to be beloved. At home he tried to cheer up the others as his mother had felt 'down' since the divorce. It seemed that his caring behaviour was not only externally motivated, but also driven by a sense of responsibility.

CHALLENGING THE BELIEFS

Working out the schemes, Roy found out he wanted to do things very well, whether related to school, his social life or his mother. He wished to regain his mother's love and, ironically, achieved the opposite. The high demands in combination with the negative image of being like his father and the fatalistic idea that he could not change his genetic make-up made life very stressful. The clarification of the underlying beliefs helped him to overcome his feelings of helplessness. Furthermore, psycho-education was given about feelings of grief, anger and powerlessness after a divorce. Although he found it difficult to feel grief, he had fewer difficulties in realising that he was angry at his mother. He decided he wanted to tell his mother that he tried his best and that he did not like her being unkind towards him. No longer fatalistic because of his genetic make-up, he was able to express his feelings towards his mother. To his surprise, his mother reacted positively. She became more pleasant and supportive and, although she still felt 'down', Roy felt less responsible for her. As time passed, Roy started organising his life better.

THE TREATMENT OUTCOME

After the treatment Roy had improved. The frequency of headache attacks diminished by more than 50% and the average duration of attacks decreased. The improvement continued at follow-up 7 months later. Although he continued to have headaches, he was less dramatic about them. He received more support from his mother, which helped him to prevent stress-inducing thoughts.

Behavioural components in psychological treatment

Behavioural management can be achieved only after sufficient knowledge of headache and pain is gained and the relationship between stress and relaxation is understood. Young patients will be guided to work at their behaviour in some form of behavioural management utilising the physical and cognitive techniques. In this way children change their thoughts and beliefs about themselves and about their pain and also try to change their way of behaving in stress-inducing situations. Behavioural management can incorporate several techniques, such as assertiveness training, stress management (or coping with stress), pain management and parental involvement. When behavioural management is mentioned as a separate treatment technique, it indicates stress management.

Assertiveness Training

Feelings of anger, grief and helplessness that are caused by events should be distinguished from those caused by other people (Osterhaus et al 1993, 1997). In considering the first, therapists help children to realise that feelings of grief and helplessness are part of life and that only the expression of these feelings may give some relief. As an important first step in dealing with feelings that are perceived as maltreatment, the therapist assists the child in changing the thought 'This is my fate' to 'I can do something about this'. In assertiveness training, participants learn to communicate in such a way as to show respect for others, while, at the same time, having respect for themselves. Children learn that being passive or aggressive towards others increases tension (and the likelihood of a headache), whereas assertive ways of communication help to avoid feelings of stress.

Given the time available in a psychological headache treatment, the therapist can only add a minimal assertive element into the therapeutic package. Therefore, the education of children on the theory of assertiveness is often limited in the group sessions, but can be tailored to the child's needs in individual sessions. Lastly, social skills training or social coping is often considered as an element of a multidimensional programme, although it is based on the same principles.

Stress Management

Stress management is an intervention method by which children are given assistance to cope with tension-producing situations, which they have recognised in earlier sessions by means of relaxation and cognitive techniques. Changing thoughts about difficult situations may help, but it is often not sufficient to change the stressfulness of a situation. Therefore, *problem solving* is necessary as an important aspect of stress management.

In the treatment of headache in academically stressed children, the objective is to identify the high standards that the children have set for themselves, which rarely make them feel successful. Children need to make their goals at a more realistic level (cognitive steps). Thereafter they can be guided and supported to solve the problem by setting targets appropriate to their abilities (stress management).

Pain Management

The purpose of pain management is to help children to cope with their pain as much as possible. This intervention technique has considerable overlap with stress management. The objective, however, is not to prevent and reduce bodily stress in general but more specifically to prevent and reduce pain and to cope with pain that is already there. It also has overlap with education on pain. In pain management training children learn (1) to prevent pain by changing their lifestyle, (2) to prevent pain by using pain control techniques such as relaxation and (3) to improve their coping and control of pain by means of adaptation.

PARENTAL INVOLVEMENT

Behavioural techniques for reducing pain in young headache patients typically consist of methods for the children themselves, but attention is also given to how parents respond to their children's pain, highlighting the importance of parental involvement (McGrath 1990, Smith 1995, Osterhaus 1998).

Children learn from their parents how to deal with pain. A history of chronic headache in the family is itself predictive of the development of headache complaints (Turkat 1982), but it should also be noted that predisposition is probably a combination of genetic, behavioural and environmental factors. Parents may teach offspring coping strategies when they experience pain. In addition, parents of young headache patients may become anxious and protective towards their children and they may feel obliged to lift their daily demands and expectations and release them from responsibilities. In this manner, they teach their children to be passive and inadvertently encourage them to adopt 'sick roles'. Children may then exaggerate their pain or their pain may increase.

Other operational learning mechanisms may also be considered. Parents can be inconsistent in their response to their child's pain, alternating between ignoring the complaint and smothering the child with attention. Research on operational learning has demonstrated that behaviours reinforced at unpredictable intervals are more often maintained and less likely to be reduced than behaviours reinforced consistently.

Thus, children are likely to report pain if their parents regularly report pain, are more attentive to them when they have pain or are inconsistently responsive to their child's pain. Children are less likely to report pain if their parents pay more attention to them when they are pain free.

Therefore, the parents' role is important in reducing pain behaviour through their parenting strategies.

Parents can be taught to reinforce desirable behaviour through contingent attention (increase the duration and intensity of parental positive social responses during pain-free intervals), to ignore non-verbal pain behaviours and to respond to verbal pain complaints in a non-rewarding, but understanding, way. The parents can also promote normalisation of the child's sleep pattern, daytime activity, school attendance and meal times (a healthy lifestyle). The second step in management includes prevention of stress and pain by delegating responsibility from parents to the child for treatment compliance, promoting self-mastery and control.

When parents suspect that external environmental factors are responsible for their child's headaches, they may unconsciously reinforce the child's anxiety towards certain 'trigger' factors that may not be the real triggers for their headaches. In these cases, parents can benefit from the knowledge that internal psychological or temperamental factors can also be involved in recurrent pain syndromes, rather than exclusively environmental stimuli.

The third step in pain management is for the child to learn to cope with pain. Parents have a key role in comforting the child during pain rather than only reinforcing it. Several studies have shown that a caring parental behaviour that was necessary to help the child during pain may be perceived as a maladaptive or overprotective behaviour (Osterhaus 1998).

Case study 3: a patient who benefited from behavioural and special therapeutic elements

CLINICAL HISTORY

Saida is a 17-year-old female who lives with her single mother. Her parents divorced during her early childhood and she did not know her father. Her grown-up brothers and sisters have left home and have their own families. The family immigrated to the Netherlands from Suriname 7 years earlier.

Saida has suffered from tension-type headache since the age of 12 years. She has one or two attacks per week. The pain is mild in intensity. The headache attacks occur between the afternoon and dinnertime and last for an average of 5 hours. The headache is bilateral and is not accompanied by any other symptoms. Adaptation to a new life in the Netherlands and worries about school are thought to be the most important triggers. She takes paracetamol for the occasional severe headache, but otherwise she prefers to be left alone and tries to relax in her room. Her mother is very supportive and gives her massages and a good pillow. Saida rarely misses school because of her headaches. The therapist did not meet Saida's mother, who does not speak Dutch well. Saida told the therapist that her mother is extremely dependent on her. Her mother is insecure and does not talk to Dutch people. Her mother does not like to be left alone and never goes to family or religious meetings without her daughter. For the same reasons, Saida always does her homework in the living room with her mother. When Saida wants to be alone in her own room, she is never alone for long, because then her mother comes to join her there, lying or sitting on Saida's bed.

THE THERAPY

Saida benefited from the group sessions. She was highly cooperative at individual sessions; she made ABC schemes in her workbook with great care; she expressed worries about school and her social life. Saida wanted to go to university, but feared she would fail. She believed that people often found her arrogant, whereas she described herself as shy and insecure.

IDENTIFICATION OF IRRATIONAL BELIEFS AND NEGATIVE FEELINGS

Saida saw herself as intelligent and good for her family, but not very gifted socially. She felt highly responsible for her mother and other family members and wanted to be loved by them. She believed that she had to be kind to the others, especially her mother, when they had problems. Her own feelings, abilities and wishes took second place. In addition, she felt unable to make 'real' friends in the Netherlands as people found her arrogant. During the group sessions this belief was challenged and the group members assured her that, if people were to get to know her better, they would understand that she was not arrogant but socially insecure. Fortunately, she was confident about her abilities, but asked too much of herself.

CHALLENGING THE BELIEFS

It was clear that an incongruent technique was needed to confront her with her impossible wish to be perfect in her care for her mother. The therapist told her that she was right to think that children are indeed responsible for their parents, even if their parents require a lot of care. The therapist asked her to do all she could to make her mother feel comfortable in the Netherlands. Initially, she agreed with the therapist, but disagreed during the next session. She appeared irritated and told the therapist that this view was exaggerated and she thought her brothers and sisters could take over some of the responsibilities, as she regularly took care of her brothers' and sisters' children. The therapist maintained the incongruent attitude and reminded Saida that her siblings already had their own families and responsibilities. She nevertheless decided to talk it over with them. Finally, her brothers and sisters helped and they took over some of the responsibilities. Saida was happy and told the therapist that her mother had been too demanding. Thus, this problem was treated not by means of ABC schemes but by a paradoxical strategy.

Saida discovered that her perception of herself as not being socially gifted was related to her social fears. She explained to the therapist that this had become worse after the immigration. She did not understand the social rules in the Netherlands and tried to 'survive' by making an arrogant stance. Dutch social codes were compared with those in a Hindu community in Suriname and she laughed at her misunderstanding of some Dutch habits. By now, Saida was ready to challenge her irrational beliefs. The therapist suggested that she might help herself by asking questions, such as Do I have to be perfect? What if my marks at school are not excellent? Is that a disaster? What if they think I am arrogant? What if I do not know how to behave? What if they laughed at me because of my accent? Why am I afraid of them? Will they all despise me? Even if they do, what difference will it make?

It is clear that it was not enough for Saida to challenge her beliefs about her social functioning. She needed some social skills training. She benefited from assertive role-playing techniques to help her manage situations such as asking something for herself and expressing her feelings. This helped her. Because her mother was less dependent on her, she had the opportunity to organise her own life better.

THE TREATMENT OUTCOME

After the treatment Saida had clinically improved and the frequency of her headache attacks had diminished by about 70%. This result remained at follow-up 7 months later.

An overview of treatment evaluation studies

It is likely that negative studies remain unpublished, and therefore scientific endorsement of psychological therapies for headache in children is tentative. Table 27.1 provides an overview of controlled studies into the effects of behavioural treatment in young headache patients. All these studies use a 50% reduction in headache activity as a criterion for clinical improvement.

A total headache score is usually calculated from the diary by summing the product of the duration and intensity of every single headache attack. This headache score is then divided by the number of weeks the diary has been kept for, which results in a weekly average or the so-called 'headache index'. Sometimes the term 'headache index' is calculated in a different manner, implying that the clinical improvement measures are incomparable. In this chapter the percentage reduction in headache activity is calculated using the following formula:

$$\frac{\text{Pretreatment index} - \text{Post-treatment index}}{\text{Pretreatment index}} \times 100\%$$

THE RELATIVE EFFICACY OF THE TREATMENT ELEMENTS

It is not possible to draw conclusions on the relative efficacies of individual therapy elements from the published studies because of major differences in sample size, age of participants, sex distribution, therapy setting and baseline complaints. The studies also employ different measurement and recruitment procedures, use different numbers of individual and group sessions and do not provide information on outcome in the control condition.

As the efficacies of the separate therapeutic strategies have not been sufficiently investigated, we should rely on the methodologically strongest studies, which happen to be the studies on combined treatment packages. The improvement percentages of these studies are sufficiently encouraging to conclude that multistrategy programmes are successful in treating young headache patients.

Practical issues in the application of research

THE SKILLS OF THE THERAPIST

An experienced therapist will be able to evaluate the clinical history, identify the child's problems and plan the management. The therapist needs to be able to motivate the child and develop an individualised treatment package that is flexible, to enable the child to learn strategies to deal with stress and pain. The clinician has to assume a concerned and supportive manner that promotes self-esteem, self-mastery and control. Periods of potentially increased stress (e.g. transitions or loss) should be anticipated and managed prospectively. If necessary (in cases of severe depression, psychiatric or family system problems), the clinician should make appropriate mental health referrals. It may be necessary at times to provide a longer individual therapy time in order to effect a change in cognitive and behavioural patterns that have already existed for years.

A supportive, accepting and positive atmosphere in group sessions can be of great importance (Osterhaus 1998). Therefore, individual and group sessions are necessary.

THE INCLUSION OF BIOFEEDBACK

The specific mechanisms of action of skin temperature biofeedback are not fully understood (Blanchard and Andrasik 1985). Several studies have shown conflicting results: 'hand cooling' rather than 'hand warming' was effective in relieving headache activity (Blanchard and Andrasik 1985), although hand warming was predictive of treatment success (Morrill and

TABLE 27.1
Controlled evaluation studies of psychological management of paediatric headache

Author(s)	Design	Number of patients (treatment groups)	Mean age range (y)	Treatment in the experimental group(s)	Number of sessions	Predominant setting	Clinical improvement post treatment
Relaxation training							
Larsson and Melin (1986)	CGS	32 (experiments 1 and 2, control)	16–18	Group relaxation training	9	Clinic	67%
				Group information contact	9	Clinic	0%
Larsson et al (1987a)	CGS	46 (experiments 1 and 2, control)	16–18	Therapist-administered relaxation training	9	School	50%
				Self-help relaxation training	1	Home	38%
Larsson et al (1987b)	CGS	36 (experiments 1 and 2, control)	16–18	Self-help relaxation training	3	Home	67%
				Problem discussion	9	School	40%
Larsson and Melin (1988)	CGS	28 (experiment, control)	16–18	Relaxation training	9	School	27%
McGrath et al (1988)	CGS	99 (experiments 1 and 2, control)	9–17 (13.1)	Relaxation training	6	Clinic	39%
				Individual problem discussion	6	Clinic	36%
Wisniewsky et al (1988)	CGS	10 (experiment, control)	12–17 (13.5)	Relaxation training	8	Clinic	60%
Larsson et al (2005)	CGS	288 (seven randomised trials over 20 years including different treatment methods)	10–18	Therapist-administered relaxation	1	School	Therapist-administered relaxation was superior to ATCO, self-monitoring or school-nurse-administered relaxation
				School-nurse-administered relaxation	1	School	
				ATCO or self-monitoring	1	Home	
Biofeedback							
Andrasik and Holroyd (1980)	CGS	39 (experiments 1, 2 and 3, control)	(19.7)	EMG feedback: decrease	7	Clinic	80%
				Placebo feedback: no change	7	Clinic	100%
				Placebo feedback: increase	7	Clinic	80%
Labbé and Williamson (1984)	CGS	28 (experiment, control)	7–16	Temperature feedback	10	Clinic	93%
Fentress et al (1986)	CGS	18 (experiments 1 and 2, control)	8–12 (10.1)	EMG feedback relaxation	9	Clinic	83%
				EMG feedback	9	Clinic	83%

Study	Type	Sample	Age	Treatment	Sessions	Setting	Outcome
Burke and Andrasik (1989)	MBAP	9 (experiments 1, 2 and 3)	10–14 (11.4)	Therapist-administered thermal feedback	10	Clinic	66%
				Self-administered thermal feedback	1	Home	66%
				Parent-administered thermal feedback	1	Home	100%
Allen and McKeen (1991)	MBAP	21 (experiments 1, 2 and 3)	7–12	Thermal feedback and parent counselling (time-lagged)	3	Home	87%
Labbé (1995)	CGS	30 (experiments 1 and 2, control)	8–18 (12)	Relaxation and thermal feedback	10	Clinic	100%
				Relaxation training	10	Clinic	90%
Bussone et al (1998)	CGS	35 (experiment, control)	11–15	Relaxation training and EMG feedback	10	Clinic	54%
Multicomponent							
Mehegan et al (1987)	MBAP	18 (experiments 1, 2, 3 and 4; time lagged)	8–12	Relaxation training, biofeedback and pain management	9	Clinic	89%
Van der Helm-Hylkema et al (1990)	CGS	20 (experiment, control)	10–19	Relaxation training, thermal biofeedback, cognitive training	8	Clinic	90%
McGrath et al (1992)	CGS	73 (experiments 1 and 2, control)	11–18	Relaxation training, cognitive training, assertiveness, problem solving, distraction strategies	8	Clinic	43%
				Relaxation and cognitive training: self-help with seven adherence telephone calls	1	Home	75%
Osterhaus et al (1993)	CGS	41 (experiment, control)	12–19	Relaxation training, thermal biofeedback, cognitive training, assertiveness, problem solving	8	School	47%
Griffith and Martin (1996)	CGS	42 (three groups; clinic based, home based or waiting list)	10–12	Relaxation and CBT	8	Clinic/home	80% for clinic 62% for home
Osterhaus et al (1997)	CGS	39 (experiment, control)	12–22	Relaxation training, biofeedback, cognitive training, assertiveness, problem solving	8	Clinic	52%
Barry and von Baeyer (1997)	CGS	29 (experiment, control)	7–12 (9.4)	Abbreviated cognitive, behaviour and parent therapy	2	Clinic	17%
Allan and Shriver (1998)	CGS	27 (self-administered and clinic based)	7–18	Biofeedback treatment group and biofeedback by parents' groups	6	Clinic/home	Significant improvement
Kroner-Herwig and Denecke (2002)	CGS	75 (therapist group, self-help group, waiting list)	10–14	Relaxation and CBT	8	Clinic/home	68–76%

CGS, controlled group study; MBAP, multiple baseline across participants; EMG, electromyography; CBT, cognitive–behavioural therapy.

Blanchard 1989). Similarly, the correlation between actual changes in EMG activity and outcome was not demonstrated (Holroyd et al 1984), as individuals who were led to believe that their feedback exercises were successful showed the most improvement. This may suggest that the effectiveness of the EMG biofeedback training is mediated by cognitive factors, and relaxation exercises may be as effective as thermal biofeedback in reducing headache.

TREATMENT OF DIFFICULT PATIENTS WHO FAILED TO RESPOND TO USUAL TECHNIQUES

Some children may fail to respond to treatment for several reasons, including school phobia or refusal and analgesic abuse. In some cases the parents may share the child's view that the child should not attend school because of headaches. In such circumstances complex family mechanisms may be operating and family therapy is recommended. In others, the mechanisms are not so clear and extreme somatisation may exist, and the behaviour of the parents may be encouraging pain. A similar problem arises when children, supported by their parents, abuse analgesics. Again, it is difficult to determine whether the basic problem is related to the child's chronic condition or to a family problem, which can be treated only by means of family therapy.

Although patients seek treatment for their headache, it is not unusual for some patients to have an ambivalent attitude towards change, either because they are attached to their own habits or, more often, because they achieve secondary gain. Incongruent or 'paradoxical' therapeutic strategies may be used for patients who are uncooperative at the start of the treatment (Van Dijk et al 1980). In the first technique the therapist 'joins the resistance' rather than attempting to break it, and in the second technique the therapist paradoxically recommends that the patient resists the change. Usually, this recommendation is seen as an 'order' and the patient becomes resistant to his or her habits. Surprisingly, this therapeutic style often results in a quick spontaneous change in the patient's behaviour.

Humour is another therapeutic technique that may help to establish and consolidate a good therapist–patient relationship. It may also encourage the child to look at their problems from a different perspective and reduce the feelings of helplessness.

Summary and conclusions

Psychological interventions for paediatric headache, generally, take the form of multistrategy packages, in which cognitive and behavioural elements are integrated. The treatment packages are different in number of sessions, the organisation of the sessions (individual or group sessions) and in the setting in which the treatment is given. Treatment packages consist of a standard part (group sessions) and an individual part (individual sessions) with the possibility to select tailor-made specific methods for the specific needs of the individual patient.

Psychological treatment of childhood headache requires a highly experienced clinician, who has excellent therapeutic skills, to motivate the child to benefit from treatment in a relatively short time. Sufficient individual time for the child and the therapist is needed to ensure enough attention is given to the specific problems and to allow for therapist guidance. The treatment can be home based with weekly telephone contact and would be expected to be more effective than group sessions only.

Children's treatment would benefit from involvement of the parents. Parents need to be educated on the negative effects of pain encouragement, and on how to support their children, but without rewarding pain.

Thermal biofeedback can be a useful tool in the treatment of migraine, but its mechanism of action is not clear. For some patients who do not benefit from the treatment, programme-specific therapeutic techniques, such as incongruent treatment and humour, are needed.

Finally, a combined programme including behavioural and cognitive elements and involving group sessions and sufficient therapist time for the individual child is superior to the more narrow approach with less therapist time.

REFERENCES

Allen KD, McKeen LR (1991) Home-based multicomponent treatment of pediatric migraine. *Headache* 31: 467–72. http://dx.doi.org/10.1111/j.1526-4610.1991.hed3107467.x

Allen KD, Shriver MD (1998) Role of parent-mediated pain behavior management strategies in biofeedback treatment of childhood migraine. *Behav Ther* 29: 477–90. http://dx.doi.org/10.1016/S0005-7894(98)80044-0

Andrasik F, Holroyd KA (1980) A test of specific and nonspecific effects in the biofeedback treatment of tension headache. *J Consult Clin Psychol* 48: 575–86. http://dx.doi.org/10.1037/0022-006X.48.5.575

Blanchard EB, Andrasik F (1985) *Management of Chronic Headaches: A Psychological Approach*. New York: Pergamom.

Barry J, von Baeyer CL (1997) Brief cognitive-behavioral group treatment for children's headache. *Clin J Pain* 13: 215–20. http://dx.doi.org/10.1097/00002508-199709000-00006

Burke EJ, Andrasik F (1989) Home- vs. clinic-based biofeedback treatment for pediatric migraine: results of treatment through one-year follow-up. *Headache* 29: 434–40. http://dx.doi.org/10.1111/j.1526-4610.1989.hed2907434.x

Bussone G, Grazzi L, D'Amico D, Leone M, Andrasik F (1998) Biofeedback-assisted relaxation training for young adolescents with tension-type headache: a controlled study. *Cephalalgia* 18: 463–7. http://dx.doi.org/10.1046/j.1468-2982.1998.1807463.x

Dryden W, Ellis A (1987) *The Practice of Rational-Emotive Therapy*. New York: Springer Verlag.

Ellis A, Harper RA (1975) *A Guide to Rational Living*. North Hollywood: Wiltshire.

Fentress DW, Masek BJ, Mehegan JE, Benson H (1986) Biofeedback and the relaxation-response training in the treatment of pediatric migraine. *Dev Med Child Neurol* 28: 139–46. http://dx.doi.org/10.1111/j.1469-8749.1986.tb03847.x

Griffiths JD, Martin PR (1996) Clinical- versus home-based treatment formats for children with chronic headache. *Br J Health Psychol* 1: 151–66. http://dx.doi.org/10.1111/j.2044-8287.1996.tb00499.x

Holroyd KA, Penzien DB, Hursey KG et al (1984) Change mechanisms in EMG biofeedback training: cognitive changes underlying improvements in tension headache. *J Consult Clin Psychol* 52: 1039–53. http://dx.doi.org/10.1037/0022-006X.52.6.1039

Jacobson E (1938) *Progressive Relaxation*. Chicago: University of Chicago Press.

Kröner-Herwig B, Denecke H (2002) Cognitive-behavioural therapy of paediatric headache. Are there any differences in efficacy between a therapist-administered group training and a self-help format? *J Psychosomatic Res* 53: 1107–14.

Labbé E (1995) Treatment of childhood migraine with autogenic training and skin temperature feedback: a component analysis. *Headache* 35: 10–13. http://dx.doi.org/10.1111/j.1526-4610.1995.hed3501010.x

Labbé EL, Williamson DA (1984) Treatment of childhood migraine using autogenic feedback training, *J Consult Clin Psychol* 52: 968–76. http://dx.doi.org/10.1037/0022-006X.52.6.968

Larsson B, Melin L (1986) Chronic headaches in adolescents: treatment in a school setting with relaxation training as compared with information-contact and self-registration. *Pain* 25: 325–36. http://dx.doi.org/10.1016/0304-3959(86)90236-8

Larsson B, Melin L (1988) The psychological treatment of recurrent headache in adolescents – short-term outcome and its prediction, *Headache* 28: 187–95. http://dx.doi.org/10.1111/j.1526-4610.1988.hed2803187.x

Larsson B, Melin L, Lamminen ML, Ulstedt EA (1987a) A school-based treatment of chronic headaches in adolescents. *J Pediatr Psychol* 12: 553–66. http://dx.doi.org/10.1093/jpepsy/12.4.553

Larsson B, Daleflod B, Håkansson L, Melin L (1987b) Therapist-assisted versus self-help relaxation treatment of chronic headaches in adolescents: a school-based intervention. *J Child Psychol Psychiatry* 28: 127–36. http://dx.doi.org/10.1111/j.1469-7610.1987.tb00657.x

Larsson B, Carlsson J, Fichtel A, Melin L (2005) Relaxation treatment of adolescent headache sufferers: results from a school-based replication series. *Headache* 45: 692–704.

McGrath PA (1990) *Pain in Children: Nature, Assessment, and Treatment*. New York: The Guilford Press.

McGrath PJ, Humphreys P, Goodman JT et al (1988) Relaxation prophylaxis for childhood migraine: a randomized placebo-controlled trial. *Dev Med Child Neurol* 30: 626–31. http://dx.doi.org/10.1111/j.1469-8749.1988.tb04800.x

McGrath PJ, Cunningham SJ, Lascelles MA, Humphreys P (1990) *Help Yourself: A Treatment for Migraine Headaches*. Ottawa: University of Ottawa Press.

McGrath PJ, Humphreys P, Keene D et al (1992). The efficacy and efficiency of a self-administerd treatment for adolescent migraine. *Pain* 49: 321–4. http://dx.doi.org/10.1016/0304-3959(92)90238-7

Mehegan JE, Masek BJ, Harrison RH, Russo DC, Leviton A (1987) A multicomponent behavioral treatment for pediatric migraine. *Clin J Pain* 2: 191–6. http://dx.doi.org/10.1097/00002508-198602030-00008

Morrill B, Blanchard EB (1989) Two studies of the potential mechanisms of action in the thermal biofeedback treatment of vascular headache. *Headache* 29: 169–76. http://dx.doi.org/10.1111/j.1526-4610.1989.hed2903169.x

Osterhaus SOL (1998) *Recurrent Headache in Youngsters: Measurement, Behavioral Treatment, Stress- and Family-Factors*. Amsterdam: G&FK.

Osterhaus SOL, Passchier J, Van der Helm-Hylkema H et al (1993) Effects of behavioral psychophysiological treatment on schoolchildren with migraine in a nonclinical setting: predictors and process variables. *J Pediatr Psychol* 18: 697–715. http://dx.doi.org/10.1093/jpepsy/18.6.697

Osterhaus SOL, Lange A, Linssen WHJP, Passchier J (1997) A behavioral treatment of young migrainous and nonmigrainous headache patients: prediction of treatment success. *Int J Behav Med* 4: 378–96. http://dx.doi.org/10.1207/s15327558ijbm0404_8

Richter NC (1984) The efficacy of relaxation training with children. *J Abnorm Child Psychol* 12: 319–44. http://dx.doi.org/10.1007/BF00910671

Schultz LC (1956) *Das Autogene Training (Koonzentrative Selbstentspannung): Versuch einer Linischparktischen Darstellung*. Stuttgart: Georg Thieme Verlag.

Smith MS (1995) Comprehensive evaluation and treatment of recurrent pediatric headache. *Pediatr Ann* 24: 450–7.

Spinhoven P (1988) Similarities and dissimilarities in hypnotic and nonhypnotic procedures for headache control: a review. *Am J Clin Hypn* 30: 183–95. http://dx.doi.org/10.1080/00029157.1988.10402731

Turkat ID (1982) An investigation of parental modeling in the etiology of diabetic illness. *Behav Res Ther* 21: 547–52. http://dx.doi.org/10.1016/0005-7967(82)90032-8

Van der Helm-Hylkema H, Orlebeke JF, Enting LA, Thijssen JHH, Van Ree J (1990) Effects of behaviour therapy on migraine and plasma endorphin in young migraine patients. *Psychoneuroendocrinology* 15: 39–45. http://dx.doi.org/10.1016/0306-4530(90)90045-B

Van Dijk R, van der Velden K, van der Hart O (1980) Een indeling van directieve interventies. In: van der Velden K, editor. *Directieve Therapie 2*. Houten: Bohn Stafleu Van Loghum.

Werder SD, Sargent JD (1984) A study of childhood headache using biofeedback as a treatment alternative. *Headache* 24: 122–6. http://dx.doi.org/10.1111/j.1526-4610.1984.hed2403122.x

Wisniewski JJ, Genshaft JL, Mulick JA, Coury DL, Hammer D (1988) Relaxation therapy and compliance in the treatment of adolescent headache. *Headache* 28: 612–17. http://dx.doi.org/10.1111/j.1526-4610.1988.hed2809612.x

28
DIETARY MANAGEMENT OF HEADACHE AND MIGRAINE

Sepideh Taheri

The relationship between headache and diet has been a subject of interest and fascination for many centuries, but conclusive evidence for such a relationship is often missing for many types of foods and drinks. Research on the subject is limited to case series and open studies, mainly in adult patients, with very few in children. In this chapter, an attempt to identify the roles of foods and chemicals in the pathogenesis and also in the treatment of headache disorders will be made. A review of the literature will be made where possible, but anecdotal evidence and cases to illustrate the complexity of the issues will be presented.

The onset of headache attacks following the consumption of certain foods and food additives is reported in 17% to 80% of patients by Millichap and Yee (2003). Others extend this relationship to include cyclical vomiting syndrome and abdominal migraine (Russell et al 2002, Li et al 2008). The list of foods that have been implicated in triggering headaches is very long, but the most commonly reported foods and drinks are given in Table 28.1. Other nutritional issues that may be implicated in the triggering of headache attacks include obesity, as seen in idiopathic intracranial hypertension, and missing meals, as seen in many children with migraine.

Caffeine
Caffeine consumption and withdrawal have been proposed as headache triggers in children and adults (Hering-Hanit and Gadoth 2003, Hagen et al 2009). In the author's experience, caffeine is probably the most common food ingredient that triggers headaches in children (Taheri 2011).

Consumption of caffeinated drinks in the form of colas and sports or energy drinks has increased exponentially in recent years (Ellison et al 1995). The caffeine content of a standard soft drink is approximately 24mg per serving [240ml (8oz)]. Energy drinks contain up to 14 times this amount – enough to result in caffeine toxicity (Committee on Nutrition and the Council on Sports Medicine and Fitness 2011). Caffeine is also present in *guarana*, which is a plant extract that is marketed to increase energy, enhance physical performance and promote weight loss. Just 1g of guarana contains approximately 40mg of caffeine. Thus, the presence of guarana in an energy drink increases the total caffeine level in the beverage (Ellison et al 1995).

TABLE 28.1
Dietary items and chemical migraine triggers

Offending food item	Chemical trigger
Cheese	Tyramine
Chocolate	Phenylethylamine, theobromine
Citrus fruits	Phenolic amines, octopamine
Hot dogs, ham, cured meats	Nitrites, nitric oxide
Dairy products, yogurt	Allergenic proteins (casein, etc.)[a]
Fatty and fried foods	Linoleic and oleic fatty acids
Asian, frozen, snack foods	Monosodium glutamate
Coffee, tea, cola	Caffeine, caffeine withdrawal
Food dyes, additives	Tartrazine, sulphites
Artificial sweetener	Aspartame
Wine, beer	Histamine, tyramine, sulphites
Fasting	Stress hormone release, hypoglycaemia

[a]Headache from ice cream is probably a cold-induced vasoconstrictor reflex response (Russell et al 2002).

The mechanism of caffeine-induced headache includes cerebral vasoconstriction after caffeine consumption and rebound cerebral vasodilation typically 24 to 48 hours after caffeine withdrawal.

Caffeine withdrawal symptoms include headache, fatigue, drowsiness, poor concentration, less desire to socialise, flu-like symptoms, irritability, depressed mood, muscle pain or stiffness, and nausea or vomiting. Gradual withdrawal of caffeine over a number of days is recommended to avoid severe withdrawal symptoms. Regular caffeine intake should be discouraged for all children, although this poses a great societal challenge because of the widespread availability of caffeine-containing substances and a lack of awareness of the potential risks.

Artificial sweeteners

Aspartame (NutraSweet) is the most widely used sugar substitute in low-calorie foods, beverages and medications. Since its introduction in 1981, many reports have shown aspartame to be a headache trigger, especially if taken in moderate to large amounts (900–3000mg/d) over a long period of time (Koehler and Glaros 1988, Lipton et al 1988, 1989, Van de Eeden et al 1994). In other studies, however, aspartame did not trigger headache more often than a placebo (Schiffman et al 1987, Leon et al 1989).

Sucralose is another artificial sweetener (Splenda) that may trigger migraine attacks (Bigal and Krymchantowski 2006, Patel et al 2006, Hirsch 2007), but in clinical practice, its role as a headache trigger is not clear, at least in the author's experience.

Case study 1

A 10-year-old female, with well-controlled insulin-dependent diabetes mellitus from the age of 5, presented with a 5-month history of daily bitemporal tension-type headache. She is a sensitive child who is stressed easily. A dietary history revealed that she drank several cups of diluted 'sugar-free' juice daily. She was advised to exclude juices containing sweeteners.

She was reviewed after 6 weeks with a headache and food diary, and reported complete resolution of headache, except on one occasion, which was within 6 hours of a self-challenge with 500ml of an aspartame-containing drink.

Monosodium glutamate

Monosodium glutamate (MSG) is a flavour-enhancing agent widely used in Chinese food and snacks such as potato crisps. It is also used in many canned, prepared and packaged foods under various descriptions including 'hydrolysed vegetable protein', 'autolysed yeast', 'sodium caseinate', 'yeast extract', 'hydrolysed oat flour' or 'calcium caseinate'. MSG (E621) is one of 10 glutamate-containing flavour-enhancing agents (E620–E629).

It may trigger headaches by direct vasoconstriction at high doses (Merrit and Williams 1990), or it may stimulate glutamate receptors or activate a neurotransmission pathway in which nitric oxide is released in endothelial cells, leading to vasodilatation (Scher and Scher 1992).

The evidence for MSG as a potential trigger for migraine in adults has been supported by some studies (Asero and Bottazzi 2007, Bush and Montalbano 2008) but not others (Raiten et al 1995). There are no studies specific for children. In the author's experience, at least 28% of children who are known to have a high daily intake of MSG-containing food, experience significant improvement in their headache on dietary exclusion, but without a control group a placebo effect cannot be excluded.

Case study 2

A 7-year-old male had near-daily tension-type headaches, episodic migraines and frequent central abdominal pain. A dietary history revealed a high daily intake of savoury snacks and food sauces.

After a 6-week MSG exclusion diet, during which he kept a headache and food diary, he reported only three headaches during the first 10 days of exclusion and nil thereafter.

Cocoa

The biogenic amines phenylethylamine and theobromine, as well as caffeine, and catechin are the main substances in chocolate (Gibb et al 1991). The evidence for their roles in headache is controversial: some clinical studies have shown a clear relationship between intake of cocoa and headache onset (Egger et al 1983, 1989), whereas others have failed to show any relationship at all (Moffett et al 1974, Marcus et al 1997). It is possible that a subgroup of migraine patients may react to cocoa, if taken in large amounts ($\geq$3–4 times per week).

Case study 3

A 3-year-old vegetarian child, with mild renal impairment secondary to haemolytic–uraemic syndrome, presented with recurrent migraines without aura, occurring approximately once or twice a week for 4 months and increasing in frequency. History, examination including blood pressure, and renal function were unremarkable. The only possible trigger factor for his headaches was daily consumption of dark chocolate, which his parents perceived to be beneficial for health.

Exclusion of chocolate for 6 weeks resulted in complete resolution of the child's headaches.

Cheese and other dairy products

Patients and doctors have long recognised dairy products, especially cheese, as headache triggers mediated by biogenic amines, but there are no controlled trials so far to confirm this.

Case study 4

A 13-year-old male attended neurology, psychology and pain services for 3 years with chronic, debilitating, frontal, tension-type, daily headaches with migrainous exacerbations two or three times a week. In the last year, he had also developed bizarre symptoms of dizziness and ataxia, especially in association with the migraine attacks.

All investigations were normal including neuroimaging. He lost nearly half a year of schooling because of the headaches. Treatment with gabapentin helped his sleeping, but gave him troublesome abdominal pains. A dietary history revealed an intake of cow's milk of at least 1 litre per day. His intake of MSG, processed meats and tomato sauce was also significant. He was advised to exclude these three foodstuffs from his diet for 6 weeks, and keep a headache/food diary.

At review, he had no improvement in his headaches, but, within 2 weeks of starting a dairy-free diet, he reported a significant reduction in the intensity of his headaches, and by 6 weeks he had complete resolution of headaches and, interestingly, of dizziness and ataxia. He was followed up for a further 9 months, during which he remained entirely symptom free, resumed full-time school attendance and was discharged from all hospital services. He did not perform a dairy challenge, as he had been anxious about precipitating another migraine.

Processed meat

Processed meats are rich in nitrites and biogenic amines and provide 3.5% to 20% of people's daily nitrite intake, of which only 2% comes from vegetables. The headache associated with nitrite consumption is termed 'hot dog headache'. Nitrite-induced headache is thought to result from the release of nitric oxide, which acts on the vascular endothelium to produce vasodilatation (Henderson and Raskin 1972, Thomsen 1997).

Case study 5

A 6-year-old male presented with frequent tension-type headaches and migraine without aura occurring approximately once a week, and sometimes exacerbated by motion in a car or bus. The only possible trigger factor identified was an excessive intake of processed red meats in the form of ham, bacon and sausages at least four times a week. His food and headache diaries, after exclusion of all processed meats for 6 weeks, showed total resolution of his headaches, including those exacerbated by motion.

Alcohol-related headaches

Wine, especially red wine, has been implicated as a potential migraine trigger in adults. Alcoholic beverages may seem an unlikely cause of headaches in children, but alcohol consumption is increasing at an alarming rate in adolescents of both sexes (National Centre on Addiction and Substance Abuse 2002). Ingested in large quantities, alcohol will lead to a hangover headache, but drinking wine, even in moderate amounts, can trigger a migraine headache in susceptible patients. Biogenic amines, including tyramine, histamine, phenolic flavonoids and sulphites, are generally invoked in the headache mechanism (Peatfield 1995). Alcohol, thus, should be considered in the assessment of the child with headache.

Biogenic amine theory of headache

Histamine and other biogenic amines are present to various degrees in many foods, and their presence increases with maturation. The formation of biogenic amines in food requires the availability of free amino acids, the presence of decarboxylase-positive microorganisms and conditions allowing bacterial growth and decarboxylase activity. Therefore, high concentrations of histamine are found mainly in products of microbial fermentation, such as aged cheese, sauerkraut, wine and processed meat (Table 28.2). Other foods, especially citrus fruits and tomatoes, are also thought to have histamine-releasing capacity (Table 28.3). Diamine oxidase (DAO) is the main enzyme for the metabolism of ingested histamine. The ingestion of histamine-rich food or of alcohol or drugs that release histamine or block DAO may provoke diarrhoea, headache, rhinoconjunctival symptoms, asthma, hypotension, arrhythmia, urticaria, pruritus, flushing and other symptoms in susceptible individuals. The evidence for biogenic amine theory of food intolerance is increasing (Jansen et al 2003, Maintz and Novak 2007). Adults with cluster headaches have significantly higher circulating plasma trace amines than healthy individuals (D'Andrea et al 2004).

TABLE 28.2
Foods rich in histamine

Food categories	Histamine mg/kg	mg/l	Recommended upper limit for histamine mg/kg	mg/l	Tyramine mg/kg	mg/l
Fish (frozen/smoked or salted/canned)			200		ND	
Mackerel	1–20/1–1788/ ND–210					
Herring	1–4/5–121/1–479					
Sardine	ND/14–150/3– 2000					
Tuna	ND/ND/1–402					
Cheese			No recommendation			
Gouda	10–900				10–900	
Camembert	0–1000				0–4000	
Cheddar	0–2100				0–1500	
Emmental	5–2500				0–700	
Swiss	4–2500				0–700	
Parmesan	10–581				0–840	
Meat			No recommendation			
Fermented sausage	ND–650				0–1237	
Salami	1–654					
Fermented ham	38–271				123–618	
Vegetables						
Sauerkraut	0–229		10		2–951	
Spinach	30–60					
Aubergine	26					
Tomato ketchup	22					
Red wine vinegar	4					
Alcohol						
White wine		ND–10		2		1–8
Red wine		ND–30		2		ND–25
Top-fermented beer		ND–14				1.1–36.4
Bottom-fermented beer		ND–17				0.5–46.8
Champagne		670				

Different values in the Histamine column come from different studies. Data taken from Maintz and Novak (2007). ND, not detected.

TABLE 28.3

Foods with suggested histamine-releasing capacities

Plant derived	Animal derived	Others
Citrus fruit	Fish	Additives
Papaya	Crustaceans	Liquorice
Strawberries	Pork	Spices
Pineapple	Egg white	
Nuts		
Peanuts		
Tomatoes		
Spinach		
Chocolate		

Data were taken from Schwelberger (2010).

Experimental and clinical evidence for the concept of histamine intolerance is needed as affected patients would benefit from a clear, evidence-based diagnostic and therapeutic regime (Kelman 2007, Schwelberger 2010), especially children.

Immunoglobin G-mediated theory of headache

Diet restriction, based on the detection of immunoglobin G (IgG) antibodies against food antigens, has been found to significantly reduce the frequency of migraine attacks (Alpay et al 2010), suggesting that inflammation plays an important role in the pathogenesis of migraine (Geppetti et al 2005). The most commonly implicated foods are listed in Table 28.4. Inflammation caused by food could create the pro-inflammatory milieu (the release of pro-inflammatory cytokines) that may enhance the other triggers, such as stress, in some patients.

All IgG subclasses, except IgG4, lead to an inflammatory response on contact with antigens. Children with coeliac disease who have headache as a presenting symptom (25%) are shown to have cerebral white matter lesions that resolve alongside the headache on adherence to a gluten-free diet (Lionetti et al 2009, Turkoglu et al 2011).

Specific IgG antibodies to suspected foods may identify food sensitivity and enable a rational modification of dietary habits, in order to prevent chronic inflammation and the onset of migraine in sensitised patients. However, more research is still needed on IgG-mediated food sensitivity.

Fasting and hypoglycaemia

Skipping meals is a common trigger for migraine (Fuenmeyor and Garcia 1984, Robbins 1994, Scharff et al 1995). The mechanism by which fasting triggers headaches may be related to alterations in serotonin and noradrenaline levels in brainstem pathways (Martin and Behbehani 2001), or the release of stress hormones such as cortisol, or possibly hypoglycaemia

TABLE 28.4
The food categories with IgG-positive test (Geppetti et al 2005)

Food	Number of patients with positive test results (*n*=30)
Spices	27
Seeds and nuts	24
Seafood	24
Starch	22
Food additives	21
Vegetables	21
Cheese	20
Fruits	20
Sugar products	20
Other additives	14
Eggs	14
Milk and milk products	14
Infusions	13
Salads	10
Mushrooms	9
Yeasts	5
Meat	5

(Hockaday and Pearce 1975, Dexter et al 1978), although the role of hypoglycaemia is not certain.

Obesity and headaches

There is strong evidence for the relationship between obesity and headaches, in both adults and children (Kinik et al 2010). A reduction in body mass index (BMI) leads to a significant reduction in headaches (Robberstad et al 2010). Several studies have also shown that calorie restriction in children and adults with idiopathic intracranial hypertension leads to a reduction and, in some cases, normalisation of intracranial pressure and a reduction or resolution of headaches (Marton et al 2008, Sinclair et al 2010, Bond et al 2011b).

The relationship between migraine and obesity may be explained through a variety of physiological, psychological and behavioural mechanisms, many of which are affected by weight loss. However, currently there is little evidence available for the pathways through which weight loss may exert an effect on migraines.

The calculation of the BMI of children with headache is an important part of the physical examination.

Treatment options

DIETARY EXCLUSION REGIMES

Frequently consumed foods (more than three or four times per week) are most likely to trigger headaches. These are often the child's favourite! Occasionally consumed foods may only trigger migraine in a small proportion of patients. Headaches triggered by food usually occur up to 24 hours after ingestion, making it difficult to pinpoint the offending substance (Martin and Behbehani 2001).

When dietary triggers are suspected, it is best to discuss the options with the child and the parents, and to decide jointly on an exclusion regime. A restrictive regime, in which multiple foods are excluded, is unlikely to be adhered to. Therefore, the recommended management is to exclude only one or possibly two foods at any one time for a period of 6 weeks, and for the parent to keep a headache and food diary indicating the child's symptoms and intake of food and drink. If symptoms resolve, causality is likely. An oral challenge with the suspected trigger is advisable if there is any doubt about the causality, but the food may have to be taken for several days for headaches to recur. If symptoms are unchanged, then the process of exclusion and review is repeated until dietary causes are exhausted. Further therapeutic options are then considered.

ROLE OF NUTRACEUTICALS IN MIGRAINE MANAGEMENT

If migraine prophylaxis is indicated, then non-toxic nutraceuticals may be considered (see suggested algorithm). The guidelines, published in 2012 by the National Institute for Health and Clinical Excellence (NICE 2012), review the evidence for the prophylactic value of several substances. The evidence is generally found to be weak and of low quality, but NICE is able to recommend the discussion of the use of butterbur (below) and riboflavin (Chapter 12) with migraine sufferers, as they may reduce migraine frequency and intensity in some people. NICE was unable, based on the evidence, to recommend other substances, but acknowledged the possible role of magnesium and feverfew (below and Chapter 12).

*Butterbur (*Petasites hybridus*) root extract*

Butterbur (*Petasites hybridus*) root extract has emerged as a potential treatment in the prevention of migraine. The butterbur plant is a perennial shrub that was used in ancient times for its medicinal properties. Plants in the genus *Petasites* are thought to act through calcium channel regulation and the inhibition of peptide leukotriene biosynthesis, which may be implicated in the inflammatory cascade associated with migraine (Sheftell et al 2000, Pearlman and Fisher 2001). Two studies in adults (Grossman and Schmidrams 2000, Lipton et al 2004) and one in children and adolescents (Pothmann and Danesch 2005) have shown a significant ($\geq$50%) reduction in migraine frequency through the use of butterbur. In all three studies, butterbur was well tolerated with only mild gastrointestinal events, predominantly eructation (burping). The recommended dose is 75mg twice daily for 1 month, then 50mg twice daily.

Other supplements, such as alpha-lipoic acid and feverfew (*Tanacetum parthenium*), have been studied with inconclusive results in adults. Their use in paediatric patients is not currently recommended (Sun-Edelstein and Mauskop 2009).

Magnesium

Magnesium may be involved in migraine pathogenesis by counteracting vasospasm, inhibiting platelet aggregation and stabilising cell membranes. Its concentration influences serotonin receptors, nitric oxide synthesis and release, inflammatory mediators and various other migraine-related receptors and neurotransmitters. Migraineurs have a low level of brain magnesium during attacks and may also have a systemic magnesium deficiency. Furthermore, magnesium deficiency may play a particularly important role in menstrual migraine (Sun-Edelstein and Mauskop 2009). A supplement of magnesium pidolate (2.25g/d) was shown to reduce headache in children (Grazzi et al 2007) with minor side effects (unpleasant taste).

Co-enzyme Q10

Co-enzyme Q10 (CoQ10) is a vitamin-like substance present in most body cells. It is a component of the electron transport chain and participates in mitochondrial aerobic cellular respiration, generating energy in the form of ATP. Reduced levels of plasma CoQ10 were detected in children and adolescents with migraine, and supplementation led to a significant reduction in headaches (Hershey et al 2007). The recommended dosage is 1 to 3mg/kg/day. The effect of CoQ10 seems to begin after the first month and to be maximal after 3 months, and therefore patients will have to be advised about this delay in action. Side effects have been reported only rarely, making CoQ10 a safe alternative to traditional prophylactic agents. The postulated mechanism of the action of CoQ10 is improvement of mitochondrial function. Mitochondrial dysfunction resulting in impaired oxygen metabolism may play a role in migraine pathogenesis (Rozen et al 2002, Sandor et al 2005).

Ginkgolide B

Ginkgolide B, a herbal constituent extract from *Ginkgo biloba* tree leaves, is a natural modulator of the action of glutamate in the central nervous system. Moreover, it is a potent antiplatelet activating factor (PAF), which in turn makes it an important mediator of inflammation. Indeed, PAF, released from platelets and leukocytes during the first phase of migraine attack, may sensitise the trigeminalvascular complex and induce pain.

Preliminary trials examining ginkgolide B in the prophylaxis of migraine have shown the extract to produce a significant reduction in migraine frequency over a 6-month period (D'Andrea et al 2009). Most of these studies have used ginkgolide (60mg Ginkgo Biloba Terpenes Phytosome) in combination with CoQ10 (11mg) and vitamin B2 (8.7mg). An open-label study in school-aged children has confirmed a significant reduction in the frequency of headaches with a ginkgolide B–CoQ10–riboflavin–magnesium complex (Esposito and Carotenuto 2011). Further randomised trials will be needed to confirm these very promising initial findings.

DIETARY MANAGEMENT OF HEADACHES IN COMORBID CONDITIONS

Several other chronic conditions encountered frequently in children are associated with headaches, either as a primary symptom, such as in idiopathic intracranial hypertension, or as part of a symptom complex, such as in attention-deficit–hyperactivity disorder, irritable bowel syndrome, abdominal migraine or coeliac disease. Evidence is emerging that suggests that modification of diet, such as exclusion of gluten in coeliac disease and moderation of intake of several of the food additives mentioned earlier in this chapter, leads to a significant reduction in headaches in children with comorbid conditions (Hadjivassiliou et al 2001, Li et al 2008, Lionetti et al 2009, Pelsser et al 2010).

Conclusion

A dietary history may form an important part of clinical assessment, especially for foods that are known to trigger migraine and are consumed frequently. A food and symptom diary may also be a useful addition. A simple exclusion diet may reduce the need for more complex therapies.

REFERENCES

Alpay K, Ertas M, Orhan EK, Ustay DK, Lieners C, Baykan B (2010) Diet restriction in migraine, based on IgG against foods: a clinical double-blind, randomised, cross-over trial. *Cephalalgia* 30: 829–37. http://dx.doi.org/10.1177/0333102410361404

Asero R, Bottazzi G (2007) Chronic rhinitis with nasal polyposis associated with sodium glutamate intolerance. *Int Arch Allergy Immunol* 144: 159–61. http://dx.doi.org/10.1159/000103229

Bigal ME, Krymchantowski AV (2006) Migraine triggered by sucralose-a case report. *Headache* 46: 515–17. http://dx.doi.org/10.1111/j.1526-4610.2006.00386_1.x

Bond DS, Roth J, Nash JM, Wing RR (2011a) Migraine and obesity: epidemiology, possible mechanisms and the potential role of weight loss treatment. *Obes Rev* 12: e362–71. http://dx.doi.org/10.1111/j.1467-789X.2010.00791.x

Bond DS, Vithiananthan S, Nash JM, Thomas JG, Wing RR (2011b) Improvement of migraine headaches in severely obese patients after bariatric surgery. *Neurology* 76: 1135–8. http://dx.doi.org/10.1212/WNL.0b013e318212able

Bush RK, Montalbano MM (2008) Asthma and food additives. In: Metcalf DD, Sampson HA, Simon RA, editors. *Food Allergy: Adverse Reactions to Foods and Food Additives*. Oxford: Blackwell Publishing, pp. 335–9.

Committee on Nutrition and the Council on Sports Medicine and Fitness (2011) Clinical report-sports drinks and energy drinks for children and adolescents: are they appropriate? *Pediatrics* 127: 1182–9. http://dx.doi.org/10.1542/peds.2011-0965

D'Andrea G, Terrazzino S, Leon A et al (2004). Elevated levels of circulating trace amines in primary headaches. *Neurology* 62: 1701–5. http://dx.doi.org/10.1212/01.WNL.0000125188.79106.29

D'Andrea G, Bussone G, Allais G et al (2009) Efficacy of Ginkgolide B in the prophylaxis of migraine with aura. *Neurol Sci* 30(Suppl 1): S121–4. http://dx.doi.org/10.1007/s10072-009-0074-2

Dexter JD, RobertsJ, Byer JA (1978) The five-hour glucose tolerance test and effect of low sucrose diet in migraine. *Headache* 18: 91–4. http://dx.doi.org/10.1111/j.1526-4610.1978.hed1802091.x

Egger J, Carter CM, Wilson J, Turner MW, Soothil JF (1983) Is migraine a food allergy? A double-blind controlled trial of oligoantigenic diet treatment. *Lancet* 2: 865–9. http://dx.doi.org/10.1016/S0140-6736(83)90866-8

Egger J, Carter CM, Soothill JF, Wilson J (1989) Oligoantigenic diet treatment of children with epilepsy and migraine. *J Pediatr* 114: 51–8. http://dx.doi.org/10.1016/S0022-3476(89)80600-6

Ellison RC, Singer MR, Moore LL, Nguyen UDT, Garrahie EL, Marmor JK (1995) Current caffeine intake of young children: amount and sources. *J Am Diet Assoc* 95: 802–4. http://dx.doi.org/10.1016/S0002-8223(95)00222-7

Esposito M, Carotenuto M (2011) Ginkgolide B complex efficacy for brief prophylaxis of migraine in school-aged children: an open-label study. *Neurol Sci* 32: 79–81. http://dx.doi.org/10.1007/s10072-010-0411-5

Fuenmayor LD, Garcia S (1984) The effect of fasting on 5-hydroxytryptamine metabolism in brain regions of the albino rat. *Br J Pharmacol* 83: 357–62. http://dx.doi.org/10.1111/j.1476-5381.1984.tb16495.x

Geppetti P, Capone JG, Trevisani M, Nicoletti P, Zagli G, Tola MR (2005) CGRP and migraine; neurogenic inflammation revisited. *J Headache Pain* 6: 61–70. http://dx.doi.org/10.1007/s10194-005-0153-6

Gibb CM, Davies PTG, Glover V, Steiner TJ, Clifford Rose F, Sandler M (1991) Chocolate is a migraine-provoking agent. *Cephalalgia* 11: 93–5. http://dx.doi.org/10.1046/j.1468-2982.1991.1102093.x

Grazzi L, Andrasik F, Usai S, Bussone G (2007) Magnesium as a preventive treatment for paediatric episodic tension-type head-ache: results at 1-year follow-up. *Neurol Sci* 28: 148–50. http://dx.doi.org/10.1007/s10072-007-0808-y

Grossman M, Schmidrams H (2000) An extract of Petasites hybridus is effective in the prophylaxis of migraine. *Int J Clin Pharmacol Ther* 38: 430–5.

Hadjivassiliou M, Grunewald RA, Lawden M, Davies-Jones GA, Powell T, Smith CM (2001) Headache and CNS white matter abnormalities associated with gluten sensitivity. *Neurology* 56: 385–8. http://dx.doi.org/10.1212/WNL.56.3.385

Hagen K, Thoresen K, Stovner LJ, Zwart JA (2009) High dietary caffeine consumption is associated with a modest increase in headache prevalence: results from the Head-HUNT Study. *J Headache and Pain* 10: 153–9. http://dx.doi.org/10.1007/s10194-009-0114-6

Henderson WR, Raskin NH (1972) "Hot-dog" headache: Individual susceptibility to nitrite. *Lancet* 2: 1162–3. http://dx.doi.org/10.1016/S0140-6736(72)92591-3

Hering-Hanit R, Gadoth N (2003) Caffeine-induced headache in children and adolescents. *Cephalalgia* 23: 332–5. http://dx.doi.org/10.1046/j.1468-2982.2003.00576.x

Hershey AD, Powers SW, Vockell AL (2007) Coenzyme Q10 deficiency and response to supplementation in pediatric and adolescent migraine. *Headache* 47: 73–80. http://dx.doi.org/10.1111/j.1526-4610.2007.00652.x

Hirsch AR (2007) Migraine triggered by sucralose—a case report. *Headache* 47: 447. http://dx.doi.org/10.1111/j.1526-4610.2007.00735.x

Hockaday JM, Pearce J (1975) Anomalies of carbohydrate metabolism. In: Pearce J, editor. *Modern Topics in Migraine*. London: William Heinemann Medical, pp. 124–37.

Jansen SC, van Dusseldorp M, Bottema KC, Dubois AE (2003) Intolerance to dietary biogenic amines: a review. *Ann Allergy Asthma Immunol* 91: 233–40. http://dx.doi.org/10.1016/S1081-1206(10)63523-5

Kelman L (2007) The triggers or precipitants of the acute migraine attack. *Cephalalgia* 27: 394–402. http://dx.doi.org/10.1111/j.1468-2982.2007.01303.x

Kinik ST, Alehan F, Erol I, Kanra AR (2010) Obesity and paediatric migraine. *Cephalalgia* 30: 105–9.

Koehler SM, Glaros A (1988) The effect of aspartame on migraine headache. *Headache* 28: 10–14. http://dx.doi.org/10.1111/j.1365-2524.1988.hed2801010.x

Leon AS, Hunninghake DB, Bell C, Rassin DK, Tephly TR (1989) Safety of long-term doses of aspartame. *Arch Intern Med* 149: 2318–24. http://dx.doi.org/10.1001/archinte.1989.00390100120026

Li BUK, Lefevre F, Chelimsky GG et al (2008). The north american society for pediatric gastroenterology, hepatology, and nutrition consensus statement on the diagnosis and management of cyclic vomiting syndrome. *J Pediatr Gastroenterol Nutr* 47: 379–93. http://dx.doi.org/10.1097/MPG.0b013e318173ed39

Lionetti E, Francavilla R, Maiuri L et al (2009). Headache in pediatric patients with celiac disease and its prevalence as a diagnostic clue. *J Pediatr Gastroenterol Nutr* 49: 202–7. http://dx.doi.org/10.1097/MPG.0b013e31818f6389

Lipton RB, Newman LC, Cohen J, Solomon S (1988) Aspartame and headache. *Neurology* 38(Suppl 1): 356.

Lipton RB, Newman LC, Cohen JS, Solomon S (1989) Aspartame as a dietary trigger of headache. *Headache* 29: 90–2. http://dx.doi.org/10.1111/j.1526-4610.1989.hed2902090.x

Lipton RB, Gobel H, Einhaupl KM, Wilks K, Mauskop A (2004) Petsites hybridus root (butterbur) is an effecctive preventive treatment for migraine. *Neurology* 63: 2240–4. http://dx.doi.org/10.1212/01.WNL.0000147290.68260.11

Maintz L, Novak N (2007) Histamine and histamine intolerance. *Am J Clin Nutr* 85: 1185–96.

Marcus DA, Scharff L, Turk D, Gourley LM (1997) A double-blind provocative study of chocolate as a trigger of headache. *Cephalalgia* 17: 855–62. http://dx.doi.org/10.1046/j.1468-2982.1997.1708855.x

Martin VT, Behbehani MM (2001) Toward a rational understanding of migraine trigger factors. *Med Clin North Am* 85: 911–41. http://dx.doi.org/10.1016/S0025-7125(05)70351-5

Marton E, Feletti A, Mazzucco GM, Longatti P (2008) Pseudotumor cerebri in pediatric age: role of obesity in the management of neurological impairments. *Nutr Neurosci* 11: 25–31. http://dx.doi.org/10.1179/147683008X301388

Merrit JE, Williams PB (1990) Vasospasm contributes to monosodium glutamate induced headache. *Headache* 30: 575–80. http://dx.doi.org/10.1111/j.1526-4610.1990.hed3009575.x

Millichap JG, Yee MM (2003) The diet factor in pediatric migraine. *Pediatr Neurol* 28: 9–15. http://dx.doi.org/10.1016/S0887-8994(02)00466-6

Moffett AM, Swash M, Scott DF (1974) Effect of chocolate in migraine: a double-blind study. *J Neurol Neurosurg Psychiatry* 37: 445–8. http://dx.doi.org/10.1136/jnnp.37.4.445

National Centre on Addiction and Substance Abuse (2002) *Report on Teen Tipplers*. New York: Columbia University.

NICE (National Institute for Health and Clinical Excellence) (2012) Diagnosis and Management of Headache in Young People and Adults – CG150. Available at: www.guidance.nice.org.uk/cg150.

Patel RM, Sarma R, Grimsley E (2006) Popular sweetener sucralose as a migraine trigger. *Headache* 46: 1303–4. http://dx.doi.org/10.1111/j.1526-4610.2006.00543_1.x

Peatfield RC (1995) Relationships between food, wine and beer-precipitated migrainous headaches. *Headache* 35: 355–7. http://dx.doi.org/10.1111/j.1526-4610.1995.hed3506355.x

Pearlman EM, Fisher S (2001) Preventive treatment for childhood and adolescent headache: role of once-daily montelukast sodium. *Cephalalgia* 21: 461.

Pelsser LM, Frankena K, Buitelaar JK, Rommelse NN (2010) Effects of food on physical and sleep complaints in children with ADHD: a randomized controlled pilot study. *Eur J Pediatr* 169: 1129–38. http://dx.doi.org/10.1007/s00431-010-1196-5

Pothmann R, Danesch U (2005) Migraine prevention in children and adolescents: results of an open study with a special butterbur root extract. *Headache* 45: 196–203. http://dx.doi.org/10.1111/j.1526-4610.2005.05044.x

Raiten DJ, Talbot JM, Fisher KD (1995) Analysis of adverse reactions to monosodium glutamate (MSG). *J Nutr* 125: 2892–906S.

Robberstad L, Dyb G, Hagen K, Stovner LJ, Holmen TL, Zwart JA (2010) An unfavorable lifestyle and recurrent headaches among adolescents: the HUNT study. *Neurology* 75: 712–17. http://dx.doi.org/10.1212/WNL.0b013e3181eee244

Robbins L (1994) Precipitating factors in migraine: a retrospective review of 494 patients. *Headache* 34: 214–16. http://dx.doi.org/10.1111/j.1526-4610.1994.hed3404214.x

Rozen TD, Oshinsky ML, Gebeline CA et al (2002) Open label trial of coenzyme Q10 as a migraine preventive. *Cephalalgia* 22: 137–41. http://dx.doi.org/10.1046/j.1468-2982.2002.00335.x

Russell G, Abu-Arafeh I, Symon DNK (2002) Abdominal migraine: evidence for existence and treatment options. *Pediatr Drugs* 4: 1–8.

Sandor PS, Di Clemente L, Coppola G et al (2005) Efficacy of coenzyme Q10 in migraine prophylaxis: a randomized controlled trial. *Neurology* 64: 713–15. http://dx.doi.org/10.1212/01.WNL.0000151975.03598.ED

Scharff L, Turk DC, Marcus DA (1995) Triggers of headache episodes and coping response of headache diagnostic groups. *Headache* 35: 397–403. http://dx.doi.org/10.1111/j.1526-4610.1995.hed3507397.x

Scher W, Scher BM (1992) A possible role for nitric oxide in glutamate (MSG)-induced Chinese restaurant syndrome, glutamate induced asthma, "hot-dog headache," pugilistic Alzheimer's disease, and other disorders. *Med Hypotheses* 38: 185–8. http://dx.doi.org/10.1016/0306-9877(92)90091-P

Schiffmann SS, Buckley CE, Sapson HA et al (1987) Aspartame and susceptibility to headache. *N Engl J Med* 317: 1181–5. http://dx.doi.org/10.1056/NEJM198711053171903

Schwelberger HG (2010) Histamine intolerance: a metabolic disease? *Inflamm Res* 59(Suppl 2): S219–21. http://dx.doi.org/10.1007/s00011-009-0134-3

Sheftell F, Rapoport A, Weeks R, Walker B, Gammerman I, Baskin S (2000) Montelukast in the prophylaxis of migraine: a potential role for leukotriene modifiers. *Headache* 40: 158–63. http://dx.doi.org/10.1046/j.1526-4610.2000.00022.x

Sinclair AJ, Burdon MA, Nightingale PG et al (2010) Low energy diet and intracranial pressure in women with idiopathic intracranial hypertension: prospective cohort study. *BMJ* 341: c2701. http://dx.doi.org/10.1136/bmj.c2701

Sun-Edelstein C, Mauskop A (2009) Foods and supplements in the management of migraine headaches. *Clin J Pain* 25: 446–52. http://dx.doi.org/10.1097/AJP.0b013e31819a6f65

Taheri S (2011) To study the effect of dietary exclusion in the treatment of childhood chronic headache disorders. International Headache Congress, poster presentation. *Cephalagia* 31(Suppl 1): 202.

Thomsen LL (1997) Investigations into the role of nitric oxide and the large intracranial arteries in migraine headache. *Cephalalgia* 17: 873–95. http://dx.doi.org/10.1046/j.1468-2982.1997.1708873.x

Turkoglu R, Tuzun E, Icoz S et al (2011) Antineuronal antibodies in migraine patients with white matter lesions. *Int J Neurosci* 121: 33–6. http://dx.doi.org/10.3109/00207454.2010.524331

Van den Eeden SK, Koepsell TD, Longstreth WT Jr, van Belle G, Daling JR, McKnight B (1994) Aspartame ingestion and headaches: a randomized crossover trial. *Neurology* 44: 1787–93. http://dx.doi.org/10.1212/WNL.44.10.1787

29
MANAGEMENT OF THE CHILD WITH HEADACHE IN GENERAL PRACTICE

David P Kernick

Introduction

Headache is the most frequent neurological symptom and the most common manifestation of pain in childhood (Goodman et al 1991). It has a high risk of developing into a chronic condition and persisting into adulthood (Guidetti and Galli 1998), with an associated risk of developing other physical and psychiatric morbidities (Fearon and Hotopf 2001).

Headache has a significant impact upon the quality of life of children (Kernick et al 2009), at a time when the social and academic demands on the child are significant. One primary care study found that 20% of schoolchildren had headache one or more times a week with an adverse impact on at least 12 days during the 3-month study period; 10% of schoolchildren had headache on at least 2 days per week and their generic quality of life scores (PedQL4) were worse than those of children with asthma, diabetes or cancer (Kernick et al 2009).

The current understanding of headache sits within a biopsychosocial framework (Andrasik et al 2005) in which other conditions, particularly anxiety and depression, are common (Egger et al 1998, Smith et al 2003). However, headache can be the presenting feature of an important pathology, brain tumours invariably being a concern for parents, patients and doctors (Morgan et al 2007). General practitioners, as the point of first contact in many healthcare systems, are in a good position to diagnose and treat headache, explore underlying concerns and identify relevant psychosocial issues.

What is happening in primary care?

There is a paucity of information on consultation behaviour and management of children's headaches in primary care. The barriers to care and the poor management of headache that have been identified in an adult population (Forward et al 1998, Dowson and Jagger 1999) are likely to be more prominent in the paediatric population, in which diagnosis is more difficult and the patient may be less able to articulate his or her problems and seek help. A UK general practice study of 1100 children aged between 3 and 11 found that only 11% of patients with migraine had ever consulted their general practitioner. The reasons parents gave for not seeking help included a belief that nothing could be done, not wanting to reinforce illness behaviour and encourage truancy from school and not realising that their child suffered from migraine (Mortimer et al 1992).

The negative health beliefs and health-seeking behaviour of parents who often have headache themselves may also be an important factor. For example, investigators in one primary care study wrote to 2500 children aged 8 to 17 and registered with a large practice, to ask them if they had troublesome headache and, if so, to invite them to an assessment from a general practitioner with an interest in headache. Only 3% of children accepted the invitation, and of these, only 66% actually attended, despite high levels of proven disability. There was a significant clinical improvement in those who did attend, using interventions well within the remit of general practice (Kernick et al 2008).

Headaches account for 4% of UK general practitioner consultations among adults (Latinovic et al 2006) compared with 0.6% in patients 18 years and under. Among the latter group, general practitioners fail to make a diagnosis at presentation in 80% of cases and, of these undiagnosed patients, only 5% will receive a diagnosis in the subsequent year (Kernick et al 2008). General practitioners refer 24% of paediatric headache consultations to secondary care compared with 4% of adult headache presentations (Latinovic et al 2006, Kernick et al 2008).

When they do present to their general practitioner, children want three answers from their physician: the cause of their headache, the cure for their headache and a reassurance that they do not have a life-threatening illness (Lewis et al 1996). From the perspective of the general practitioner the aims of headache management are to

- establish a diagnosis;
- exclude serious pathology and address concerns of the patient and parents;
- refer the patient to secondary care when the diagnosis is in doubt;
- treat a diagnosed primary headache;
- explore relevant psychosocial issues; and
- liaise with the school nurse when relevant.

Making the diagnosis

Migraine is the most common troublesome headache in the paediatric population. A family history of migraine is a strong predictor of migraine, particularly in children and adolescents, and can be a helpful pointer towards a diagnosis. Fifty per cent of adolescent migraineurs will have a positive family history, and this number is 74% in children (Eidlitz-Markus et al 2008). The variety of symptoms that accompany migraine is greater in children than in adults and includes pain elsewhere in the body, dizziness and general malaise, nausea and vomiting. These symptoms may occur in the absence of headache, particularly in children with a hereditary predisposition to migraine.

There are a number of factors that lead to diagnostic difficulties for general practitioners. Primary headache often does not conform to International Headache Society criteria and general practitioners may be unaware that migraine in children differs from that in adults in that attacks can be shorter and the headache can be bilateral (Hershey et al 2005). Younger children may also have difficulty in describing their pain. There can also be a large overlap between migraine and tension-type headache with a number of intermediate forms (Zebenholzer et al

291

TABLE 29.1
Migraine screening test

A positive answer to two of the following three questions has a high positive predictive value for migraine:

Do you feel nauseated or sick in your stomach during headache?

Does light bother you during your headaches (more than when you do not have a headache)?

Do your headaches limit your ability to work, study or perform necessary activities for at least 1d?

2000). Clinical features of both migraine and tension-type headache are experienced by 20% of headache sufferers and 15% will describe significant variability in attacks (Rossi et al 2001). Simple screening tools for migraine that have a high predictive value are available for use in adolescents (Zarifoglum 2007) (see Table 29.1).

Fundoscopy is the minimum requirement for an examination when a child presents with headache, but, if the presentation is atypical, a more extensive examination should include at least testing of the cranial nerves. Measurement of blood pressure is rarely, if ever, helpful but may help to reassure an anxious parent. A full blood count and renal function may be undertaken when a diagnostic picture has not emerged, but these are more useful as delaying tactics rather than for establishing a diagnosis.

Who should be referred when the child presents with headache?
Although there are a number of causes of secondary headache, the patient, family and general practitioner are always concerned that the headache may reflect a brain tumour. Nevertheless, despite advances in neuroimaging, the timely diagnosis of childhood brain tumours remains problematic.

A large case–control study, with a 1-year follow-up, in children who presented to their general practitioner with headache found a risk of a primary brain tumour of 0.03% against a background risk in healthy individuals of 0.004% (Gilles 1991). Among children in whom the general practitioner was able to make a diagnosis of a primary headache, there were no primary tumours.

General practitioners should be aware of factors that are associated with an increased risk of a brain tumour: a personal or family history of a brain tumour, leukaemia or sarcoma; prior therapeutic central nervous system irradiation; neurofibromatosis and tuberous sclerosis.

Although an early diagnosis of brain tumour will facilitate management and reduce functional impact, the problem of identification of incidental pathology and the unnecessary anxiety it incurs is an important factor and should not be overlooked (Hayward 2003). Rates of abnormalities that do not alter management are quoted between 3.7% and 20% (Wöber-Bingöl et al 1996, Lewis and Dorbad 2000, Schwedt et al 2006). Spending more time during a consultation discussing a patient's concerns may reduce the need for unnecessary referral.

Table 29.2 shows guidance for general practitioners when a brain tumour is suspected.

TABLE 29.2

Guidance for general practitioners when a brain tumour is suspected

Immediate referral – red flag presentations

These presentations need urgent referral whether a primary headache can be diagnosed or not. Children who have a brain tumour may deteriorate rapidly and concerns should be discussed with a secondary healthcare professional the same day

An abnormal neurological sign or symptom occurring with a headache, including:

Confusion or disorientation during a headache

Visual abnormalities (check acuity, fields, movements and fundoscopy; if uncertain, request urgent eye check)

Abnormal head position (may be in response to double vision or neck pain)

Motor abnormalities (check fine and gross motor skills, gait and balance)

Cerebellar dysfunction (nystagmus, ataxia, intention tremor)

Persistent headaches (continuous or recurrent for ≥4wk) that wake a child from sleep *or* occur on waking

A persistent headache (may present subtly, e.g. holding head and crying) occurring at any time in a child younger than 4y

Persistent (continuous or recurrent for ≥2wk) vomiting with a headache

Review within 4wk – orange flag presentations

These presentations need review within 4wk; if a primary headache diagnosis cannot be made, these children should be referred. Orange flags include

Headache with behavioural changes

Headache with deterioration in school work

Headache with growth arrest or abnormal puberty

A persistent unilateral or occipital headache

Headache with polyuria and polydipsia (exclude diabetes insipidus)

Persistent headache in a child with a personal or family history of NF1, tuberous sclerosis, brain tumour, leukaemia, sarcoma or early-onset breast cancer

Recent change in headache characteristics in a previously diagnosed primary headache

Reassure – yellow flags

A yellow flag is a primary headache from diagnosis to 1y. Patients should be monitored every 3mo (including assessment of vision, motor skills, growth, development and pubertal status). In the absence of orange or red flags at the end of this period, it is unlikely that the headache is a result of a brain tumour. This does not preclude long-term follow-up to ensure optimum headache management

NF1, neurofibromatosis 1.

General practitioner treatment of primary headache

The exploration of dietary and trigger factors is important and is covered more extensively in other chapters. Trigger factors can be subtle and children have a low threshold for stress, often have irregular sleep patterns, and may have dietary irregularities, especially in terms of missed meals and lack of hydration. A high-fibre cereal snack taken at regular intervals is helpful, as is a regular intake of fluid and avoidance of caffeinated drinks. The general practitioner is well placed to explore psychosocial issues that may have an impact on management, but this area is not always dealt with satisfactorily (Martinez et al 2006).

The majority of headaches can be managed with drugs appropriate to primary care. However, there is a tendency for parents and practitioners to administer small doses of analgesia and delay treatment until the headache is established and severe enough to warrant treatment. For effective pain relief, analgesics should be given early in their optimum doses: 10 to 20mg/kg every 6 to 8 hours (maximum 60mg/kg/day) for paracetamol and 10mg/kg every 6 to 8 hours for ibuprofen are appropriate for both migraine and tension-type headache, but the potential for medication overuse headache should always be considered in frequent users.

In some children with migraine, nausea and vomiting are troublesome symptoms for which early treatment with domperidone may help and improve the response to painkillers. Although oral triptans are safe, owing to the high placebo response in childhood trials which can approach 60%, efficacy and therefore licence has not been obtained. Nasal sumatriptan 10mg has been shown to be effective and safe in adolescents and is licensed in those above 12 years.

Prevention is indicated by frequent episodes of headache that interfere with the quality of life and education. Pizotifen is the drug of choice for migraine in general practice and works well in children. Weight gain can be a problem. Propranolol can be useful, but when the emphasis is on tension-type headache, amitriptyline is the drug of choice. Other drugs, including antiepileptics, are best left to specialist practice. Preventative treatment should be used for at least 2 months at optimum dose before it can be judged as effective or unhelpful. Table 29.3 shows appropriate doses for use in primary care.

The general practitioner's role in tackling the burden of headache in schools
Most migraines occur during typical school hours (Winner et al 2003). A Swedish study found that, in a 6-month period, 17% of schoolchildren visited a school nurse with weekly or more frequent headache, with 12% experiencing headache less frequently. Although the importance of interventions in school settings is recognised, access to health care is variable (Brink and Nader 1981). In many schools, there is not a school nurse and the first point of contact is the

TABLE 29.3
Preventative drugs used in children's migraine (see also Chapter 12)

Drug	Dose	
	Under 12y	12–18y
Pizotifen	0.5–1.0mg/d	1.5–3.0mg/d
	Single dose at night	Single dose at night
Propranolol	0.2–0.5mg/kg TDS	20–40mg TDS
	Max 4.0mg/kg/d	Max 160mg/d
Amitriptyline		Up to 50mg/night

TDS, three times per day.

school first-aider. If children have a headache, invariably they are sent straight home or they are thought to be attempting to avoid lessons and not taken seriously.

Communication between schools and general practitioners is also poor. One study found that only 3% of headache cases seen by the school nurse were discussed with or referred to the child's physician (Dimario 1992). General practitioners have an important role to play in raising the problem of headache in their local schools and ensuring good lines of communication with school nurses.

Conclusion

The general practitioner is the first point of contact for the majority of headache presentations and most headaches can be adequately managed in this setting with drugs well within the remit of the practitioner. However, consultation rates are low and only a minority of presentations reach a diagnostic threshold. Diagnostic uncertainty, concern over serious pathology and lack of clinical confidence result in high rates of referral to secondary care, which in many cases may be inappropriate. Improved education in primary care, which includes the school setting, has the potential to significantly reduce the burden of headache in the community.

REFERENCES

Andrasik F, Flor H, Turk D (2005) An expanded view of psychological aspects in head pain: the biopsychosocial model. *Neurol Sci* 26(Suppl 2): 87–91. http://dx.doi.org/10.1007/s10072-005-0416-7

Brink S, Nader P (1981) Utilisation of school and primary health care resources for common health problems of school children. *Pediatrics* 68: 700–4.

Dimario F (1992) Childhood headaches: a school nurse perspective. *Clin Pediatr (Phila)* 31: 279–82. http://dx.doi.org/10.1177/000992289203100503

Dowson A, Jagger S (1999) The UK migraine patient survey: quality of life and treatment. *Cur Med Res Opin* 15: 241–53. http://dx.doi.org/10.1185/03007999909116495

Egger H, Angold A, Costello E (1998) Headaches and psychopathology in children and adolescents. *J Am Acad Child Adolesc Psychiatry* 37: 951–8. http://dx.doi.org/10.1097/00004583-199809000-00015

Eidlitz-Markus T, Vorali O, Haimi-Cohen Y, Zeharia A (2008) Symptoms of migraine in a paediatric population by age group. *Cephalalgia* 28: 1259–63. http://dx.doi.org/10.1111/j.1468-2982.2008.01668.x

Fearon P, Hotopf M (2001) Relation between headache in childhood and physical and psychiatric symptoms in adulthood: national birth cohort study. *BMJ* 322: 1–6. http://dx.doi.org/10.1136/bmj.322.7295.1145

Forward SP, McGrath PJ, McKinnon D, Brown T, Swann J, Currie EL (1998) Medication patterns of recurrent headache sufferers: a community study. *Cephalalgia* 18: 146–51. http://dx.doi.org/10.1046/j.1468-2982.1998.1803146.x

Gilles F (1991) The epidemiology of headache among children with brain tumour. *J Neurooncol* 10: 31–46. http://dx.doi.org/10.1007/BF00151245

Goodman J, McGrath P (1991) The epidemiology of pain in children and adolescents: a review. *Pain* 46: 247–64. http://dx.doi.org/10.1016/0304-3959(91)90108-A

Guidetti V, Galli F (1998) Evolution of headache in childhood and adolescents: an 8-year follow-up. *Cephalalgia* 18: 449–54. http://dx.doi.org/10.1046/j.1468-2982.1998.1807449.x

Hayward R (2003) VOMIT (Victims of Modern Imaging Technology) – an acronym for our times. *BMJ* 326: 1273. http://dx.doi.org/10.1136/bmj.326.7401.1273

Hershey A, Winner P, Cabbouche M et al (2005) Use of ICHD II criteria in the diagnosis of pediatric migraine. *Headache* 45: 1288–97. http://dx.doi.org/10.1111/j.1526-4610.2005.00260.x

Kernick D, Stapley S, Goadsby P, Hamilton W (2008) What happens to new onset headache presented to primary care? A case-cohort study using electronic primary care records. *Cephalalgia* 28): 1188–95.

Kernick D, Reinhold D, Campbell J (2009) Impact of headache on young people in a school population. *Br J Gen Pract* 59: 678–81. http://dx.doi.org/10.3399/bjgp09X454142

Latinovic R, Gulliford M, Ridsdale L (2006) Headache and migraine in primary care: consultation, prescription and referral rates in a large population. *J Neurol Neurosurg Psychiatry* 77: 385–7. http://dx.doi.org/10.1136/jnnp.2005.073221

Lewis D, Dorbad D (2000) The utility of neuroimaging in the evaluation of children with migraine or chronic daily headache who have normal neurological examinations. *Headache* 40: 629–32. http://dx.doi.org/10.1046/j.1526-4610.2000.040008629.x

Lewis D, Middlebrook M, Mehallick L, Rauch T, Deline C, Thomas E (1996) Paediatric headache, what do children want? *Headache* 36: 224–30. http://dx.doi.org/10.1046/j.1526-4610.1996.3604224.x

Martinez R, Reynolds S, Howe A (2006) Factors that influence the detection of psychological problems in adolescents attending general practices. *Br J Gen Pract* 256: 594–9.

Morgan M, Jenkins L, Ridsdale L (2007) Patient pressure for referral for headache: a qualitative study of GPs referral behaviour. *Br J Gen Pract* 57: 29–35.

Mortimer M, Kay J, Jarron A (1992) Childhood migraine in general practice: clinical features and characteristics. *Cephalalgia* 12: 238–43. http://dx.doi.org/10.1046/j.1468-2982.1992.1204238.x

Rossi L, Cortinovis I, Menegazzo L, Brunelli G, Bossi A, Macchi M (2001) Classification criteria and distinction between migraine and tension type headache in children. *Dev Med Child Neurol* 43: 45–51. http://dx.doi.org/10.1017/S001216220100007X

Schwedt T, Guo Y, Rothner A (2006) Benign imaging abnormalities in children and adolescents with headache. *Headache* 46: 387–98. http://dx.doi.org/10.1111/j.1526-4610.2006.00371.x

Smith MS, Martin-Herz SP, Womack WM, Marsigan J (2003) Comparative study of anxiety, depression, somatisation, functional disability and illness attribution in adolescents with chronic fatigue or migraine. *Pediatrics* 111: 376–81. http://dx.doi.org/10.1542/peds.111.4.e376

Winner P, Rothner A, Putman D, Asgharnegad M (2003) Demographic and migraine characteristics of adolescents with migraine: Glaxo Wellcome clinical trials database. *Headache* 43: 451–7. http://dx.doi.org/10.1046/j.1526-4610.2003.03089.x

Wöber-Bingöl C, Wöber C, Prayer D et al (1996) Magnetic Resonance Imaging for recurrent headache in childhood and adolescence. *Headache* 36: 83–90. http://dx.doi.org/10.1046/j.1526-4610.1996.3602083.x

Zarifoglum M, Karli N, Taskapihouglu O (2007) Can ID migraine be used as a screening test for adolescent migraine. *Cephalalgia* 28: 65–71.

Zebenholzer K, Wober C, Kienbacher C, Wober-Bingol C (2000) Migrainous disorder and headache as a tension type not fulfilling the criteria: a follow up study of children and adolescents. *Cephalalgia* 20: 611–16. http://dx.doi.org/10.1046/j.1468-2982.2000.00090.x

30
SPECIALIST CLINICS FOR THE CHILD WITH HEADACHE

Stewart MacLeod and Ishaq Abu-Arafeh

Headache is a common condition and many children with headache do not seek medical advice. Children and their parents use over-the-counter, simple analgesics to treat headache without consulting a doctor (Oates et al 1993, Sheftell 1997) and quite often the treatment is appropriate (Goldstein et al 1999). However, the treatment given to children by parents and carers may be inappropriate (Simon and Weinkle 1997, Du and Knopf 2009), using less than optimum doses. In general, at least 40% of adolescents and schoolchildren, over the age of 11 years, use over-the-counter painkillers to treat their own headache (Dengler and Roberts 1996, Chambers et al 1997). Families may seek advice on the management of their children's headaches from different healthcare professionals including school nurses, general practitioners, paediatricians, psychologists, psychiatrists, opticians, ophthalmologists, ear, nose and throat surgeons, and others.

For the vast majority of children, headache is either infrequent or mild to moderate and therefore treatment measures with simple analgesics at home are adequate. In the UK, general practitioners are the first port of call for parents and children seeking medical help in the treatment of headache. For those children attending primary care, Chapter 29 gives a detailed management plan, explains the roles of general practitioners and outlines the referral criteria for secondary care.

Purpose of the headache clinic
Headache clinics for children are provided within secondary or tertiary care for children who have failed to respond to treatment at primary care or require special investigations and specialist treatment or where there is some diagnostic difficulty in classifying the nature of the headache. In some children the headache disorders can be complex, attacks are frequent and/or prolonged and symptoms are severe, and the impact on a child's life and education is immense. Over the past 15 years, the authors' clinic has seen a change in the referral pattern with more and more children with chronic daily headache (CDH) being referred for assessment and treatment. Currently, around one-third of the children attending the authors' headache clinic have CDH.

As has been clearly demonstrated across many chapters of this book and elsewhere, headache in children has its own differences and particulars from headache in adults, and therefore the adult services for people with headache would not be appropriate for the care of children with complex paediatric presentations, complex family interactions and the limited range of medications available for use in this age group. For all the above reasons, management of children's headache requires expertise and resources that can only be provided by a specialist headache service for children. In recognition of these needs, the number of specialist headache clinics for children has grown steadily around the world over the past 10 to 20 years, especially in major European and North American paediatric centres.

The functions of the specialist headache clinics have expanded. In addition to providing optimum care for children and their families, headache clinics also help in raising the standards and quality of health care. Specialist clinics are the ideal environment for the development of clinical care pathways and management guidelines. Specialist clinics may also promote clinical research and appropriate use of resources. Multidisciplinary teamwork would be best delivered in such an environment, bringing experts from neurology, psychiatry, psychology, nursing and supporting services together for the benefit of headache sufferers. Experience from headache clinics for adults and clinics for children with epilepsy (Robinson et al 2000), asthma (Temmink et al 2001), cystic fibrosis (Collins et al 1999) and diabetes mellitus (Haines and Swift 1997) have shown similar benefits to patients.

Staffing of a specialist headache clinic

The expertise needed in the assessment and management of the child with headache and the support given to the family should reflect the biopsychosocial nature of headache disorders. The biopsychosocial model is highly relevant and keeps in focus the different needs of the child and the family (Seshia et al 2008).

Paediatricians are most suited to look after children with headache as they are able to have adequate communication with children and their families and provide a holistic approach to the child's physical and emotional needs, and paediatricians can also recognise the child's developmental abilities in describing abstract ideas such as pain.

Paediatric neurologists also have important roles in specialist headache clinics in addressing and planning the investigation of children with possible secondary headaches and in interpreting the results of investigations.

Child and adolescent psychiatrists and *clinical psychologists* are able to diagnose and address the common psychiatric comorbidities of headache such as mood changes, depression, anxiety, poor sleeping habits and poor tolerance of pain. The input of an experienced psychiatrist/psychologist will allow a better understanding of the child's needs and will also provide specialist treatment for some children, such as cognitive–behavioural therapy, biofeedback and relaxation.

An *experienced paediatric dietitian* will be able to help some children to avoid food trigger factors and provide support during the planning of an exclusion diet. Dietetic support is essential in gaining full compliance with dietary exclusion and in providing a balanced diet with no risk of dietary deficiencies.

Children's nurses with expertise in childhood headache can provide continuity of care and support for children at home and also at school by making frequent contact with the children, their families and their school teachers.

Preclinic assessment

The practical assessment and management of the child with headache takes place at several stages, from the time of first contact with primary care, through to the referral process to secondary and tertiary care. The assessment of the child starts even before he or she attends the clinic when information has been given by the referring physician or the parents on the nature of their concerns.

The child and his or her parents usually have their own concerns and anxieties and possibly theories on aetiology, investigation and treatment. The primary care physicians usually make their own assessment on management and treatment (see Chapter 29). If a further referral to secondary or tertiary care were initiated, the information given by the referring physician would enable the headache clinic team to determine the urgency of the referral. An appropriate referral process indicates a successful relationship between primary and secondary care and utilisation of clinical care pathways and guidelines.

Urgent assessment would be given to children with symptoms and signs suggestive of raised intracranial pressure (effortless vomiting, vision disturbances, acquired squint, hypertension or papilloedema) or posterior fossa dysfunction (ataxia, nystagmus, torticollis or intention tremor). On receipt of the referral request, these children and their families should be contacted immediately and preferably by telephone.

Early assessment is given to children under the age of 5 years and those with a recent onset of severe frequent headaches. These children are usually seen within 4 weeks of the referral date.

Children with long-standing infrequent headache and who are otherwise well and healthy are seen at the clinic on a routine appointment basis.

Children requiring early or routine assessment are sent, with their appointment cards, a simple headache questionnaire to collect information about the nature of the headache (Appendix 30.1) and a headache diary to fill in details of future attacks (Appendix 30.2). The questionnaire is designed to gather information on the child's general health and symptoms between attacks and the diary gives details of the actual symptoms during headache attacks. The information, if filled in appropriately, may be good enough to make an accurate diagnosis of the most likely cause of the headache. It would also allow the physician to understand the impact of the headache on the child and the family and also the concerns of the parents. Children and parents are asked to bring the completed questionnaire and the diaries to the clinic appointment for the attending physician to include in the full assessment of the child.

Clinic assessment

The first clinic consultation is of prime importance. Children and their parents are mainly seeking information on the cause, the treatment and the prognosis of the headache. The patients must therefore feel that their complaints are being taken seriously and that they are being listened to carefully. Children should be given the opportunity to speak for themselves and encouraged to describe their own symptoms. The ultimate aim is to classify the headache accurately from the history and examination, perform investigations if appropriate and initiate management strategies. For these reasons, the first appointment needs to be uninterrupted and not less than 30 to 40 minutes in duration.

The history should be comprehensive and headache focused and should cover details of the actual headache, associated features and other medical history (Appendix 30.3). Questions should be designed to explore the duration of the illness, the frequency of attacks, the duration of attacks, the severity of the pain, the quality of the pain and the site of maximal intensity over the head (Chapters 8 and 9).

Enquiry should be made into possible trigger factors and aura symptoms. Associated symptoms, including anorexia, nausea, vomiting, pallor, dizziness, visual disturbances, abdominal pain, motor or sensory symptoms and light, noise or smell intolerance, should be documented. Children would also be asked about possible exacerbating (walking and exertion) and relieving factors (rest, sleep and analgesics). Information would also be collected on previously taken medication (including dosages) to treat acute attacks and medications used for prophylaxis. The response to and side effects of the treatment would also be recorded. Information is also recorded on relevant past medical history, family history (particularly of headache), school performance, social and after school activities, personality traits and hobbies.

GENERAL PAEDIATRIC ASSESSMENT
This will include a full general paediatric history and physical examination to identify or exclude any systemic illness that may have contributed to headache. Medical paediatric history should include systemic review, use of over-the-counter medications, past medical history, developmental and emotional issues, and family and social history.

General paediatric examination should include the measurement and plotting on growth charts of weight, height and head circumference and the measurement of blood pressure. General paediatricians will help in optimising the treatment of systemic illnesses, if present, such as chronic respiratory conditions (asthma, hay fever, sinus diseases, etc.), allergies, constipation and others.

PAEDIATRIC NEUROLOGY ASSESSMENT
Neurological assessment is an integral part of the assessment of the child with headache and should include a detailed examination for signs of increased intracranial pressure, cerebellar dysfunction and focal neurological deficits. Neurological examination should include the assessment of cranial nerves and particularly the inspection of optic discs.

EMOTIONAL AND BEHAVIOURAL ASSESSMENT
Screening for emotional and behavioural difficulties can be part of the general and neurological assessment and, if positive, a full assessment by a clinical psychologist will help to identify issues and offer help and treatment.

ASSESSMENT OF THE IMPACT OF HEADACHE
It is important to document the impact of the headache on the child and family. This should include details about school absenteeism and interference with social activities, such as peer relationships and sporting activities. Simple questioning is usually sufficient but various quantitative tools are available such as PedMIDAS (short and easy to use but applicable only to

migraine). PedQoL4 is more comprehensive and may be time-consuming, but is very useful for some patients (see Chapter 7).

Diagnostic tests
In a minority of children, investigations may be needed. Any investigation should be employed judiciously and rationally to help to confirm or refute a suspected diagnosis and there is no place for indiscriminate or routine use. The range of tests is relatively limited to neuroimaging, electroencephalography or lumbar puncture. The second and third tests would be indicated if an epileptic phenomenon or benign intracranial hypertension, respectively, is suspected. However, neuroimaging with either computed tomography (CT) or magnetic resonance imaging (MRI) is the most commonly employed investigation. MRI is preferable as it allows better resolution of the brain (particularly the posterior fossa) and better visualisation of the cerebral vasculature and CT carries a significant radiation burden. However access to MRI, particularly on an urgent basis, may be limited. Very young children may also require anaesthesia for MRI.

Neuroimaging is indicated in all children with chronic and recurrent headache who have concomitant symptoms and signs that might suggest an underlying brain pathology, including recent focal neurological deficits, cerebellar dysfunction and signs of raised intracranial pressure and symptoms suggestive of complicated or hemiplegic migraine.

Neuroimaging might also be considered in situations in which the headache fails to fit a clear pattern of a recognised primary headache disorder, where there has been a recent change in the pattern of the headache, an alteration in the child's personality or marked deterioration in school performance. In addition, neuroimaging should be seriously considered for children under the age of 5 years, particularly if an adequate description of the headache symptoms is not forthcoming and examination is inadequate.

A normal brain scan can be reassuring (to families and clinicians), but it is important to warn families about the relatively high incidence of non-specific unrelated abnormalities seen in scans, particularly with MRI.

Management of the child with headache

HEADACHE EDUCATION
Verbal and written information will help with a better understanding of the headache disorder and better adherence to management advice and treatment. Children and their parents can access reliable information about migraine and other types of headache, the impact of migraine on a child's life and treatment options from good web-based resources. Both the Migraine Trust (www.migrainetrust.org) and Migraine Action (www.migraine.org.uk) have specific leaflets and resources for children. Migraine Action has produced information for parents and children of different ages, school nurses, youth leaders and others.

ADVICE ON HEALTHY LIFESTYLE
An integral part of managing chronic headache of any type is the adoption of a lifestyle that reduces the frequency and severity of headache. Advice is given to maintain a good eating routine with at least three regular meals per day, including breakfast, lunch and dinner. The

regularity of meals is probably more important than the quantity of food consumed, so, if the child is resistant to taking breakfast or lunch, a small amount of food is better than none. Children should avoid sugar-rich snacks and replace them with foods containing complex starch, such as cereals and fruits.

Adopting a good pattern of sleep, by going to bed at a certain time, appropriate to the child's age and family, and waking up at a good time in the morning, allows the child to feel fresh, take breakfast and prepare for school. Sleep deprivation can trigger headache attacks and good sleep may prevent headache recurrence.

Children with sedentary lifestyles and those who spend too much time in front of television and computer screens may be at higher risk of headache attacks. Children who take regular exercise and participate regularly in sports are less prone to headache. Apart from their overall positive impact on a child's health, sports and exercise are also important in reducing the risk of headache and should be encouraged with good periods of rest after exercise.

SUPPORT IN THE APPROPRIATE USE OF MEDICATIONS

The education of the child and the family should include the roles of rescue treatment and preventative treatment.

Rescue treatment should be available for the child at all times including during school. The dose should be calculated according to weight and given as early as possible after the onset of headache. The most appropriate route of drug administration should be given according to each child's attack profile and response to available medications. The nasal route can be used for those with early-onset nausea and vomiting in the course of a migraine attack or in those for whom oral medications are unsuccessful. In children with medication overuse headache, complete abstinence from pain killers should be encouraged, planned and adhered to.

The use of preventative treatment should be explained in full and in particular the medicine should be used as prescribed daily, whether the child has a headache or not. In many cases parents and children may confuse the role of preventative medications and may use them as painkillers. The role of these medications should be made very clear from the outset and any misunderstanding should be addressed. Children and parents should be given an indication of what to expect from preventative treatment. Although complete remission of symptoms is desirable, unfortunately it is not always achievable. A reduction in the number, severity and/ or duration of attacks is a more realistic objective. The treatment course should continue for at least 2 to 3 months at appropriate dose before it is judged ineffective. If effective, the medications can be used for 6 to 12 months before being discontinued and sustained improvement may continue after cessation of treatment. Preventative treatment can be restarted if headache relapses after discontinuation of treatment.

The side effects of preventative medication should also be discussed and a plan to stop medication should be made if certain side effects become unacceptable.

FOLLOW-UP VISITS

For some patients and parents the purpose of the consultation is to confirm a diagnosis made in primary care, to confirm the appropriateness of the management line or to reassure them of the absence of a serious underlying disease. In these situations, the first clinic visit may achieve the purpose and follow-up is required only if there is a change in the character of the headache or the patient or parents have further concerns.

In the majority of the authors' patients (80%) a second visit is required to confirm the clinical information collected at the first consultation and to confirm the normality of physical examination (Callaghan and Abu-Arafeh 2001). The second visit is particularly important for children less than 5 years of age, if headache diaries were not filled in or were not representative of the child's pattern of headache attacks and if neurological examination was incomplete.

In a small number of patients, frequent clinic visits may be needed to assess headache management, especially for those with chronic daily headache disruptive to their education, social and family life, and participation in sports and leisure activities. Repeated visits may be necessary on introducing preventative medications in order to assess side effects and response to treatment, and adjust the dose.

MULTIDISCIPLINARY MANAGEMENT OF DIFFICULT CASES
Children with atypical headaches that require further evaluation may need to attend the clinic on several occasions, but only rarely is an admission to hospital necessary.

Children with a definite diagnosis of the type of headache, but who failed to respond to the simple management plan, may need the involvement of more than one member of the clinic team. A headache nurse specialist can provide valuable input to the management of childhood headache, not only within the confines of the clinic setting, but in the wider setting of the home and school (Scham 1995). The nurse reviews the headache education programme with the child and the parents and may visit the family at home. There is also a place for wider discussion on a healthy lifestyle, healthy eating, sleep, rest, leisure activity, sport and exercise. The nurse might also carry out school visits, where appropriate, and offer teaching staff general advice on headache aetiology and management, including the possible trigger factors that can be avoided and the relieving factors that can be provided. The nurse could discuss the availability and use of both analgesics and rescue therapies within school hours.

School-based relaxation exercises and training for children with chronic headache can also be facilitated or administered by the headache specialist nurse (Larsson and Carlsson 1996). There is value in educating school nurses about childhood headache and the management strategies available.

An essential member of the clinic team is the clinical psychologist. For those children with chronic daily headache, episodic tension-type headache or mixed headaches, the input of a clinical psychologist can be invaluable. Children with excessive anxiety, behavioural problems and chronic disabling or life-threatening disorders may constitute a difficult group that would benefit from such an input. In the authors' clinic, around 10% of patients are assessed by and receive help from clinical psychologists, allowing the authors to understand the children's concerns and their families' anxieties. Such understanding is essential in order to facilitate the implementation of behaviour modification, conflict-solving, biofeedback and relaxation exercises. Psychiatric involvement can also on occasions be required, but probably in not more than 2% of the clinic population.

A dietitian can also play a role in the management team. The introduction of an exclusion diet may be helpful in the management of migraine. A dietitian with an interest in exclusion diets may help some children in identifying the types of foods that may trigger their attacks of migraine. The dietitian will explain to the parents the value of dietary management and supervise the treatment. One item of food will be excluded at a time for long enough to assess the effects of its withdrawal. If the exclusion diet is successful in reducing the attacks of headache, the food item will be reintroduced to reassess the recurrence of symptoms and confirm the diagnosis. The dietitian would also help the child and the parents to identify the ingredients of ready-made foods in order to identify the trigger item. Occasionally, some children may require a special 'ketogenic' diet to control severe headaches.

REFERENCES

Callaghan M, Abu-Arafeh I (2001) Clinical spectrum and causes of headache in all children attending a specialist headache clinic. *Dev Med Child Neurol* 42(Suppl 85): 24.

Chambers CT, Reid GJ, McGrath PJ, Finley GA (1997) Self-administration of over-the-counter medication for pain among adolescents. *Arch Pediatr Adolesc Med* 151: 449–55. http://dx.doi.org/10.1001/archpedi.1997.02170420019003

Collins CE, MacDonald-Wicks L, Rowe S, O'Loughlin EV, Henry RL (1999) Normal growth in cystic fibrosis associated with a specialised centre. *Arch Dis Child* 81: 241–6. http://dx.doi.org/10.1136/adc.81.3.241

Dengler R, Roberts H (1996) Adolescents use of prescribed drugs and over-the-counter preparations. *J Public Health Med* 18: 437–42. http://dx.doi.org/10.1093/oxfordjournals.pubmed.a024542

Du Y, Knopf H (2009) Self-medications among children and adolescents in Germany: results of national health survey for children and adolescents (KiGGS). *Br J Clin Pharmacol* 68: 599–608. http://dx.doi.org/10.1111/j.1365-2125.2009.03477.x

Goldstein J, Hoffman HD, Armellino JJ et al (1999) Treatment of severe, disabling migraine attacks in an over-the-counter population of migraine sufferers: results from three randomized, placebo-controlled studies of the combination of acetaminophen, aspirin, and caffeine. *Cephalalgia* 19: 684–91. http://dx.doi.org/10.1046/j.1468-2982.1999.019007684.x

Haines LC, Swift PG (1997) Report of the 1994 BPA/BDA Survey of Services for Children with Diabetes: Changing patterns of care. *Diabet Med* 14: 693–7. http://dx.doi.org/10.1002/(SICI)1096-9136(199708)14:8<693::AID-DIA412>3.0.CO;2-T

Larsson B, Carlsson JA (1996) School-based, nurse-administered relaxation training for children with chronic tension-type headache. *J Pediatr Psychol* 21: 603–14. http://dx.doi.org/10.1093/jpepsy/21.5.603

Oates LN, Scholz MJ, Hoffert MJ (1993) Polypharmacy in a headache centre population. *Headache* 33: 436–8. http://dx.doi.org/10.1111/j.1526-4610.1993.hed3308436.x

Robinson RO, Edwards M, Madigan C, Ledgar S, Boutros A (2000) Audit of a children's epilepsy clinic. *Dev Med Child Neurol* 42: 387–91. http://dx.doi.org/10.1017/S0012162200000700

Scham I (1995) The role of the nurse clinician in recurrent childhood headache. *Axone* 16: 83–6.

Seshia SS, Phillips DF, von Baeyer CL (2008) Childhood chronic daily headache: a biopsychosocial perspective. *Dev Med Child Neurol* 50: 541–5. http://dx.doi.org/10.1111/j.1469-8749.2008.03013.x

Sheftell FD (1997) Role and impact of over-the-counter medications in the management of headache. *Neurol Clin* 15: 187–98. http://dx.doi.org/10.1016/S0733-8619(05)70303-0

Simon HK, Weinkle DA (1997) Over-the-counter medications. Do parents give what they intend to give? *Arch Pediatr Adolesc Med* 151: 654–6. http://dx.doi.org/10.1001/archpedi.1997.02170440016003

Temmink D, Francke AL, Hutten JB, Spreeuwenberg P, van der Zee J, Abu-Saad HH (2001) Content and outcomes of Dutch nurse clinics for children with asthma. *J Asthma* 38: 73–81. http://dx.doi.org/10.1081/JAS-100000024

Appendix 30.1 Headache questionnaire

To help us understand the nature of your headache and give you the appropriate advice when you attend the clinic, we would be grateful if you can fill the short questionnaire below today.

Name:	Sex:
Date of birth:	Date of first clinic appointment:

How long has your child had headache for?	
How many times does your child get headache per month?	
How long is each attack of headache from start till full recovery (hours)?	
How long is the shortest?	
How long is the longest?	
How long is the usual attack?	

		Yes	No
How ill is your child during attacks of headache?	Lies in bed		
	Stops some activities		
	Continues as normal		
Does your child return to normal health between attacks?			

What are your main concerns that made you or your doctor request this appointment?

1	
2	
3	

What treatment has been tried, so far, **to relieve pain** and what was the response?

Name of treatment	Useful	Not useful	Any side effect

What treatment has been tried, so far, **to prevent attacks** and what was the result?

Name of treatment	Useful	Not useful	Any side effect

What other non-drug treatment has been used e.g. diet, homeopathy, etc.?

Name of treatment	Useful	Not useful	Any side effect

Appendix 30.2 Headache diary

Name: Date of birth: Sex: Address:

Attack number	1	2	3	4	5	6
Date						
Time started						
Time resolved						
Severity of headache*						
Type of headache**						
Site of maximal pain on head						
What may have started it off?						
Symptoms preceding headache						
During headache attacks						
Loss of appetite						
Nausea or feeling sick						
Vomiting						
Does light make it worse?						
Does noise make it worse?						
Is it worse on walking?						
Other symptoms						
Does rest make it better?						
Does sleep make it better?						
Is it better after painkillers?						
What do you take?						

*Severity: Write 1 if headache is not interfering with normal activities
                 Write 2 if headache is interfering with some activities
                 Write 3 if headache is interfering with all activities
**Type of pain: Choose one of the following or your own descriptions:
                 throbbing, hitting, banging, tightness, pressure, squeezing, sharp, stabbing, dull
                 or can't describe

Appendix 30.3 Headache clinical data

Hospital Unit Number:	Date of birth:	Date of clinic attendance:
Full post code:	Age:	Date of referral:
Clinic doctor: 1. Consult, 2. Registrar	Sex: 1= male, 2= female	Waiting time:

Code	Source of referral:	Referral marked:	Past acute therapy	Past prophylaxis	Diet tried
1	GP	Not marked	Paracetamol	Pizotifen	No
2	A&E	Urgent	Ibuprofen	Propranolol	Yes, what?
3	Local paediatricians	Non-urgent	Diclofenac	None	
4	District paediatricians		Triptans	Others, specify	
5	Others, specify		Others, specify		

Referral reason:	Tumour worry	Missing school	Failed treatment	Uncertain diagnosis
	Symptoms change	Increase frequency	Others, specify	For reassurance

Duration of illness (months):	Frequency of attacks/month: Number of attacks so far: < 5, or >5	Duration of attacks (hours): **Usual:** **Shortest:**

Clinical features of types of headache I or II if present (tick the appropriate response):

Severity of pain:	I II	Site of pain:	I II	Quality of pain:	I II	Aura symptoms:	I II
Normal activities	☐☐	Whole head	☐☐	Dull	☐☐	None	☐☐
Stop some activity	☐☐	Forehead	☐☐	Just "sore"	☐☐	Visual	☐☐
Stop all activities	☐☐	Unilateral	☐☐	Throbbing	☐☐	Sensory	☐☐
		Top of head	☐☐	Sharp	☐☐	Motor	☐☐
		Back of head	☐☐	Pressure/ tightness	☐☐	Mood changes	☐☐
		Others	☐☐	Others	☐☐	Speech defect	☐☐
Trigger factors:	I II	**Other symptoms:**	I II		I II	**Relieving factors:**	I II
None known	☐☐	None	☐☐	Abdominal pain	☐☐	Rest	☐☐
Missing meal	☐☐	Anorexia	☐☐	Unilat. weakness	☐☐	Sleep	☐☐
Missing sleep	☐☐	Nausea	☐☐	Visual defects	☐☐	Paracetamol	☐☐
Stress/excitement	☐☐	Vomiting	☐☐	Sensory symptoms	☐☐	Ibuprofen	☐☐
Food (**sure**)	☐☐	Light intolerance	☐☐	Confusion	☐☐	Vomiting	☐☐
Food (**suspected**)	☐☐	Noise intolerance	☐☐	Speech defects	☐☐	None	☐☐
Others	☐☐	Worse on walking	☐☐	Vertigo	☐☐	Others	☐☐
		Pallor	☐☐	Others	☐☐		

Between attacks:	Completely well	Constant headache	Other symptoms
Present associated illnesses:			
Past illnesses:			
Personality as described by parents:			

Schoolwork	School attended	Problems at school	Other activities	Family illnesses
Above average	Mainstream	None known	None	None
Average	Special school	Bullying	Too busy	Severe headache
Below average	Others	Others	Too hard work	Other headache
Learning support			Other stresses	Other, what?

Examination	Specify any abnormalities ……..		
Other comments	What investigations before referral? CT/MRI Ophthalmology Others		
Diagnosis:	Migraine without aura	Migraine with aura	Probable Migraine
	Chronic tension-type headache	Episodic tension-type headache	Probable TTH
	Chronic daily headache	Chronic migraine	Analgesia induced
	Secondary headache	Others:	
Treatment:	Reassurance	Lifestyle advice	Withdraw pain killers
Acute treatment	Simple analgesics as required	Triptans as required	Others
Preventative	Pizotifen	Propranolol	Amitriptyline	Topiramate	Others
Plan:	Discharge	Review	Refer psychology	CT or MRI	

31
DRAWING AS AN EXPRESSION OF MIGRAINE SYMPTOMS IN CHILDREN: CAN A PICTURE REALLY PAINT A THOUSAND WORDS?

Vicky Quarshie

Introduction

The aim of this chapter is not to teach clinicians how to become expert art therapists and how to analyse a child's drawings, but to illustrate the abilities of children to provide a non-verbal communication of their feelings and, in particular, of how they perceive the migraine attacks and how headache and migraine affect them, and to illustrate how these drawings help in the clinical assessment and the diagnosis.

A brief look at the history of images used to convey headache pain will be explored and evidence from other disciplines in relation to the usefulness of children's drawings as a diagnostic and therapeutic tool will be presented. Current research evidence within this area in relation to children's headaches will be explored and some case presentations made.

It is hoped that the utilisation of children's drawings will add another tool to the traditional assessment and diagnostic methods. Making plain paper and coloured pencils available to children at the consulting room may prove to be a further asset to the diagnostic toolkit.

Early evidence of headache drawings

Chapter 2 reviewed in detail the history of headache and showed how drawings and inscriptions have provided an insight into how ancient civilisations expressed their knowledge of headache. It is very likely that mankind has been troubled by headache since the dawn of civilisation, as seen in evidence of trephination on human Neolithic skulls dating from 7000 to 3000 BC and also in early cave drawings (Lyons and Petrucelli 1978). The discovery of the *Ebers Papyrus*, dated circa 1200 BC, based on medical documents from 2500 BC, described Ancient Egyptians' role in the early management of headache, migraine, neuralgia and shooting head pains (Critchly 1967). A cartoon drawing has been created of the interpretation, depicting a crocodile made of clay, with sacred grain within its mouth, and an eye of faience, bound to the head of a patient with a strip of fine linen with the names of the gods written on it and the physician praying.

Hildegard von Bingen, or Saint Hildegard (1098–1179), was a highly creative German abbess who had visions from a young age, which she documented in her work. A review of the images of her visions suggested that the images gave a clear indication that she suffered from migraine attacks (Sacks 1970). It is possible that Hildegard expressed both religious beliefs and migraine auras within her art.

Evidence that children's drawings can contribute to diagnosis and therapy

CAN A PICTURE REALLY PAINT A THOUSAND WORDS?

In recent years, the focus of child health-related research has seen a marked shift from seeking information about children's health to seeking and obtaining information directly from them (Carter 2002). This approach, of course, requires that methods to extract this information should be developmentally appropriate for the children, to enable them to effectively express and communicate their experiences. According to the United Nations Convention on the Rights of the Child, children should be encouraged and enabled to make their views known on issues that affect them (Bellamy 2003).

Drawing is often referred to as the universal language of childhood. Children are always dabbling with art in one form or another, whether with crayons, coloured pencils, pen, water colours or even oil paints in some cases. We have all marvelled at people, including our friends, who can draw and paint and wished that we could be like them, instead of being able only to draw a man like a potato or as a series of lines with a circle for a head. For most, as we move on in life, we leave painting behind us, and the only painting that we ever do now is of our gates, and the walls of our houses.

Children's artwork could be the initial starting point of the therapeutic communication and interaction between the child and clinician and could act as a vehicle that takes both on a journey of increased interaction and deepens the therapeutic relationship (Winncott 1971). It is also noted that artistic expression is a developmentally appropriate means of communication for children, it can serve as a valuable tool for children to express their experiences (Rubin 1984) and may enhance the therapeutic process (Malchiodi 1999).

Further studies, aimed to measure if indeed drawing facilitates children's communication of their perceptions and feelings (Gross and Haynes 1998), found that children who were asked to draw while giving their account reported much more information and detail than those giving a verbal account only. A subsequent study showed similar results when a group of children were interviewed using both methods. This approach is very similar to the 'draw and write' method (Pridmore and Lansdown 1997). Therefore, drawing may help children organise the order of the story and assist with the process of memory retrieval (Gross and Haynes 1998), possibly not dissimilar to the process whereby adults use headache diaries to recall their headache experience, and possibly act as a prompt to disclose more than they would with a verbal account alone.

A simple method of using artwork is to establish a rapport called 'illuminative artwork'. In this method, the individual is asked to provide artwork on a topic or a theme; the facilitator does not impose his or her own interpretation on the work but encourages the individual to use the artwork as a communication tool. When specific aspects are raised, a focused exploration can continue to establish their particular significance and to address the issues raised (Spouse 2000). Children typically view drawing as a non-threatening and enjoyable activity (Malchiodi 1999). Furthermore, children, particularly very young ones, may not have the cognitive ability to express themselves in words and usually express themselves more naturally and spontaneously through actions such as drawing, which can help to externalise thoughts, anxieties, emotions and experiences often too painful to speak out loud. Think about your own children. How often, when offered the day's artistic masterpiece when collecting a child from preschool or nursery, have you been completely clueless with regards to the image represented on the paper until you have asked for an explanation of the picture and been given a detailed summary? It is this communication that is important, and the drawing stimulates the dialogue that then makes the marks on the paper comprehensible. Malchiodi (1999) argues that drawings expediently bring pertinent issues of the individual child to the surface to be addressed, thus accelerating the therapeutic treatment process for the child. In the current healthcare climate, this has additional benefit when there is limited time allocated to follow-up and review appointments.

EVIDENCE THAT CHILDREN'S DRAWINGS CAN AID HEADACHE DIAGNOSIS AND THERAPY

The question that remains is not what is it that migraineurs see but, rather, what is it that they draw. A large study (possibly the first) reported on the effectiveness of children's drawings, describing their headaches, as an aid in the differential headache diagnosis (Stafstrom et al 2002). The study, comprising 226 children consulting for headache, employed a similar method to that described as 'illuminative artwork' (Spouse 2000). While waiting for their consultation, each participating child was given a blank piece of white A4 paper and a pencil with an eraser. The only instruction they were given was: 'please draw a picture of yourself having a headache'. If the child requested additional instructions, he or she was asked 'where is your pain?', 'what does your pain feel like?' and 'are there any other changes or symptoms that happen before or during your headache that you can show me in a picture?'.

Some children chose to provide additional information with written words and explanation; however, this was not requested, encouraged or discouraged. No time restraint was imposed on the exercise; however, most children completed the task within a few minutes.

The exercise was completed while the examiner spoke with the parent/carer with regards to the child's medical history; however, the headache was not discussed until the drawing was completed. To avoid bias, the drawing was then set aside and not viewed by the examining neurologist. The usual routine clinical examination was then continued, the child evaluated, a diagnosis made using International Headache Society criteria and the management plan explained. For the purpose of the study, a diagnosis of either migraine or non-migraine headache was given solely on the clinical findings. Following this process, the child was then asked to explain the drawing and notes were made based on these explanations.

Phase 2 of the study involved the drawings being independently reviewed by two experienced clinicians: paediatric neurologists who were blinded to the clinical histories. Each was asked to evaluate each drawing and, based upon their own clinical experience, decide if the pictures contained features more consistent with migraine or non-migraine headache.

The results of the study demonstrated that, compared with the clinical interview and examination, which are regarded as the criterion standard for making a diagnosis, the headache drawings had a 93.1% sensitivity, 82.7% specificity and 87.1% positive predictive value for migraine, in that the drawings contained an artistic representation of a migrainous feature, such as throbbing/pounding pain, which was often depicted by something hitting the head repeatedly or by a sharp object. Symptoms of gastric stasis were identifiable within 7.2% of the drawings; graphic images of nausea of vomiting into the toilet were unmistakable. Visual symptoms included drawings of white flashes or coloured spots moving across the visual field; as no coloured pencils were provided, many children added words to the drawings to explain this. Photophobia was often represented by closed eyes, lamps being turned off or a blanket or cloth pulled over the eyes. Images depicting the desire to keep still or lie down were consistently positive indicators within the drawings of a diagnosis of migraine. Interestingly one child with a strong paternal family history of hemiplegic migraine drew pins sticking into one half of the face – this was supported by his verbal account of experiencing the sensation of pins and needles beginning in one half of the face then moving down into the arm and leg.

Children with headaches diagnosed as non-migraine tended to draw compression around the head, represented, for example, by a band or something squeezing the head, very similar to the accounts given by adults often given a diagnosis of muscular tension headache. Similar results were replicated in a study of 124 children (Wojaczynska-Stanek et al 2008); however, the children in this study were given the choice of pens and coloured pencils. It was observed within the study that black and red were colours predominantly used to portray pain, as noted in an earlier work (Unruh et al 1983). It would therefore appear that offering the use of colour within the drawing process could quite possibly enhance the process and offer further insight into the child's experience.

Of course the drawing is not suggested as a replacement for the clinical interview and examination; however, it can provide a useful insight into the child's headache experience. Children's headache drawings can reveal much more than the quality and location of their pain. Depressive illness related to the pain experience can be represented within the drawings, displayed as anger, crying and helplessness (Lewis et al 1996).

A later study, which examined serial pictures drawn by children with a migraine diagnosis throughout their treatment, concluded that the process of children drawing their headache experience could also be utilised in subsequent follow-up appointments to monitor the effectiveness of treatment and clinical status (Stafstrom et al 2005).

Case study 1

An 8-year-old female presented with a 2-year history of infrequent headaches lasting between 1 and 4 hours. The headaches are generally relieved by sleep, cool packs on the head and occasionally ibuprofen suspension. She often complains of accompanying abdominal pain, nausea and occasionally vomiting. During episodes she is lethargic and prefers to keep still and lie down. During episodes she is very pale and her eyes appear heavy and tired.

Her mother, a nurse herself, has migraine with aura and had abdominal migraine as a child.

The mother, who was aware of the usefulness of drawings as a way for children to communicate their emotions and experiences, asked her daughter while she was drawing one day if she could draw a picture of what her headache feels like and was very surprised with the picture the child presented to her and what she explained (see interpretation of the drawing overleaf).

Patient's interpretation of the drawing

The young girl explained that she drew a line down the centre of the face because the headache only occurred on that side of her head (indicating the left side). The background area was left white because inside her head it felt like a really brightly lit, white room. She explained that the right side of the face was smiling as normal – this is how she feels when she does not have the headache.

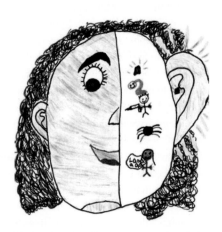

She drew five small separate pictures on the left side of the face to describe how she felt before the start of pain: a flashing police light in her vision, a spider crawls inside her head and moves around and then the spider turns into a snake weaving about, with a continued perception of movement inside the head. At the same time she feels that everything is very loud and that people are very noisy and shouting around her; hence she had drawn her left ear to be much bigger than the right – the yellow lines represent sound around the ear.

The young girl, keen to explain her symptoms, became very animated and excited. She was able to convey her actual experience with much enthusiasm, and she explained that the drawing in the centre of the left side of the face is of somebody with a hammer banging inside her head. Then, with eyes wide and arms outstretched, she stated that it then felt as if she had swallowed a whole person, who was banging inside her head and shouting, trying to get out, which she demonstrated quite excitedly and then asked, *'Now do you understand?'*.

Case study 2

A 7-year-old male presented with episodic headaches. His verbal description of headache was that his head hurt all over (indicated with his hands) and that he felt sick. His parents described him as very pale, quiet and lethargic, preferring to lie down instead of his usual non-stop active play with his older sister.

The parents also reported episodes of projectile vomiting during the initial headache phase. At age 4 to 5 years, he had episodes of tummy aches lasting for about an hour or two with no other symptoms of gastric disturbance, from which he would make a complete recovery. The parents also recalled on one occasion their child had mentioned seeing some moving blue light dots on his bedroom curtains, which are actually plain pale blue. This was not recalled to be associated with an episode of headache or any other symptoms, but it was memorable as the child had spent several minutes trying to point and show them where the dots were. To describe his headache he drew a face (see interpretation of the drawing opposite).

Patient's interpretation of the drawing

He explained that the left side of the 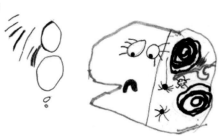 drawing is actually the front of his head and his face is frowning because he feels sad when he experiences the headache, and the images to the right of the drawing are actually sensations that he feels at the back of his head and inside his head. He described a sensation of spiders and insects crawling inside his head as well as the sensation of a hammer repeatedly hitting the inside of his head, accompanied by a sensation of spinning within his head.

He explained the circles and lines at the left of the picture as shiny blobs and lines he sees in front of his eyes, sometimes before the start of a headache.

Case study 3

A female adolescent with some mild learning difficulties and memory problems, congenital hypertonia and gross motor delay presented with a 3-year history of persistent headaches prior to attending the clinic. During the initial consultation she was accompanied by her mother, and a diagnosis of possible chronic migraine with and without aura was made and a treatment plan was formulated and discussed.

During two subsequent review consultations, she was again accompanied by her mother, whom she relied upon heavily to provide information, as she said she could not remember events or information about headache frequency and symptoms experienced, owing to her memory problems.

The mother tried to prompt her daughter, encouraging her to provide information herself to promote her daughter's autonomy; however, she only became more anxious during the consultation. The clinician had earlier in the consultation established that the patient enjoyed drawing at college but because of her health she had felt too unwell to go. She was asked if she thought she could draw her headache and what she experienced during an episode. At the next review clinic she brought drawings on six sheets of A4 paper (see the following interpretations of the drawings).

Interpretation of the drawings

The main feature of the drawings is that many of the objects have been drawn twice. This feature can be attributed to the fact that the patient often experiences double vision, which is not always associated with headache; it is often worse in the evening and it can fluctuate, coming and going during the evening. It can also occur before a headache and the patient stated that sometimes when she is looking at people it looks like they 'have two heads'.

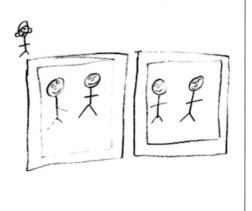

Interpretation of the drawing

This picture depicts wavy lines in front of her eyes and this can sometimes develop before the headache occurs. It never lasts for more than an hour and stays in the same place.

The image is also there when she has her eyes closed and these lines can be of different colours, but particularly pink.

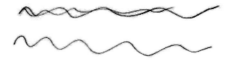

Interpretation of the drawing

The explanation given for this picture is that sometimes when looking at an object, it appears to be in one position and then the object appears to move to a different angle. She stated that this can happen during the headache phase and she has noticed that she has bumped into things, particularly door frames.

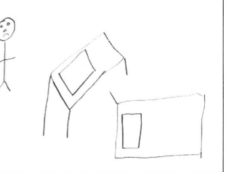

Interpretation of the drawing

A girl watching television and the people on the screen appear of normal size, although the particular programme was of a guitarist and she stated that the guitar looked significantly bigger. She states this can often happen with people who appear to be a lot taller than her – they look like giants when walking past her.

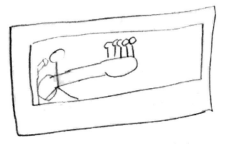

    She states this can happen particularly when she is experiencing the headache.

    This is a manifestation of Alice in Wonderland syndrome as described in Chapter 10.

Interpretation of the drawing

Again depicts some visual disturbance whereby the buttons on the remote control can merge together.

Interpretation of the drawing

Lying in bed she states that she feels that she is falling over backwards even when she is laid flat on her back in bed and she has a sensation that her legs go over the back of her head. She states this can be present during the headache and can occur intermittently for up to a period of 1 hour and she tries to lie still during this time.

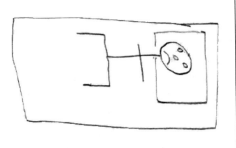

Summary

There is increasing evidence within this arena to suggest that the artwork of migraine sufferers can provide a useful insight into their experience of the attacks and the condition. Poldoll and Robinson (1999) reviewed artwork produced by migraine sufferers and identified that migraineurs who draw and paint their headache experience often find it easier to express and communicate their experience more effectively, particularly in relation to aura and surreal feelings and emotions.

Several forms of visual phenomena are often depicted. Photopsia is often depicted as bright flashes of light, similar to the effect of an old-fashioned camera flash bulb, fortification spectra are often depicted as bright shimmering jagged lines across the visual field and metamorphopsia is represented as a distortion of images in size, shape and colour.

This has often been termed 'Alice in Wonderland syndrome' and is named after the events described in Lewis Carrol's book *Through the Looking-Glass, and What Alice Found There*, as the visual effects often include partial loss of vision, ranging from blank spots in the visual field or drawings appearing as if the artist is looking through a tunnel.

These findings are often consistent with the growing body of literature relating to the migraine drawings produced by children and certainly the individuals within the case studies presented; all of the patients found it easier to draw and communicate their experiences than provide a verbal account alone.

It could be argued that through this method, significantly more information is obtained to support the clinical diagnosis, and this method aids the therapeutic relationship between the individual and the clinician.

To reiterate, it is not being suggested that a drawing can replace the clinical assessment; however, it is hoped that the clinicians reading this will now consider adding this simple, quick, cost-effective assessment tool to their diagnostic toolkit.

REFERENCES

Bellemy C (2003) *The State of the World's Children*. New York: UNICEF.

Carter B (2002) Chronic pain in childhood and the medical encounter: professional ventriloquism and hidden voices. *Qual Health Res* 12: 28–41.

Critchley M (1967) Migraine: from cappadocia to queen square. In: Smith R, editor. *Background to Migraine, Volume1*. London: Heinemann, p. 20.

Gross J, Haynes H (1998) Drawing facilitates children's verbal reports of emotionally laden events. *J Exp Psychol Appl* 4: 163–79.

Lewis DW, Middlebrook MT, Mehallick L, Manning Rauch T, Deline C, Thomas EF (1996) Pediatric headaches: What do the children want? *Headache* 36: 224–30. http://dx.doi.org/10.1046/j.1526-4610.1996.3604224.x

Lyons A, Petrucelli RJ (1978) *Medicine: An Illustrated History*. New York: Harry N. Abrams, Inc, pp. 113–15.

Malchiodi, C (1999) Understanding somatic and spiritual aspects of children's art expressions. In: Malchiodi C, editor. *Medical Art Therapy with Children*. London: Jessica Kingsley, pp. 173–96.

Poldoll K, Robinson D (1999) Out-of-body experiences and related phenomena in migraine art. *Cephalalgia* 19: 886–96.

Pridmore P, Lansdown R (1997) Exploring children's perceptions of health: does drawing really break down barriers? *Health Educ J* 56: 219–30. http://dx.doi.org/10.1177/001789699705600302

Rubin J (1984) *Child Art Therapy: Understanding and Helping Children Grow through Art*, 2nd edn. New York: Von Nostrand Reinhold.

Sacks O (1970) *Migraine* (revised edition). New York: Vintage Books.

Spouse J (2000) An impossible dream? Images of nursing held by pre-registration students and their effect on sustaining motivation to become nurses. *J Adv Nurs* 32: 730–9. http://dx.doi. org/10.1111/j.1365-2648.2000.01534.x

Stafstrom CE, Rostasy K, Minsteret A (2002) The usefulness of children's drawings in the diagnosis of headache. *Pediatrics* 109: 460–72. http://dx.doi.org/10.1542/peds.109.3.460

Stafstrom CE, Goldenholz SR, Dulli DA (2005) Serial headache drawings by children with migraine: correlation with clinical headache status. *J Child Neurol* 20: 809–13. http://dx.doi.org/10.1177/0883073805020 0100501

Unruh A, McGrath P, Cunningham SJ, Humphreys P (1983) Children's drawings of their pain. *Pain* 17: 385–92. http://dx.doi.org/10.1016/0304-3959(83)90170-7

Winnicott D (1971) *Playing and Reality*. New York: Basic Books.

Wojaczyńska-Stanek K, Koprowski R, Wróbel Z, Gola M (2008) Headache in children's drawings. *J Child Neurol* 23: 184–91. http://dx.doi.org/10.1177/0883073807307985

INDEX

Notes
As the subject of this book is childhood headache, entries have been kept to a minimum under these two terms. Readers are advised to look under more specific terms as well as specific diseases/disorders. Page numbers in *italics* refer to material in figures, whilst those numbers in **bold** refer to material in tables. *vs* indicates a comparison or differential diagnosis. Abbreviations used: DHE, dihydroergotamine; ICHD-II, International Classification of Headache Disorders, 2nd edition; MRI, magnetic resonance imaging; SUNCT, short-lasting unilateral neuralgiform headache attacks with conjunctival injection and tearing.

Other titles from Mac Keith Press www.mackeith.co.uk

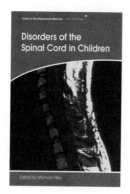

Disorders of the Spinal Cord in Children
Michael Pike (Ed)

Clinics in Developmental Medicine
2013 ▪ 272pp ▪ hardback ▪ 978-1-908316-80-6
£110.00 / €129.30 / $170.00

This book offers comprehensive coverage of paediatric spinal cord disorders, their clinical assessment, appropriate investigations, medical and neurosurgical management, and neuro-rehabilitation. Future prospects for spinal cord regeneration and repair are discussed. This text will be particularly useful for paediatric neurologists, neuro-surgeons and oncologists as well as rehabilitation physicians and therapists.

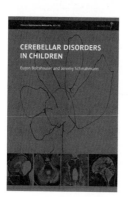

Cerebellar Disorders in Children
Eugen Boltshauser and Jeremy Schmahmann (Eds)

Clinics in Developmental Medicine No. 191-192
2012 ▪ 456pp ▪ hardback ▪ 978-1-907655-01-2
£125.00 / €150.00 / $200.00

This clinically orientated text by an international group of experts is the first definitive reference book on disorders of the cerebellum in children. It presents a wealth of practical clinical experience backed up by a strong scientific basis for the information and guidance given. This book will be an invaluable resource for all those caring for children affected by cerebellar disorders, including malformations, genetic and metabolic disorders, acquired cerebellar damage, vascular disorders, and acute ataxias.

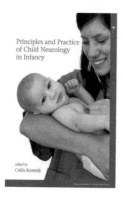

Principles and Practice of Child Neurology in Infancy
Colin Kennedy (Ed)

A practical guide from Mac Keith Press
2012 ▪ 384pp ▪ softback ▪ 978-1-908316-35-6
£29.95 / €38.10 / $49.50

This handbook of neurological practice in infants is designed to be of practical use to all clinicians, but particularly those in under-resourced locations. Seventy per cent of children with disabilities live in resource-poor countries and most of these children have neurological impairments. This book presents recommendations for investigations and treatments based on internationally accepted good practice that can be implemented in most settings.

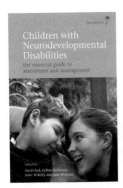

Children with Neurodevelopmental Disabilities:
the essential guide to assessment and management
Arnab Seal, Gillian Robinson, Anne M. Kelly
and Jane Williams (Eds)

2013 ▪ 744pp ▪ softback ▪ 978-1-908316-62-2
£65.00 / €78.00 / $154.95

A comprehensive textbook on the practice of paediatric neurodisability,
written by practitioners and experts in the field. Using a problem-
oriented approach, the authors give best-practice guidance, and centre on
the needs of the child and family, working in partnership with multidisciplinary, multi-agency teams. Drawing on evidence-based practice,
the authors provide a ready reference for managing common problems
encountered in the paediatric clinic.

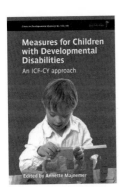

Measures for Children with Developmental Disabilities
An ICF-CY approach
Annette Majnemer (Ed)

Clinics in Developmental Medicine No. 194-195
2012 ▪ 552pp ▪ hardback ▪ 978-1-908316-45-5
£150.00 / €186.00 / $235.00

This title presents and reviews outcome measures across a wide range
of attributes that are applicable to children and adolescents with
developmental disabilities. It uses the children and youth version of
the International Classification of Functioning, Disability and Health
(ICF-CY) as a framework for organizing the various measures into
sections and chapters. Each chapter coincides with domains within the
WHO framework of Body Functions, Activities and Participation and
Personal and Environmental Factors.

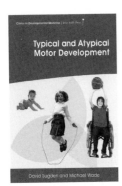

Typical and Atypical Motor Development
David Sugden and Michael Wade

Clinics in Developmental Medicine
2013 ▪ 400pp ▪ hardback ▪ 978-1-908316-55-4
£145.00 / €180.00 / $234.95

Sugden and Wade, leading authors in this area, comprehensively cover
motor development and motor impairment, drawing on sources in
medicine and health-related studies, motor learning and developmental
psychology. A theme that runs through the book is that movement
outcomes are a complex transaction of child resources, the context in
which movement takes place, and the manner in which tasks are
presented.

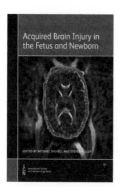

Acquired Brain Injury in the Fetus and Newborn
Michael Shevell and Steven Miller (Eds)

International Review of Child Neurology Series
2012 ▪ 330pp ▪ hardback ▪ 978-1-907655-02-9
£125.00 / €155.00 / $195.00

Given the tremendous advances in the understanding of acquired neonatal brain injury, this book provides a timely review for the practising neurologist, neonatologist and paediatrician. The editors take a pragmatic approach, focusing on specific populations encountered regularly by the clinician. They offer a 'bench to bedside' approach to acquired brain injury in the preterm and term newborn infant. The contributors, all internationally recognized neurologists and scientists, provide readers with a state-of-the art review in their area of expertise.

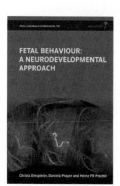

Fetal Behaviour: A Neurodevelopmental Approach
Christa Einspieler, Daniela Prayer, Heinz F.R. Prechtl

Clinics in Developmental Medicine No. 189
2012 ▪ 212pp ▪ hardback ▪ 978-1-898683-87-92
£70.00 / €84.00 / $109.95

Fetal behaviour and movements not only give an insight into the developing brain, as an expression of neural activity, but are also necessary for the further development of neural structure and of other organs. This book presents an account of our current understanding of fetal behaviour as obtained through the assessment of fetal movements and behavioural states. The approach is based on the premises of developmental neurology, and provides important clues for the recognition of the age-specific functional repertoire of the nervous system. The companion DVD contains 26 videos using both ultrasound and dynamic MRI to illustrate the text.

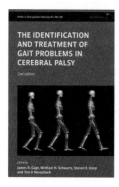

The Identification and Treatment of Gait Problems in Cerebral Palsy, 2nd edition
James R. Gage, Michael H. Schwartz, Steven E. Koop and Tom F. Novacheck (Eds)

Clinics in Developmental Medicine No. 180-181
2009 ▪ 660pp ▪ hardback ▪ 978-1-898683-65-0
£125.00 / €150.00 / $209.00

The only book to deal specifically with the treatment of gait problems in cerebral palsy, this comprehensive, multi-disciplinary volume will be invaluable for all those working in the field of cerebral palsy and gait. The book is accompanied by a DVD containing a teaching video on normal gait and a CD-ROM containing videos of all case examples used in the book.

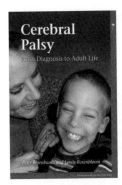

Cerebral Palsy: From Diagnosis to Adult Life
Peter Rosenbaum and Lewis Rosenbloom

A practical guide from Mac Keith Press
2012 ▪ 224pp ▪ softback ▪ 978-1-908316-50-9
£29.95 / €36.10 / $50.00

This book has been designed to provide readers with an understanding of cerebral palsy as a developmental as well as a neurological condition. It details the nature of cerebral palsy, its causes and its clinical manifestations. Using clear, accessible language (supported by an extensive glossary) the authors have blended current science with metaphor to explain the biomedical underpinnings of cerebral palsy.

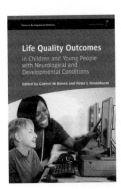

Life Quality Outcomes in Children and Young People with Neurological and Developmental Conditions
Gabriel M. Ronen and Peter L. Rosenbaum (Eds)

Clinics in Developmental Medicine
2013 ▪ 394pp ▪ hardback ▪ 978-1-908316-58-5
£95.00 / €120.70 / $149.95

Healthcare professionals need to understand their patients' views of their condition and its effect on their health and well-being. This book builds on the World Health Organization's concepts of 'health', 'functioning' and 'quality of life' for young people with neuro-disabilities: it emphasises the importance of engaging with patients in the identification of both treatment goals and their evaluation. Uniquely, it enables healthcare professionals to find critically reviewed outcome-related information.

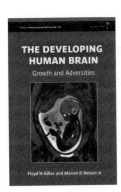

The Developing Human Brain
Floyd H. Gilles and Marvin D. Nelson Jr

Clinics in Developmental Medicine No. 193
2012 ▪ 416pp ▪ hardback ▪ 978-1-908316-41-7
£110.00 / €132.00 / $170.50

This book treats the embryonic and fetal brain as an exciting way to explore growth and aberrations of the most complicated structure in the human body, focusing on the second half of gestation and the neonatal period. It is a unique resource, with its emphasis on quantitative methods and more than 200 pathological and radiological images.

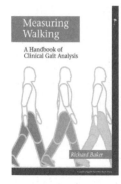

Measuring Walking: A Handbook of Clinical Gait Analysis
Richard Baker

A practical guide from Mac Keith Press
2013 ▪ 248pp ▪ softback ▪ 978-1-908316-66-0
£49.95 / €60.00 / $84.95

This book is a practical guide to instrumented clinical gait analysis covering all aspects of routine service provision. It reinforces what is coming to be regarded as the conventional approach to clinical gait analysis. Data capture, processing and biomechanical interpretation are all described with an emphasis on ensuring high quality results. There are also chapters on how to set up and maintain clinical gait analysis services and laboratories.

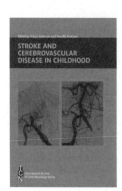

Stroke and Cerebrovascular Disease in Childhood
Vijeya Ganesan, Fenella Kirkham (Eds)

International Review of Child Neurology Series
2011 ▪ 248pp ▪ hardback ▪ 978-1-898683-34-6
£145.00 / €174.00 / $199.95

The field of stroke and cerebrovascular disease in children is one in which there has been much recent research activity, leading to new clinical perspectives. This book for the first time summarizes the state of the art in this field. A team of eminent clinicians, neurologists and researchers provide an up-to-the-minute account of all aspects of stroke and cerebrovascular disease in children, ranging from a historical perspective to future directions, through epidemiology, the latest neuroimaging techniques, neurodevelopment, comorbidities, diagnosis, and treatment.

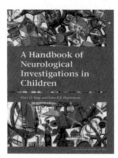

A Handbook of Neurological Investigations in Children
Mary D. King and John B. P. Stephenson

A practical guide from Mac Keith Press
2009 ▪ 400pp ▪ softback ▪ 978-1-898683-69-8
£39.95 / €48.00 / $73.95

The management and treatment of neurological disorders in children depend on establishing the diagnosis, which usually requires investigation, but the number of possible investigations is now very large indeed. This book sets out the investigations that are really needed to establish the cause of neurological disorders. Its problem-oriented approach starts with the patient's presentation, not the diagnosis, with more than 60 case vignettes to illustrate clinical scenarios.

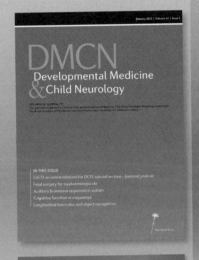
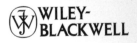